NEW HAVEN FREE PUBLIC LIBRARY

3 5000 09278 4924

THE HEALTH CARE SYSTEM

For Reference
Do Not Take
From the Library

OFFICIALLY WITHDRAWN
NEW HAVEN FREE PUBLIC LIBRARY

D1418225

OFFICIALLY WITHDRAWN
NEW HAVEN FREE PUBLIC LIBRARY

FREE PUBLIC LIBRARY
133 ELM STREET
NEW HAVEN, CT 06510

ISSN 1543-2556

THE HEALTH CARE SYSTEM

Barbara Wexler

INFORMATION PLUS® REFERENCE SERIES
Formerly Published by Information Plus, Wylie, Texas

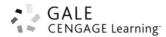

GALE
CENGAGE Learning™

Detroit • New York • San Francisco • New Haven, Conn • Waterville, Maine • London

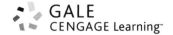

The Health Care System

Barbara Wexler

Kepos Media, Inc., Paula Kepos and Janice Jorgensen, Series Editors

Project Editors: Kathleen J. Edgar, Elizabeth Manar, Kimberly McGrath

Rights Acquisition and Management: Robyn Young

Composition: Evi Abou-El-Seoud, Mary Beth Trimper

Manufacturing: Cynde Lentz

© 2011 Gale, Cengage Learning

ALL RIGHTS RESERVED. No part of this work covered by the copyright herein may be reproduced, transmitted, stored, or used in any form or by any means graphic, electronic, or mechanical, including but not limited to photocopying, recording, scanning, digitizing, taping, Web distribution, information networks, or information storage and retrieval systems, except as permitted under Section 107 or 108 of the 1976 United States Copyright Act, without the prior written permission of the publisher.

This publication is a creative work fully protected by all applicable copyright laws, as well as by misappropriation, trade secret, unfair competition, and other applicable laws. The authors and editors of this work have added value to the underlying factual material herein through one or more of the following: unique and original selection, coordination, expression, arrangement, and classification of the information.

For product information and technology assistance, contact us at
Gale Customer Support, 1-800-877-4253.
For permission to use material from this text or product,
submit all requests online at **www.cengage.com/permissions.**
Further permissions questions can be e-mailed to
permissionrequest@cengage.com

Cover photograph: Image copyright Anetta, 2011. Used under license from Shutterstock.com.

While every effort has been made to ensure the reliability of the information presented in this publication, Gale, a part of Cengage Learning, does not guarantee the accuracy of the data contained herein. Gale accepts no payment for listing; and inclusion in the publication of any organization, agency, institution, publication, service, or individual does not imply endorsement of the editors or publisher. Errors brought to the attention of the publisher and verified to the satisfaction of the publisher will be corrected in future editions.

Gale
27500 Drake Rd.
Farmington Hills, MI 48331-3535

ISBN-13: 978-0-7876-5103-9 (set)   ISBN-10: 0-7876-5103-6 (set)
ISBN-13: 978-1-4144-4864-0   ISBN-10: 1-4144-4864-3

ISSN 1543-2556

This title is also available as an e-book.
ISBN-13: 978-1-4144-7525-7 (set)
ISBN-10: 1-4144-7525-X (set)
Contact your Gale sales representative for ordering information.

Printed in the United States of America
1 2 3 4 5 6 7 15 14 13 12 11

TABLE OF CONTENTS

PREFACE

The Health Care System is part of the *Information Plus Reference Series*. The purpose of each volume of the series is to present the latest facts on a topic of pressing concern in modern American life. These topics include the most controversial and studied social issues of the 21st century: abortion, capital punishment, care for the elderly, child abuse, crime, energy, the environment, immigration, minorities, national security, social welfare, women, youth, and many more. Even though this series is written especially for high school and undergraduate students, it is an excellent resource for anyone in need of factual information on current affairs.

By presenting the facts, it is the intention of Gale, Cengage Learning to provide its readers with everything they need to reach an informed opinion on current issues. To that end, there is a particular emphasis in this series on the presentation of scientific studies, surveys, and statistics. These data are generally presented in the form of tables, charts, and other graphics placed within the text of each book. Every graphic is directly referred to and carefully explained in the text. The source of each graphic is presented within the graphic itself. The data used in these graphics are drawn from the most reputable and reliable sources, such as from the various branches of the U.S. government and from private organizations and associations. Every effort has been made to secure the most recent information available. Readers should bear in mind that many major studies take years to conduct and that additional years often pass before the data from these studies are made available to the public. Therefore, in many cases the most recent information available in 2011 is dated from 2008 or 2009. Older statistics are sometimes presented as well, if they are landmark studies or of particular interest and no more-recent information exists.

Even though statistics are a major focus of the *Information Plus Reference Series*, they are by no means its only content. Each book also presents the widely held positions and important ideas that shape how the book's subject is discussed in the United States. These positions are explained in detail and, where possible, in the words of their proponents. Some of the other material to be found in these books includes historical background, descriptions of major events related to the subject, relevant laws and court cases, and examples of how these issues play out in American life. Some books also feature primary documents or have pro and con debate sections that provide the words and opinions of prominent Americans on both sides of a controversial topic. All material is presented in an even-handed and unbiased manner; readers will never be encouraged to accept one view of an issue over another.

HOW TO USE THIS BOOK

The U.S. health care system is a multifaceted establishment consisting of health care providers, patients, and treatment facilities, just to name a few components. This book examines the state of the nation's health care system, the education and training of health care providers, and the various types of health care institutions. The ever-increasing cost of health care, prevalence of insurance, mental health care, and a comparison of health care throughout the world are also covered.

The Health Care System consists of nine chapters and three appendixes. Each chapter is devoted to a particular aspect of the health care system in the United States. For a summary of the information covered in each chapter, please see the synopses provided in the Table of Contents. Chapters generally begin with an overview of the basic facts and background information on the chapter's topic, then proceed to examine subtopics of particular interest. For example, Chapter 5: The Increasing Cost of Health Care begins by describing the U.S. health care expenditures as a percentage of the gross domestic product and how they relate to the consumer price index.

Next, the chapter considers several forecasts and projections of health care expenditures. This is followed by an analysis of health care spending and the sources of funds. Then a discussion of the factors contributing to rising health care costs is provided. The chapter details how the health care reform legislation enacted in 2010 will influence health care spending, a discussion of prescription drug costs, the future of Medicare and Medicaid, and the costs of long-term care and mental health treatment. It concludes with a discussion of the costs of medical and health service research and the rationing of medical care. Readers can find their way through a chapter by looking for the section and subsection headings, which are clearly set off from the text. They can also refer to the book's extensive index if they already know what they are looking for.

Statistical Information

The tables and figures featured throughout *The Health Care System* will be of particular use to readers in learning about this issue. These tables and figures represent an extensive collection of the most recent and important statistics on the health care system, as well as related issues—for example, graphics cover the rate of home health care usage, the number of emergency department visits, the national health expenditure amounts, the percent of people without health insurance, and public opinion on the state of the health care system. Gale, Cengage Learning believes that making this information available to readers is the most important way to fulfill the goal of this book: to help readers understand the issues and controversies surrounding the health care system in the United States and reach their own conclusions.

Each table or figure has a unique identifier appearing above it, for ease of identification and reference. Titles for the tables and figures explain their purpose. At the end of each table or figure, the original source of the data is provided.

To help readers understand these often complicated statistics, all tables and figures are explained in the text. References in the text direct readers to the relevant statistics. Furthermore, the contents of all tables and figures are fully indexed. Please see the opening section of the index at the back of this volume for a description of how to find tables and figures within it.

Appendixes

Besides the main body text and images, *The Health Care System* has three appendixes. The first is the Important

Names and Addresses directory. Here, readers will find contact information for a number of government and private organizations that can provide further information on aspects of the health care system. The second appendix is the Resources section, which can also assist readers in conducting their own research. In this section, the author and editors of *The Health Care System* describe some of the sources that were most useful during the compilation of this book. The final appendix is the index. It has been greatly expanded from previous editions and should make it even easier to find specific topics in this book.

ADVISORY BOARD CONTRIBUTIONS

The staff of Information Plus would like to extend its heartfelt appreciation to the Information Plus Advisory Board. This dedicated group of media professionals provides feedback on the series on an ongoing basis. Their comments allow the editorial staff who work on the project to make the series better and more user-friendly. The staff's top priority is to produce the highest-quality and most useful books possible, and the Information Plus Advisory Board's contributions to this process are invaluable.

The members of the Information Plus Advisory Board are:

- Kathleen R. Bonn, Librarian, Newbury Park High School, Newbury Park, California

- Madelyn Garner, Librarian, San Jacinto College, North Campus, Houston, Texas

- Anne Oxenrider, Media Specialist, Dundee High School, Dundee, Michigan

- Charles R. Rodgers, Director of Libraries, Pasco-Hernando Community College, Dade City, Florida

- James N. Zitzelsberger, Library Media Department Chairman, Oshkosh West High School, Oshkosh, Wisconsin

COMMENTS AND SUGGESTIONS

The editors of the *Information Plus Reference Series* welcome your feedback on *The Health Care System*. Please direct all correspondence to:

Editors
Information Plus Reference Series
27500 Drake Rd.
Farmington Hills, MI 48331-3535

CHAPTER 1
THE U.S. HEALTH CARE SYSTEM

When asked to describe the U.S. health care system, most Americans would probably offer a description of just a single facet of a huge, complex interaction of people, institutions, and technology. Like snapshots, each account offers an image, frozen in time, of one of the many health care providers and the settings in which medical care is delivered. Examples of these include:

- Physician offices: for many Americans, health care may be described as the interaction between a primary care physician and a patient to address minor and urgent medical problems, such as colds, allergies, or back pain. A primary care physician (usually a general practitioner, family practitioner, internist, or pediatrician) is the frontline caregiver—the first practitioner to evaluate and treat the patient. Routine physical examinations, prevention management actions such as immunization and health screening to detect disease, and treatment of acute and chronic diseases commonly take place in physicians' offices.

- Medical clinics: these settings provide primary care services comparable to those provided in physicians' offices and may be organized to deliver specialized support such as prenatal care for expectant mothers, well-baby care for infants, or treatment for specific medical conditions such as hypertension (high blood pressure), diabetes, or asthma.

- Hospitals: these institutions contain laboratories, imaging centers (also known as radiology departments, where x-rays and other imaging studies are performed), and other equipment for diagnosis and treatment, as well as emergency departments, operating rooms, and highly specialized personnel.

Medical care is also provided through many other venues, including outpatient surgical centers, school health programs, pharmacies, worksite clinics, and voluntary health agencies such as Planned Parenthood, the American Red Cross, and the American Lung Association.

IS THE U.S. HEALTH CARE SYSTEM AILING?

Even though medical care in the United States is often considered the best available, some observers feel the system that delivers it is fragmented and in serious disarray. This section offers some of the many opinions about the challenges of the present health care system and how to improve it. In "The Health Care Crisis and What to Do about It" (2006, http://www.nybooks.com/articles/archives/2006/mar/23/the-health-care-crisis-and-what-to-do-about-it/), Robin Wells and Paul Krugman describe the nation's health care system as "a system in which the government pays directly or indirectly for more than half of the nation's health care, but the actual delivery both of insurance and of care is undertaken by a crazy quilt of private insurers, for-profit hospitals, and other players who add cost without adding value."

Regina E. Herzlinger of the Harvard Business School agrees with Wells and Krugman. In *Who Killed Health Care?: America's $2 Trillion Medical Problem and the Consumer-Driven Cure* (2007), she contends that the current U.S. health care system is in crisis because it is incorrectly organized around the motives, methods, and preferences of health care providers and payers instead of the needs of health care consumers. Herzlinger argues that the present orientation of the U.S. health care system is dangerously eroding patient welfare and driving costs so high that medical care is inaccessible for millions of Americans.

Herzlinger proposes streamlining the system by eliminating insurance companies, which she believes only serve as "middlemen" between physicians and patients. She also recommends:

- Mandatory health insurance with subsidies provided for people who cannot afford to purchase it

- Establishment of small medical facilities that provide comprehensive health care services

- A national system of medical records that ensures confidentiality as well as provider access to medical information

- Compulsory performance reviews of all hospitals and health care organizations

Herzlinger asserts that in a consumer-driven model of health care delivery, providers would compete on the basis of quality, services would be timely, coordinated, and cost effective, and innovation would be encouraged and rewarded.

Albert Fuchs, a practicing physician, offers another scathing indictment of the health care system in "Dollars to Doughnuts Diagnosis" (*Los Angeles Times*, April 16, 2008). Like Hurzlinger, he blames insurance companies for creating high-volume medical practices and compromising the time physicians can spend with patients. By dropping all of his insurance plans and seeing patients on a fee-for-service basis (paid for at the time of each visit, procedure, or treatment that is delivered), Fuchs claims he can devote more time to his patients. He also believes that eliminating insurance companies from the health care equation will cause prices to drop. Fuchs asserts, "When doctors break free from the shackles of insurance companies, they can practice medicine the way they always hoped they could. And they can get back to the customer service model in which the paramount incentive is providing the best care."

In *A Second Opinion: Rescuing America's Healthcare—A Plan for Universal Coverage Serving Patients over Profit* (2007), Arnold S. Relman of Harvard Medical School explains how the commercialization of medicine harms both physicians and patients. Relman opines that the profit motive "increases costs; it may also jeopardize quality or aggravate the system's inequity." He favors a single-payer insurance program that is supported by a progressive health care tax to finance a delivery system in which all hospitals would be not-for-profit and most physicians would be salaried employees.

The previously described ideas are just a few of the wide variety of ways in which people have proposed improvements to the existing health care system in the United States. Besides individual ideas, several large-scale reforms have been proposed by recent presidential administrations, including proposals by the Clinton administration during the early 1990s and more recently by the Obama administration. Despite these efforts, health care reform efforts in the United States have met with limited success.

Reforming the U.S. Health Care System

Derek Bok of Harvard University observes in "The Great Health Care Debate of 1993–94" (1998, http://www.upenn.edu/pnc/ptbok.html) that while in 1993 it appeared that President Bill Clinton (1946–) might successfully enact sweeping reform of the health care system, by September 1994 the legislation his administration had championed was dead. Bok attributes the demise of the legislation to divisive special interest groups and to inadequate efforts of educating the public, which resulted in confusion and misunderstanding of the provisions of the legislation and opposition to it. Bok asserts that because many Americans mistakenly assumed that eliminating excess health care costs generated by fraud and waste would not free up enough money to provide coverage for all of the uninsured, they opposed the Clinton initiative, which they deemed too costly. Bok also recounts that even as public sentiment appeared to be opposed to the Clinton plan, a poll asking respondents to evaluate various health plans without disclosing their sponsors found that 76% of respondents favored the Clinton initiative.

Health care reform was a key issue again during the 2008 presidential election. During his campaign, Senator Barack Obama (1961–) resolved to fix health care by expanding coverage of the uninsured and helping Americans afford coverage and care. Shortly after being inaugurated as president, he announced his intentions to make his campaign resolve a reality. After a year of bitter partisan (adhering to one party) conflict, the Patient Protection and Affordable Care Act (PPACA) was signed by President Obama and became law on March 23, 2010. A few days later this act was amended by the Health Care and Education Reconciliation Act, which became law on March 30, 2010.

Together the PPACA and the Health Care and Education Reconciliation Act aim to expand coverage, contain health care costs, and improve the health care delivery system. More specifically, the PPACA requires most U.S. citizens and legal residents to have health insurance and promises the creation of health insurance exchanges and other mechanisms to enable people with low incomes and small businesses to purchase insurance coverage. Starting in 2014 all employers except those with fewer than 50 employees will be required to offer coverage; failing to do so will result in penalties. The PPACA also expands Medicaid and the Children's Health Insurance Program to ensure that these public programs cover eligible people. It also strengthens Medicare prescription drug benefits. Furthermore, it eliminates lifetime and annual limits on coverage.

THE COMPONENTS OF THE HEALTH CARE SYSTEM

The health care system consists of all personal medical care services—prevention, diagnosis, treatment, and rehabilitation (services to restore function and independence)—plus the institutions and personnel that provide these services and the government, public, and private organizations and agencies that finance service delivery.

The health care system may be viewed as a complex consisting of three interrelated components: health care consumers (people in need of health care services), health care providers (people who deliver health care services—the professionals and practitioners), and the institutions and organizations of the health care system (the public and private agencies that organize, plan, regulate, finance, and coordinate services) that provide the systematic arrangements for delivering health care. The institutional component includes hospitals, clinics, and home-health agencies; the insurance companies and programs that pay for services, such as Blue Cross/Blue Shield, managed care plans such as health maintenance organizations, and preferred provider organizations; and entitlement programs such as Medicare and Medicaid (federal and state government public assistance programs). Other health care institutions are the professional schools that train students for careers in medical, public health, dental, and allied health professions, such as nursing and laboratory technology. Also included are agencies and associations that research and monitor the quality of health care services; license and accreditation providers and institutions; local, state, and national professional societies; and the companies that produce medical technology, equipment, and pharmaceuticals.

Much of the interaction among the three components of the health care system occurs directly between individual health care consumers and providers. Other interactions are indirect and impersonal, including immunization programs or screenings to detect disease, which are performed by public health agencies for whole populations. Regardless, all health care delivery relies on interactions among all three components. The ability to benefit from health care depends on an individual's or group's ability to gain entry to the health care system. The process of gaining entry to the health care system is referred to as access, and many factors can affect access to health care. This chapter provides an overview of how Americans access the health care system.

ACCESS TO THE HEALTH CARE SYSTEM

In the 21st century access to health care services is a key measure of the overall health and prosperity of a nation or a population, but access and availability were not always linked to good health status. In fact, many medical historians assert that until the beginning of the 20th century, a visit with a physician was as likely to be harmful as it was helpful. Only since the early 20th century has medical care been considered a positive influence on health and longevity.

There are three aspects of accessibility: consumer access, comprehensive availability of services, and supply of services adequate to meet community demand. Quality health care services must be accessible to health care consumers when and where they are needed. The health care provider must have access to a full range of facilities, equipment, drugs, and services provided by other practitioners. The institutional component of health care delivery—the hospitals, clinics, and payers—must have timely access to information to enable them to plan an adequate supply of appropriate services for their communities.

Consumer Access to Care

Access to health care services is influenced by a variety of factors. Characteristics of health care consumers strongly affect when, where, and how they access services. Differences in age, educational attainment, economic status, race, ethnicity, cultural heritage, and geographic location determine when consumers seek health care services, where they go to receive them, their expectations of treatment, and the extent to which they wish to participate in decisions about their own medical care.

People have different reasons for seeking access to health care services. Their personal beliefs about health and illness, motivations to obtain care, expectations of the care they will receive, and knowledge about how and where to receive care vary. For an individual to have access to quality care, there must be appropriately defined points of entry into the health care system. For many consumers, a primary care physician is their portal to the health care system. Besides evaluating and addressing the patient's immediate health care need, the primary care physician also directs the consumer to other providers of care such as physician specialists or mental health professionals.

Some consumers access the health care system by seeking care from a clinic or hospital outpatient department, where teams of health professionals are available at one location. Others gain entry by way of a public health nurse, school nurse, social worker, or pharmacist, who refers them to an appropriate source, site, or health care practitioner.

Comprehensive Availability of Health Care Services

Historically, the physician was the exclusive provider of all medical services. Until the 20th century the family doctor served as physician, surgeon, pharmacist, therapist, adviser, and dentist. He carried all the tools of his trade in a small bag and could easily offer state-of-the-art medical care in the patient's home, because hospitals had little more to offer in the way of equipment or facilities. In the 21st century it is neither practical nor desirable to ask one practitioner to serve in all these roles. It would be impossible for one professional to perform the full range of health care services, from primary prevention of disease and diagnosis to treatment and rehabilitation. Modern physicians and other health care practitioners must have access to a comprehensive array of trained personnel, facilities, and equipment so that they can, in turn, make them accessible to their patients.

Even though many medical problems are effectively treated in a single office visit with a physician, even simple diagnosis and treatment relies on a variety of ancillary (supplementary) services and personnel. To make the diagnosis, the physician may order an imaging study such as an x-ray or ultrasound that is performed by a radiology technician and interpreted by a radiologist (physician specialist in imaging techniques). Laboratory tests may be performed by technicians and analyzed by pathologists (physicians who specialize in microscopic analysis and diagnosis). More complicated medical problems involve teams of surgeons and high-tech surgical suites that are equipped with robotic assistants and rehabilitation programs in which physical and occupational therapists assist patients to regain function and independence.

Some health care services are more effectively, efficiently, and economically provided to groups rather than to individuals. Immunization to prevent communicable diseases and screening to detect diseases in their earliest and most treatable stages are examples of preventive services best performed as cooperative efforts of voluntary health organizations, medical and other professional societies, hospitals, and public health departments.

Access Requires Enough Health Care Services to Meet Community Needs

For all members of a community to have access to the full range of health care services, careful planning is required to ensure both the adequate supply and distribution of needed services. To evaluate community needs and effectively allocate health care resources, communities must gather demographic data and information about the social and economic characteristics of the population. They must also monitor the spread of disease and the frequency of specific medical conditions over time. All these population data must be considered in relation to available resources, including health care personnel; the distribution of facilities, equipment, and human resources (the available health care workforce); and advances in medicine and technology.

For example, a predicted shortage of nurses may prompt increased spending on nursing education; reviews of nurses' salary, benefits, and working conditions; and the cultivation of nonnursing personnel to perform specific responsibilities previously assigned to nurses. Similarly, when ongoing surveillance anticipates an especially virulent influenza (flu) season, public health officials, agencies, and practitioners intensify efforts to provide timely immunization to vulnerable populations such as older adults. Government agencies such as the Centers for Disease Control and Prevention (CDC), the National Institutes of Health, state and local health departments, professional societies, voluntary health agencies, and universities work together to research, analyze, and forecast health care needs. Their recommendations allow health care planners, policy makers, and legislators to allocate resources so that supply keeps pace with demand and to ensure that new services and strategies are developed to address existing and emerging health care concerns.

A REGULAR SOURCE OF HEALTH CARE IMPROVES ACCESS

According to the CDC, the determination of whether an individual has a regular source (i.e., a regular provider or site) of health care is a powerful predictor of access to health care services. Generally, people without regular sources have less access or access to fewer services, including key preventive medicine services such as prenatal care, routine immunization, and health screening. Many factors have been found that contribute to keeping individuals from having regular sources of medical care, with income level being the best predictor of unmet medical needs or problems gaining access to health care services.

Kathleen M. Heyman, Patricia M. Barnes, and Jeannine S. Schiller of the National Center for Health Statistics (NCHS) analyze the 2009 National Health Interview Survey (NHIS), an annual nationwide survey of about 55,000 people in the United States, in *Early Release of Selected Estimates Based on Data from the January–September 2009 National Health Interview Survey* (March 2010, http://www.cdc.gov/nchs/data/nhis/earlyrelease/earlyrelease201003.pdf). The researchers find that from 1997 to September 2009 the percentage of people of all ages with a usual source of medical care did not substantially vary—ranging from a high of 87.9% in 2003 to a low of 85.4% for the period January to September 2009. (See Figure 1.1.)

Still, from 1998 to September 2009 the percentage of people who needed medical care but did not obtain it because of financial barriers to access increased each year. The annual percentage of people who experienced this lack of access to medical care rose from 4.2% in 1998 to 7% for the period January to September 2009. (See Figure 1.2.)

Heyman, Barnes, and Schiller reveal that people aged 18 to 24 years were the least likely to have a regular source of care, but the likelihood of having a regular source of medical care increased among people aged 25 years and older. (See Figure 1.3.) Children under the age

FIGURE 1.1

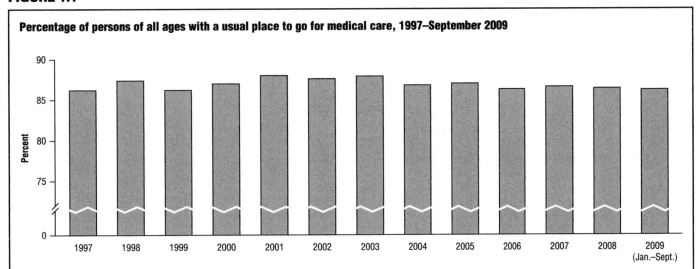

Percentage of persons of all ages with a usual place to go for medical care, 1997–September 2009

Notes: The usual place to go for medical care does not include a hospital emergency room. The analyses excluded persons with an unknown usual place to go for medical care (about 1.5% of respondents each year).

SOURCE: K. M. Heyman, P. M. Barnes, and J. S. Schiller, "Figure 2.1. Percent of Persons of All Ages with a Usual Place to Go for Medical Care: United States, 1997–September 2009," in *Early Release of Selected Estimates Based on Data from the January–September 2009 National Health Interview Survey*, National Center for Health Statistics, March 2010, http://www.cdc.gov/nchs/data/nhis/earlyrelease/earlyrelease201003.pdf (accessed May 3, 2010)

FIGURE 1.2

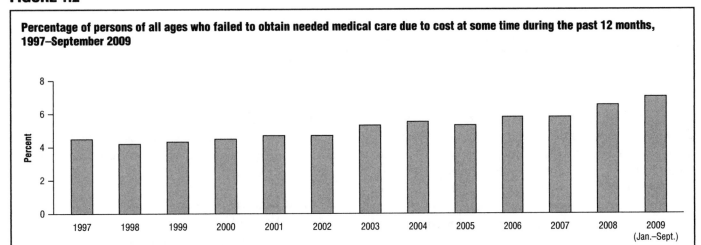

Percentage of persons of all ages who failed to obtain needed medical care due to cost at some time during the past 12 months, 1997–September 2009

Notes: The analyses excluded persons with unknown responses to the question on failure to obtain needed medical care due to cost (about 0.2% of respondents each year).

SOURCE: K. M. Heyman, P. M. Barnes, and J. S. Schiller, "Figure 3.1. Percentage of Persons of All Ages Who Failed to Obtain Needed Medical Care Due to Cost at Some Time during the Past 12 Months: United States, 1997–September 2009," in *Early Release of Selected Estimates Based on Data from the January–September 2009 National Health Interview Survey*, National Center for Health Statistics, March 2010, http://www.cdc.gov/nchs/data/nhis/earlyrelease/earlyrelease201003.pdf (accessed May 3, 2010)

of 18 were more likely than adults aged 18 to 64 years to have a usual place to go for medical care. Among adults (aged 18 to 64 years), women were more likely than men to have a usual place to seek medical care. Heyman, Barnes, and Schiller indicate that not having a regular health care provider is a greater predictor of delay in seeking care than insurance status. Health care consumers with a regular physician or a source of health care services are less likely to use the hospital emergency department to obtain routine nonemergency medical care and are less likely to be hospitalized for preventable illnesses.

In *Access to and Utilization of Medical Care for Young Adults Aged 20–29 Years: United States, 2008* (February 2010, http://www.cdc.gov/nchs/data/databriefs/db29.pdf), Robin A. Cohen and Barbara Bloom of the NCHS reiterate that health insurance status is a key determinant of access to medical care. The researchers report

FIGURE 1.3

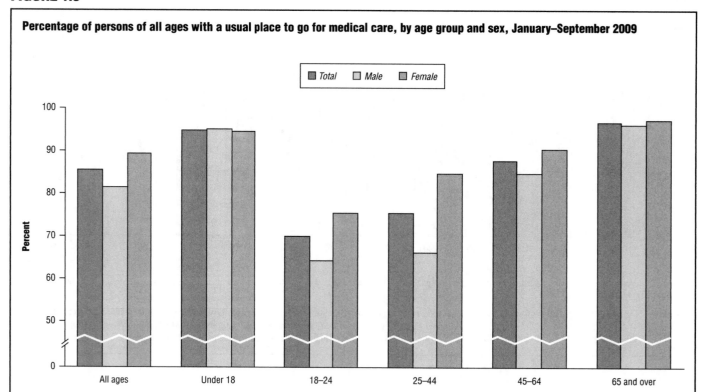

Percentage of persons of all ages with a usual place to go for medical care, by age group and sex, January–September 2009

Notes: The usual place to go for medical care does not include a hospital emergency room. The analyses excluded 105 persons (0.6%) with an unknown usual place to go for medical care.

SOURCE: K. M. Heyman, P. M. Barnes, and J. S. Schiller, "Figure 2.2. Percentage of Persons of All Ages with a Usual Place to Go for Medical Care, by Age Group and Sex: United States, January–September 2009," in *Early Release of Selected Estimates Based on Data from the January–September 2009 National Health Interview Survey*, National Center for Health Statistics, March 2010, http://www.cdc.gov/nchs/data/nhis/earlyrelease/earlyrelease201003.pdf (accessed May 3, 2010)

that nearly 13 million young adults (aged 20 to 29 years) did not have health insurance coverage in 2008 and that young adults without insurance (21%) were four times more likely to have unmet medical needs than young adults with private insurance (5%). About one-quarter (24%) of uninsured young women and one-fifth (19%) of uninsured young men had unmet medical needs.

The National Association of Community Health Centers (NACHC) is a nonprofit organization that represents the interests of federally supported and other federally qualified health centers and serves as an information source about health care for poor and medically underserved populations in the United States. The NACHC reports in *Primary Care Access: An Essential Building Block of Health Reform* (March 2009, http://www.nachc.com/client/documents/pressreleases/PrimaryCareAccessRPT.pdf) that in 2009, 60 million Americans of all income levels, race, and ethnicity were "medically disenfranchised" (at risk of inadequate access to basic medical services). This was an increase of 4 million Americans without access since the NACHC's previous report, which was issued in March 2007. The NACHC asserts that besides the uninsured and low-income populations,

which are disproportionately affected, people lack access for a variety of reasons such as scarcity of health care resources, geographically inaccessible services, and health care that is culturally sensitive.

Race and Ethnicity Continue to Affect Access to Health Care

According to Heyman, Barnes, and Schiller, Hispanic adults continue to be less likely to have a regular source for medical care than non-Hispanic white and non-Hispanic African-American adults. After adjusting for age and gender, 77.5% of Hispanics had a usual source of medical care, compared with 87.3% of non-Hispanic whites and 85% of non-Hispanic African-Americans. (See Figure 1.4.) Hispanics and non-Hispanic African-Americans are more likely than non-Hispanic whites to suffer financial barriers to access. After adjusting for age and gender, 8.6% of Hispanics and 8.7% of non-Hispanic African-Americans were unable to obtain needed medical care because of financial barriers, compared with 6.3% of non-Hispanic whites. (See Figure 1.5.) Health educators speculate that language barriers and the lack of information about the availability of health care services may serve to widen this gap.

FIGURE 1.4

FIGURE 1.5

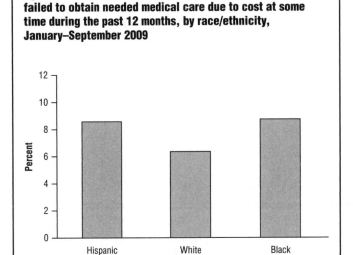

Age- and sex-adjusted percentage of persons of all ages with a usual place to go for medical care, by race/ethnicity, January–September 2009

Notes: The usual place to go for medical care does not include a hospital emergency room. The analyses excluded 105 persons (0.6%) with an unknown usual place to go for medical care. Estimates are age-sex adjusted using the projected 2000 U.S. population as the standard population and using five age groups: under 18 years, 18–24 years, 25–44 years, 45–64 years, and 65 years and over.

SOURCE: K. M. Heyman, P. M. Barnes, and J. S. Schiller, "Figure 2.3. Age-Sex-Adjusted Percentage of Persons of All Ages with a Usual Place to Go for Medical Care, by Race/Ethnicity: United States, January–September 2009," in *Early Release of Selected Estimates Based on Data from the January–September 2009 National Health Interview Survey*, National Center for Health Statistics, March 2010, http://www.cdc.gov/nchs/data/nhis/earlyrelease/earlyrelease201003.pdf (accessed May 3, 2010)

Age- and sex-adjusted percentage of persons of all ages who failed to obtain needed medical care due to cost at some time during the past 12 months, by race/ethnicity, January–September 2009

Notes: The analyses excluded 78 persons (0.1%) with unknown responses to the question on failure to obtain needed medical care due to cost. Estimates are age-sex adjusted using the projected 2000 U.S. population as the standard population and using three age groups: under 18 years, 18–64 years, and 65 years and over.

SOURCE: K. M. Heyman, P. M. Barnes, and J. S. Schiller, "Figure 3.3. Age-Sex-Adjusted Percentage of Persons of All Ages Who Failed to Obtain Needed Medical Care Due to Cost at Some Time during the Past 12 Months, by Race/Ethnicity: United States, January–September 2009," in *Early Release of Selected Estimates Based on Data from the January–September 2009 National Health Interview Survey*, National Center for Health Statistics, March 2010, http://www.cdc.gov/nchs/data/nhis/earlyrelease/earlyrelease201003.pdf (accessed May 3, 2010)

Women Face Additional Obstacles

According to the Kaiser Family Foundation, in *Health Reform: Implications for Women's Access to Coverage and Care* (December 2009, http://www.kff.org/womenshealth/upload/7987.pdf), women fare worse than men in terms of access to health care services. Kaiser notes that just 50% of women receive health coverage via employment, compared with 57% of men. Because women are more likely to be covered as a dependent on their spouse's plan, they are at greater risk of losing their coverage if their spouse becomes unemployed, dies, or divorces them.

Kaiser observes that women are at an increased risk of being uninsured because many are unemployed or employed in low-wage or part-time positions without health benefits. Women are more likely than men to work part time to serve as family caregivers for their children and older family members. Women who are poor, have low incomes, and less than a high school education are uninsured at higher rates than other groups, as are single mothers, young women, and Hispanic and Native American women.

Heyman, Barnes, and Schiller also document gender-based disparities in access. Women aged 18 to 64 years

and those aged 65 years and older were more likely than men to have failed to obtain needed medical care because of financial barriers to access. (See Figure 1.6.)

Children Need Better Access to Health Care, Too

Barbara Bloom, Robin A. Cohen, and Gulnar Freeman of the NCHS analyzed data from the 2008 NHIS to look at selected health measures, including children's access to care, and compiled their findings in *Summary Health Statistics for U.S. Children: National Health Interview Survey, 2008* (December 2009, http://www.cdc.gov/nchs/data/series/sr_10/sr10_244.pdf). Among other factors, Bloom, Cohen, and Freeman's analysis focuses on the unmet health care needs of children under the age of 18, poverty status, insurance coverage, and usual place of medical care.

The researchers note that in 2008, 5% of children in the United States did not have a regular source of medical care. Non-Hispanic African-American children (95%) and non-Hispanic white children (96%) were more likely to have a regular source of care, compared with Hispanic children (91%). Bloom, Cohen, and Freeman also reveal a relationship between not having a usual source of medical care and family structure,

FIGURE 1.6

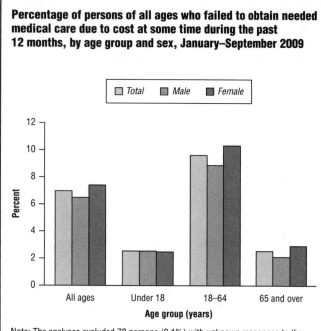

Percentage of persons of all ages who failed to obtain needed medical care due to cost at some time during the past 12 months, by age group and sex, January–September 2009

Note: The analyses excluded 78 persons (0.1%) with unknown responses to the question on failure to obtain needed medical care due to cost.

SOURCE: K. M. Heyman, P. M. Barnes, and J. S. Schiller, "Figure 3.2. Percentage of Persons of All Ages Who Failed to Obtain Needed Medical Care Due to Cost at Some Time during the Past 12 Months, by Age Group and Sex: United States, January–September 2009," in *Early Release of Selected Estimates Based on Data from the January–September 2009 National Health Interview Survey*, National Center for Health Statistics, March 2010, http://www.cdc.gov/nchs/data/nhis/earlyrelease/earlyrelease201003.pdf (accessed May 3, 2010)

family income, poverty status, and health insurance coverage. The likelihood of lacking a regular source of care was higher among poor and near-poor families of all races and ethnic groups. (See Table 1.1.)

Having health insurance and the type of health insurance also predicted whether a child had a regular source of care. In 2008 children with no health insurance (4.8 million out of a total of 6.6 million children aged 18 years and younger, or 72%) were less likely to have a usual place for health care than children with private health insurance (41.5 million out of 42.6 million, or 97%). (See Table 1.1.)

Bloom, Cohen, and Freeman also find that in 2008 more than twice as many children with private health insurance (35.1 million) received health care in a physician's office than children with Medicaid or other public health insurance (12.9 million). (See Table 1.1.) Children without health insurance were more likely to receive routine health care in an emergency department than were children with private or public health insurance.

In 2008, 9.1% of U.S. children had no health insurance coverage. (See Table 1.2.) Of those children who were uninsured, 14% lived in families with incomes of

less than $35,000 per year and 13.5% lived in families with an income of $35,000 to $49,999, compared with 4% of children in households with incomes of $75,000 to $99,999. Children from poor and near-poor families were more likely to be uninsured, have unmet medical needs, and delayed care due to costs more frequently than children from families that were not poor. Health professionals are especially concerned about delayed or missed medical visits for children because well-child visits provide an opportunity for early detection of developmental problems and timely treatment of illnesses and ensure that children receive the recommended schedule of immunizations.

According to Bloom, Cohen, and Freeman, there was significant geographic variation in insurance status, which was strongly linked to children's access to health care services. The percentage of children in the South (10.7%) and West (9.5%) who were uninsured in 2008 was higher than the percentage of uninsured children in the Midwest (8.2%) and the Northeast (6%). (See Table 1.2.)

How to Reduce Disparities in Access to Care

Health care researchers believe many factors contribute to differences in access, including cultural perceptions and beliefs about health and illness, patient preferences, availability of services, and provider bias. They recommend special efforts to inform and educate minority health care consumers and to increase understanding and sensitivity among practitioners and other providers of care. Besides factual information, minority consumers must overcome the belief that they are at a disadvantage because of their race or ethnicity. Along with action to dispel barriers to access, educating practitioners, policy makers, and consumers can help reduce the perception of disadvantage.

For decades, health care researchers have documented sharp differences in the ability of ethnic and racial groups to access medical services. The federal government has repeatedly called for an end to these disparities. Even though some observers believe universal health insurance coverage is an important first step in eliminating disparities, there is widespread concern that the challenge is more complicated and calls for additional analysis and action.

In "Health Disparities: A Case for Closing the Gap" (June 12, 2009, http://www.healthreform.gov/reports/healthdisparities/disparities_final.pdf), Michael Halle, Caya B. Lewis, and Meena Seshamani of the U.S. Department of Health and Human Services assert that "despite consistent increases in spending, disparities among demographic groups persist. Low-income Americans and racial and ethnic minorities experience disproportionately higher rates of disease, fewer treatment options, and reduced access to care." The researchers

TABLE 1.1

Selected measures of health care access for children under age 18, by selected characteristics, 2008

Selected characteristic	All children under 18 years	Has usual place of health care[a]		Location of usual place of health care[b]					
		No	Yes	Clinic	Doctor's office	Emergency room	Hospital outpatient	Some other place	Doesn't go to one place most often
				Number in thousands[c]					
Total[d] (crude)	73,859	3,869	69,935	16,925	51,496	334	715	238	171
Sex									
Male	37,750	2,094	35,625	8,855	26,068	197	277	100*	95*
Female	36,109	1,775	34,310	8,069	25,428	136	437	138*	76*
Age									
0–4 years	20,800	695	20,101	5,309	14,404	100	233	32*	†
5–11 years	28,250	1,503	26,723	6,406	19,820	149*	244	25*	60*
12–17 years	24,809	1,670	23,111	5,210	17,271	85	237	180*	110*
Race									
One race[e]	71,151	3,750	67,350	16,324	49,557	321	697	224	171
White	55,555	2,893	52,622	12,163	39,511	189	380	202	143
Black or African American	11,337	594	10,732	2,925	7,367	123	268	†	†
American Indian or Alaska Native	1,178	115*	1,063	639	400	—	†	—	—
Asian	2,911	135	2,777	546	2,179	†	†	†	†
Native Hawaiian or other Pacific Islander	170	†	156*	†	99*	†	†	—	—
Two or more races[f]	2,708	118*	2,585	601	1,939	†	18*	†	—
Black or African American and white	1,023	†	955	193	750	†	†	—	—
American Indian or Alaska Native and white	540	—	540	160*	361	—	†	†	—
Hispanic or Latino origin[g] and race									
Hispanic or Latino	15,803	1,370	14,393	5,548	8,361	137*	242	†	65*
Mexican or Mexican American	10,766	1,136	9,604	4,066	5,268	87*	135	†	†
Not Hispanic or Latino	58,056	2,499	55,542	11,377	43,135	196	473	213	106*
White, single race	41,294	1,638	39,656	7,196	31,929	64*	194	177*	78*
Black or African American, single race	10,837	559	10,267	2,747	7,114	117	241	†	†
Family structure[h]									
Mother and father	52,026	2,499	49,506	10,871	37,727	185	404	198	105*
Mother, no father	17,287	1,043	16,225	4,771	10,946	119	277	40*	36*
Father, no mother	2,377	154	2,223	568	1,605	†	†	—	†
Neither mother nor father	2,169	172	1,982	713	1,218	†	†	—	†
Parent's education[i]									
Less than high school diploma	9,255	939	8,307	4,011	3,889	111	208	†	36*
High school diploma or GED[j]	15,437	1,135	14,285	3,819	10,016	75	277	†	61*
More than high school	46,749	1,586	45,150	8,293	36,250	132*	214	181	54*
Family income[k]									
Less than $35,000	21,285	1,609	19,645	7,575	11,336	184	410	†	70*
$35,000 or more	47,483	2,012	45,454	8,305	36,484	150	239	174*	82*
$35,000–$49,999	10,230	812	9,417	2,467	6,725	74*	80*	†	†
$50,000–$74,999	12,980	710	12,266	2,640	9,431	22*	51*	†	†
$75,000–$99,999	8,719	172	8,534	1,404	7,013	†	72*	†	—
$100,000 or more	15,555	318	15,237	1,794	13,315	†	36*	59*	†
Poverty status[l]									
Poor	12,329	932	11,374	4,657	6,260	112	263	†	50*
Near poor	15,298	1,438	13,857	4,500	8,920	129*	210	†	52*
Not poor	40,140	1,129	38,991	6,131	32,425	84*	151	127*	54*
Health insurance coverage[m]									
Private	42,600	1,075	41,502	5,948	35,132	59*	122	139*	76*
Medicaid or other public	22,515	843	21,657	8,206	12,857	124*	412	26*	†
Other	1,784	78*	1,705	717	849	—	106*	†	—
Uninsured	6,625	1,847	4,764	1,953	2,457	151	71*	†	77*
Place of residence									
Large MSA[n]	37,997	1,880	36,090	7,714	27,443	191	487	131*	93*
Small MSA[n]	23,849	1,318	22,503	5,790	16,306	96*	162	71*	52*
Not in MSA[n]	12,012	670	11,342	3,420	7,746	47*	66*	†	†

explain that the economic downturn and the resulting high rates of unemployment serve to exacerbate the situation.

Halle, Lewis, and Seshamani note the huge discrepancy in health insurance coverage: more than one out of three Hispanics and Native Americans are uninsured, compared with one out of eight whites. They point out that low-income Hispanic children are three times more likely to forgo annual checkups than white children and that half of all Hispanics do not have a primary care physician, compared with just 20% of whites. There are

TABLE 1.1

Selected measures of health care access for children under age 18, by selected characteristics, 2008 [CONTINUED]

Selected characteristic	All children under 18 years	Has usual place of health care[a] No	Has usual place of health care[a] Yes	Location of usual place of health care[b] Clinic	Doctor's office	Emergency room	Hospital outpatient	Some other place	Doesn't go to one place most often
Region					Number in thousands[c]				
Northeast	12,269	276	11,992	1,873	9,835	†	174	†	†
Midwest	17,911	836	17,071	4,757	11,968	93*	191	†	†
South	25,855	1,684	24,131	4,619	18,985	172	222	45*	63*
West	17,824	1,072	16,741	5,676	10,709	49*	129	132*	41*
Current health status									
Excellent or very good	61,394	3,152	58,192	13,175	43,810	274	522	213	158
Good	11,225	649	10,572	3,322	6,975	54*	168	†	†
Fair or poor	1,206	68*	1,137	428	676	†	†	—	†

*Estimates with an asterisk have a relative standard error of greater than 30% and less than or equal to 50% and should be used with caution as they do not meet the standard of reliability or precision.
†Estimates with a relative standard error greater than 50% are indicated with a dagger, but data are not shown.
—Quantity zero.
[a]Having a usual place of health care is based on the question, "Is there a place that [child's name] USUALLY goes when [he/she] is sick or you need advice about [his/her] health?"
[b]Location of usual place of health care is based on the question, "What kind of place is it/What kind of place does [child's name] go to most often—clinic or health center, doctor's office or health maintenance organization, hospital emergency room, hospital outpatient department or some other place?"
[c]Unknowns for the columns are not included in the frequencies, but they are included in the "All children under 18 years" column.
[d]Total includes other races not shown separately and children with unknown family structure, parent's education, family income, poverty status, health insurance, or current health status. Additionally, numbers within selected characteristics may not add to totals because of rounding.
[e]In accordance with the 1997 standards for federal data on race and Hispanic or Latino origin, the category "One race" refers to persons who indicated only a single race group. Persons who indicated a single race other than the groups shown are included in the total for "One race" but are not shown separately due to small sample sizes. Therefore, the frequencies for the category "One race" will be greater than the sum of the frequencies for the specific groups shown separately. Persons of Hispanic or Latino origin may be of any race or combination of races.
[f]The category "Two or more races" refers to all persons who indicated more than one race group. Only two combinations of multiple race groups are shown due to small sample sizes for other combinations. Therefore, the frequencies for the category "Two or more races" will be greater than the sum of the frequencies for the specific combinations shown separately.
[g]Persons of Hispanic or Latino origin may be of any race or combination of races. Similarly, the category "Not Hispanic or Latino" refers to all persons who are not of Hispanic or Latino origin, regardless of race. The tables in this report use the complete new Office of Management and Budget race and Hispanic origin terms, and the text uses shorter versions of these terms for conciseness. For example, the category "Not Hispanic or Latino black or African American, single race" in the tables is referred to as "non-Hispanic black" in the text.
[h]Family structure refers to parents living in the household. "Mother and father" can include biological, adoptive, step, in-law, or foster relationships. Legal guardians are classified in "Neither mother nor father."
[i]Parent's education is the education level of the parent with the higher level of education, regardless of that parent's age.
[j]GED is General Educational Development high school equivalency diploma.
[k]The categories "Less than $35,000" and "$35,000 or more" include both persons reporting dollar amounts and persons reporting only that their incomes were within one of these two categories. The indented categories include only those persons who reported dollar amounts. Because of the different income questions used in 2007 and beyond, income estimates may not be comparable with those from earlier years.
[l]Poverty status is based on family income and family size using the U.S. Census Bureau's poverty thresholds for the previous calendar year. "Poor" persons are defined as below the poverty threshold. "Near poor" persons have incomes of 100% to less than 200% of the poverty threshold. "Not poor" persons have incomes that are 200% of the poverty threshold or greater. Because of the different income questions used in 2007 and beyond, poverty ratio estimates may not be comparable with those from earlier years.
[m]Classification of health insurance coverage is based on a hierarchy of mutually exclusive categories. Persons with more than one type of health insurance were assigned to the first appropriate category in the hierarchy. Persons under age 65 years and those aged 65 years and over were classified separately due to the prominence of Medicare coverage in the older population. The category "Private" includes persons who had any type of private coverage either alone or in combination with other coverage. For example, for persons aged 65 years and over, "Private" includes persons with only private or private in combination with Medicare. The category "Uninsured" includes persons who had no coverage as well as those who had only Indian Health Service coverage or had only a private plan that paid for one type of service such as accidents or dental care.
[n]MSA is metropolitan statistical area. Large MSAs have a population size of 1,000,000 or more; small MSAs have a population size of less than 1,000,000. "Not in MSA" consists of persons not living in a metropolitan statistical area.

SOURCE: Barbara Bloom, Robin Cohen, and Gulnur Freeman, "Table 11. Frequencies of Having a Usual Place of Health Care and Frequency Distributions of Location of Usual Place of Health Care for Children with a Usual Place of Health Care for Children under 18 Years of Age, by Selected Characteristics: United States, 2008," in "Summary Health Statistics for U.S. Children: National Health Interview Survey, 2008," *Vital Health Stat Series*, series 10, no. 244, 2009, http://www.cdc.gov/nchs/data/series/sr_10/sr10_244.pdf (accessed May 3, 2010)

also comparable discrepancies in routine care and prevention. Halle, Lewis, and Seshamani conclude that health care reform that makes care more affordable and accessible will go a long way to reducing the higher rates of disease that racial and ethnic minorities experience.

AHRQ Report Documents Disparities in Access

In July 2003 the Agency for Healthcare Research and Quality (AHRQ) released its first *National Healthcare Disparities Report* (http://www.ahrq.gov/qual/nhdr03/nhdr2003.pdf), a report requested by Congress that documented racial health disparities including access

to care. Among other things, the report cited the finding that African-Americans and low-income Americans have higher mortality rates for cancer than the general population because they are less likely to receive screening tests for certain forms of the disease and other preventive services. Even though the report asserted that differential access may lead to disparities in quality and observed that opportunities to provide preventive care are often missed, it conceded that knowledge about why disparities exist is limited.

The AHRQ report generated fiery debate in the health care community and among legislators and painted a rather bleak view of disparities. The report called

TABLE 1.2

Age-adjusted percentages of selected measures of health care access for children under age 18, by selected characteristics, 2008

Selected characteristic	All children under 18 years	Uninsured for health care[a]	Unmet medical need[b]	Delayed care due to cost[c]	Uninsured for health care[a]	Unmet medical need[b]	Delayed care due to cost[c]
		Number in thousands[d]			Percent[e]		
Total[f] (age-adjusted)	73,858	6,634	2,045	3,506	9.1	2.8	4.8
Total[f] (crude)	73,858	6,634	2,045	3,506	9.0	2.8	4.8
Sex							
Male	37,749	3,360	950	1,694	9.0	2.5	4.5
Female	36,108	3,274	1,095	1,811	9.1	3.0	5.0
Age[g]							
0–4 years	20,911	1,538	366	764	7.4	1.8	3.7
5–11 years	28,176	2,498	776	1,330	8.9	2.8	4.7
12–17 years	24,771	2,597	903	1,412	10.6	3.7	5.7
Race							
One race[h]	71,310	6,450	1,974	3,398	9.1	2.8	4.8
White	55,603	5,282	1,497	2,752	9.6	2.7	5.0
Black or African American	11,415	851	394	535	7.6	3.5	4.7
American Indian or Alaska Native	1,154	125*	55*	69*	11.1	5.1*	6.4*
Asian	2,979	187	28*	41*	6.3	0.9*	1.4*
Native Hawaiian or other Pacific Islander	159	†	—	—	—	—	—
Two or more races[i]	2,547	184	†	108*	7.5	3.1*	4.5*
Black or African American and white	969	108*	†	39*	11.8*	—	4.5*
American Indian or Alaska Native and white	504	46*	†	†	8.9*	—	—
Hispanic or Latino origin[j] and race							
Hispanic or Latino	15,802	2,638	663	959	17.2	4.3	6.2
Mexican or Mexican American	10,765	1,893	469	631	18.2	4.5	6.0
Not Hispanic or Latino	58,055	3,996	1,382	2,547	6.9	2.4	4.4
White, single race	41,323	2,759	884	1,861	6.7	2.1	4.5
Black or African American, single race	10,929	808	386	522	7.5	3.5	4.8
Family structure[k]							
Mother and father	52,429	4,416	1,260	2,372	8.5	2.4	4.6
Mother, no father	16,944	1,614	678	908	9.5	4.0	5.3
Father, no mother	2,273	319	62	156	13.1	2.4	6.8
Neither mother nor father	2,212	285	44*	70	12.4	2.0*	3.1
Parent's education[l]							
Less than high school diploma	9,011	2,050	316	455	23.2	3.6	5.2
High school diploma or GED[m]	15,892	1,746	674	888	11.1	4.3	5.6
More than high school	45,541	2,447	998	2,084	5.4	2.2	4.6
Family income[n]							
Less than $35,000	20,277	2,733	912	1,225	14.0	4.7	6.3
$35,000 or more	45,395	3,218	982	2,014	7.1	2.1	4.4
$35,000–$49,999	9,832	1,321	498	914	13.5	5.1	9.3
$50,000–$74,999	12,472	1,061	335	605	8.5	2.7	4.9
$75,000–$99,999	8,351	332	108	310	4.0	1.3	3.7
$100,000 or more	14,741	504	40*	185	3.4	0.3*	1.2
Poverty status[o]							
Poor	11,781	1,469	431	572	12.9	3.8	5.1
Near poor	14,460	2,254	747	1,201	15.9	5.3	8.4
Not poor	38,674	1,953	631	1,359	5.1	1.6	3.5
Health insurance coverage[p]							
Private	42,845	—	549	1,303	—	1.3	3.0
Medicaid or other public	22,082	—	515	839	—	2.5	4.0
Other	1,762	—	†	29*	—	—	—
Uninsured	6,634	6,634	947	1,304	100	14.0	19.4
Place of residence							
Large MSA[q]	38,962	3,287	1,058	1,774	8.5	2.7	4.6
Small MSA[q]	23,064	2,015	689	1,117	8.8	3.0	4.9
Not in MSA[q]	11,832	1,332	298	615	11.4	2.5	5.2

for detailed data to support quality improvement initiatives and observed that "community-based participatory research has numerous examples of communities working to improve quality overall, while reducing healthcare disparities for vulnerable populations."

Highlights from the National Healthcare Disparities Report 2009

In *National Healthcare Disparities Report 2009* (March 2010, http://www.ahrq.gov/qual/nhdr09/nhdr09.pdf), the AHRQ tracks the measures of access to care that the

TABLE 1.2

Age-adjusted percentages of selected measures of health care access for children under age 18, by selected characteristics, 2008

[CONTINUED]

Selected characteristic	All children under 18 years	Selected measures of health care access					
		Uninsured for health care[a]	Unmet medical need[b]	Delayed care due to cost[c]	Uninsured for health care[a]	Unmet medical need[b]	Delayed care due to cost[c]
Region		Number in thousands[d]			Percent[e]		
Northeast	12,338	735	178	343	6.0	1.4	2.8
Midwest	17,438	1,424	504	919	8.2	2.9	5.3
South	26,173	2,781	788	1,365	10.7	3.0	5.2
West	17,909	1,694	576	879	9.5	3.2	4.9
Current health status							
Excellent or very good	60,869	5,102	1,328	2,562	8.5	2.2	4.2
Good	11,557	1,346	590	797	11.7	5.1	6.9
Fair or poor	1,314	168	128	146	12.8	9.5	10.8

*Estimates with an asterisk have a relative standard error of greater than 30% and less than or equal to 50% and should be used with caution as they do not meet the standard of reliability or precision.

†Estimates with a relative standard error greater than 50% are indicated with a dagger, but data are not shown.

—Quantity zero.

[a]Uninsured for health care is based on the following question in the family core section of the survey: "[Are you/Is anyone] covered by health insurance or some other kind of health care plan?"

[b]Unmet medical need is based on the following question in the family core section of the survey: "During the past 12 months, was there any time when [you/someone in the family] needed medical care, but did not get it because [you/the family] couldn't afford it?"

[c]Delayed health care due to cost is based on the following question in the family core section of the survey: "During the past 12 months, [have/has] [you/anyone in the family] delayed seeking medical care because of worry about the cost?"

[d]Unknowns for the columns are not included in the frequencies, but they are included in the "All children under 18 years" column.

[e]Unknowns for the column variables are not included in the denominators when calculating percentages.

[f]Total includes other races not shown separately and children with unknown family structure, parent's education, family income, poverty status, health insurance, or current health status. Additionally, numbers within selected characteristics may not add to totals because of rounding.

[g]Estimates for age groups are not age adjusted.

[h]In accordance with the 1997 standards for federal data on race and Hispanic or Latino origin the category "One race" refers to persons who indicated only a single race group. Persons who indicated a single race other than the groups shown are included in the total for "One race" but are not shown separately due to small sample sizes. Therefore, the frequencies for the category "One race" will be greater than the sum of the frequencies for the specific groups shown separately. Persons of Hispanic or Latino origin may be of any race or combination of races.

[i]The category "Two or more races" refers to all persons who indicated more than one race group. Only two combinations of multiple race groups are shown due to small sample sizes for other combinations. Therefore, the frequencies for the category "Two or more races" will be greater than the sum of the frequencies for the specific combinations shown separately.

[j]Persons of Hispanic or Latino origin may be of any race or combination of races. Similarly, the category "Not Hispanic or Latino" refers to all persons who are not of Hispanic or Latino origin, regardless of race. The tables in this report use the complete new Office of Management and Budget race and Hispanic origin terms, and the text uses shorter versions of these terms for conciseness. For example, the category "Not Hispanic or Latino black or African American, single race" in the tables is referred to as "non-Hispanic black" in the text.

[k]Family structure refers to parents living in the household. "Mother and father" can include biological, adoptive, step, in-law, or foster relationships. Legal guardians are classified in "Neither mother nor father."

[l]Parent's education is the education level of the parent with the higher level of education, regardless of that parent's age.

[m]GED is General Educational Development high school equivalency diploma.

[n]The categories "Less than $35,000" and "$35,000 or more" include both persons reporting dollar amounts and persons reporting only that their incomes were within one of these two categories. The indented categories include only those persons who reported dollar amounts. Because of the different income questions used in 2007 and beyond, income estimates may not be comparable with those from earlier years.

[o]Poverty status is based on family income and family size using the U.S. Census Bureau's poverty thresholds for the previous calendar year. "Poor" persons are defined as below the poverty threshold. "Near poor" persons have incomes of 100% to less than 200% of the poverty threshold. "Not poor" persons have incomes that are 200% of the poverty threshold or greater. Because of the different income questions used in 2007 and beyond, poverty ratio estimates may not be comparable with those from earlier years.

[p]Classification of health insurance coverage is based on a hierarchy of mutually exclusive categories. Persons with more than one type of health insurance were assigned to the first appropriate category in the hierarchy. Persons under age 65 years and those aged 65 years and over were classified separately due to the prominence of Medicare coverage in the older population. The category "Private" includes persons who had any type of private coverage either alone or in combination with other coverage. For example, for persons aged 65 years and over, "Private" includes persons with only private or private in combination with Medicare. The category "Uninsured" includes persons who had no coverage as well as those who had only Indian Health Service coverage or had only a private plan that paid for one type of service such as accidents or dental care.

[q]MSA is metropolitan statistical area. Large MSAs have a population size of 1,000,000 or more; small MSAs have a population size of less than 1,000,000. "Not in MSA" consists of persons not living in a metropolitan statistical area.

Notes: Estimates were based on responses about all children in the family, not only the sample child. Estimates are age adjusted using the projected 2000 U.S. population as the standard population and using age groups 0–4 years, 5–11 years, and 12–17 years.

SOURCE: Barbara Bloom, Robin Cohen, and Gulnur Freeman "Table 15. Frequencies and Age-Adjusted Percentages (with Standard Errors) of Selected Measures of Health Care Access for Children under 18 Years of Age, by Selected Characteristics: United States, 2008," in "Summary Health Statistics for U.S. Children: National Health Interview Survey, 2008," *Vital Health Stat Series*, series 10, no. 244, 2009, http://www.cdc.gov/nchs/data/series/sr_10/sr10_244.pdf (accessed May 3, 2010)

first report, *National Healthcare Disparities Report*, identified in 2003. These measures include factors that facilitated access, such as having a primary care provider, and factors that were barriers to access, such as having no health insurance. The AHRQ's principal findings are:

- Disparities in access persist and many are not decreasing. The AHRQ notes that disparities related to race, ethnicity, and socioeconomic status still exist in terms of

access to the health care system. Table 1.3 shows the factors that account for disparities in access among members of racial and ethnic minorities, and Table 1.4 shows how socioeconomic variables (income, education, and insurance status) serve to enable or deter access. For example, in 2007 African-Americans, Native Americans or Alaskan Natives, and Hispanics continued to experience worse access to care than whites, and poor people and those without insurance had less access to care

TABLE 1.3

Racial and ethnic differences in factors that influence access to care, 2007

Core report measure	Racial difference[a]					Ethnic difference[b]
	Black	Asian	NHOPI	AI/AN	>1 race	Hispanic
Health insurance coverage						
People under age 65 with health insurance	=	=	=	↓	=	↓
People under age 65 who were uninsured all year	=	=	=	=	=	↓
Usual source of care						
People with a specific source of ongoing care	=	=		=	=	↓
People with a usual primary care provider	↓	↓	=	=	=	↓
People without a usual source of care who indicated a financial or insurance reason for not having a source of care	↑	=			=	↓
Patient perceptions of need						
People who were unable to get or delayed in getting needed care	=	↑		↓	↓	↑

Notes: NHOPI = Native Hawaiian or other Pacific Islander; AI/AN = American Indian or Alaska Native.
[a]Compared with whites.
[b]Compared with non-Hispanic whites.

Key to symbols used in access to health care tables:

= Group and comparison group have about same access to health care.

↑ Group has better access to health care than the comparison group.

↓ Group has worse access to health care than the comparison group.

Blank cell: Reliable estimate for group could not be made.

SOURCE: "Table 3.1a. Racial and Ethnic Differences in Facilitators and Barriers to Health Care," in *National Healthcare Disparities Report 2009*, U.S. Department of Health and Human Services, Agency for Healthcare Research and Quality, March 2010, http://www.ahrq.gov/qual/nhdr09/nhdr09.pdf (accessed May 3, 2010)

TABLE 1.4

Socioeconomic factors that influence access to health care, 2007

Core report measure	Income difference[a]			Educational difference[b]		Insurance difference[c]
	<100%	100–199%	200–399%	<HS	HS grad	Uninsured
Health insurance coverage						
People under age 65 with health insurance	↓	↓	↑	↓	↓	
People under age 65 who were uninsured all year	↓	↓	↑	↓	↓	
Usual source of care						
People with a specific source of ongoing care	↓	↓	↑	↓	↓	↓
People with a usual primary care provider	↓	↓	↓	↓	=	↓
People without a usual source of care who indicated a financial or insurance reason for not having a source of care	↓	↓	↑	↓	↓	↓
Patient perceptions of need						
People who were unable to get or delayed in getting needed care	↓	↓	↓	↓	↓	↓

HS = High school.
[a]Compared with persons with family incomes 400% of federal poverty thresholds or above.
[b]Compared with persons with any college education.
[c]Compared with persons under 65 with any private health insurance.

Key to symbols used in access to health care tables:

= Group and comparison group have about same access to health care.

↑ Group has better access to health care than the comparison group.

↓ Group has worse access to health care than the comparison group.

Blank cell: Reliable estimate for group could not be made.

SOURCE: "Table 3.1b. Socioeconomic Differences in Facilitators and Barriers to Health Care," in *National Healthcare Disparities Report 2009*, U.S. Department of Health and Human Services, Agency for Healthcare Research and Quality, March 2010, http://www.ahrq.gov/qual/nhdr09/nhdr09.pdf (accessed May 3, 2010) than those with higher incomes. (See Table 1.3 and Table 1.4.) For Hispanics, all disparities in access were found to have worsened.

- Even though some disparities are diminishing, many groups continue to face disparities in access. Socioeconomic status accounts for some differences in health insurance coverage of racial and ethnic groups but not all. Hispanics of every income and educational level remained less likely than their non-Hispanic peers to have health insurance. African-Americans and Native Americans or Alaskan Natives who had attended college were much less likely than whites who had attended college to have health insurance.

- No group had attained the goal of 100% of Americans covered by health insurance set forth in *Healthy People 2010* (November 2000, http://www.healthypeople.gov/ document/tableofcontents.htm), the set of national health objectives that aim to identify and reduce the most significant preventable threats to health.

HEALTH CARE REFORM PROMISES TO IMPROVE ACCESS

Even though the goal of achieving universal health care coverage by 2010 was not met that year, the enactment of health care legislation promised to help the United States make great strides toward expanding coverage and access to health care for many more Americans. The Health Care and Education Reconciliation Act was signed by President Obama in March 2010. The landmark legislation was the culmination of a yearlong struggle and marked the realization of one of the president's key domestic priorities. It has been hailed as the most sweeping social legislation since the enactment of Social Security in 1935 and Medicare and Medicaid in 1965. The act promises to improve access to care by extending health care coverage to millions of uninsured Americans and by preventing health insurance companies from denying coverage to people with preexisting medical conditions or dropping them when they develop costly medical problems.

The months leading up to this historic moment were tense, so much so that the future of the PPACA remained in jeopardy until Congress passed it. The U.S. Senate approved its version of the health care reform bill, the Patient Protection and Affordable Care Act, in December 2009 in a 60–39 vote that adhered to party lines. Every Republican senator opposed the bill even though it was much more conservative than the corresponding bill, the Service Members Home Ownership Tax Act, in the U.S. House of Representatives. The House bill contained a public insurance option—a government-run health insurance company—and stronger sanctions for employers who failed to provide insurance for their workers. The Senate bill replaced the public insurance option with the

creation of insurance exchanges—regulated marketplaces where insurance companies can compete to gain the business of individuals and small companies purchasing health insurance. The intent of these exchanges is to guarantee that insurance offerings are both comprehensive in terms of coverage and competitively priced.

Because there were no Republican supporters of the legislation, House Democrats worked feverishly to secure the 216 votes necessary to pass the bill. Last-minute accommodations were made to secure the votes, most notably by inserting language that ensured that the longstanding ban on using federal funds for abortion would not be overturned. Because it was a budget bill, it could be approved under reconciliation, a process that requires a majority to pass and is not subject to filibuster (the use of obstructive tactics to prevent adoption of a measure favored by the majority).

The Health Care and Education Reconciliation Act, which was intended to enable the PPACA to be amended, was introduced by Representative John M. Spratt Jr. (1942–; D-SC) on March 17, 2010, and the House passed the bill on March 21. The Senate amended the bill and passed its amended version on March 25. Fifty-six Democrats voted in favor of the bill and a bipartisan (two-party) group of 43 senators voted against it. The amended bill was then returned to the House, where it was passed on March 30 in a vote of 220 in favor and 207 not in favor.

ACCESS TO MENTAL HEALTH CARE

Besides the range of barriers to access faced by all Americans trying to access the health care system, people seeking mental health care face unique challenges, not the least of which is that they are even less able than people in good mental health to successfully navigate the fragmented mental health service delivery system. Furthermore, because people with serious mental illness frequently suffer from unemployment and disability, they are likely to join the ranks of the impoverished, uninsured, and homeless, which only compounds access problems. Finally, the social stigmas (deeply held negative attitudes) that promote discrimination against people with mental illness are a powerful deterrent to seeking care.

The social stigmas attached to being labeled "crazy" prevent some sufferers of mental illness from seeking and obtaining needed care. Myths about mental illness persist, especially the mistaken beliefs that mental illness is a sign of moral weakness or that an affected individual can simply choose to "wish or will away" the symptoms of mental illness. People with mental illness cannot just "pull themselves together" and will themselves well. Without treatment, symptoms can worsen and persist for months or even years.

People with mental illness experience other types of social stigmas as well. They may face discrimination in the workplace, in school, and in finding housing. Thwarted in their efforts to maintain independence, people suffering from mental illness may become trapped in a cycle characterized by feelings of worthlessness and hopelessness and may be further isolated from the social and community supports and treatments most able to help them recover.

Disparities in Access to Mental Health Care

The principal barriers to access of mental health care are the cost of services, the fragmented organization of these services, and the social stigmas toward mental illness. These obstacles may act as deterrents for all Americans, but for racial and ethnic minorities they are compounded by language barriers, ethnic and cultural compatibility of practitioners, and geographic availability of services.

The AHRQ finds in *National Healthcare Disparities Report 2009* that when compared with whites, minorities have less access to care and are less likely to receive needed services. For example, according to the AHRQ, the disparities between African-Americans and whites in the receipt of specific mental health services were worsening in 2007. (See Table 1.5.)

Furthermore, the AHRQ observes that along with race, economics also affect access to mental health care.

TABLE 1.5

Disparities between African Americans and whites over time, 2007

Topic	Improving	Worsening	Same
HIV and AIDS	**New AIDS causes per 100,000 population age 13 and over**		
Maternal and child health	Children ages 19–35 months who received all recommended vaccines Children ages 3–6 with a vision check		Children ages 2–17 given advice about exercise Children ages 2–17 given advice about healthy eating Children ages 2–17 who had a dental visit
Mental health and substance abuse		Adults age 18 and over with past-year major depressive episode who received treatment for the depression in the past year People age 12 and over who needed treatment for any illicit drug use or alcohol problem who received such treatment in the past year	Suicide deaths per 100,000 population
Respiratory diseases	Adults age 65 and over who ever received pneumococcal vaccination	**Hospital patients with pneumonia who received recommended care**	Tuberculosis patients who completed a curative course of treatment within 1 year of initiation of treatment
Lifestyle modification			Current smokers age 18 and over given advice to quit smoking Adults with obesity given advice about exercise
Functional status preservation and rehabilitation		Home health care patients whose ability to walk or move around improved	
Supportive and palliative care	Short-stay nursing home residents with pressure sores		Long-stay nursing home residents who were physically restrained High-risk long-stay nursing home residents with pressure sores Home health care patients who were admitted to the hospital
Patient safety	**Postoperative complications** **Central venous catheter-associated adverse events**	Adults age 65 and over who received potentially inappropriate prescription medications **Appropriate timing of antibiotics received by adult Medicare patients having surgery**	Failure to rescue
Timeliness	Emergency department visits in which patients left without being seen Adults who can sometimes or never get care for illness or injury as soon as wanted		
Patient centeredness			Poor provider-patient communication—children Poor provider-patient communication—adults
Access	People under age 65 with health insurance	**People without a usual source of care due to a financial or insurance reason**	People under age 65 uninsured all year People who have a specific source of ongoing care People who have a usual primary care provider People who were unable to get or delayed in getting needed medical care, dental care, or prescription medications

Note: Measures in bold indicate improvement or worsening at a rate of greater than 5% per year.

SOURCE: "Table 4.4. Change in Black-White Disparities over Time: Specific Measures," in *National Healthcare Disparities Report 2009*, U.S. Department of Health and Human Services, Agency for Healthcare Research and Quality, March 2010, http://www.ahrq.gov/qual/nhdr09/nhdr09.pdf (accessed May 3, 2010)

For example, poverty may be both a risk factor for mental health problems and a consequence of poor mental health. Table 1.5 shows that the adults with major depression who were more likely to have received treatment were white and had middle or high incomes.

IS ACCESS A RIGHT OR A PRIVILEGE?

The AHRQ and other health care researchers and policy makers observe that having health insurance does not necessarily ensure access to medical care. They contend that many other factors, including cost-containment measures put in place by private and public payers, have reduced access to care. Nonetheless, reduced access affects vulnerable populations—the poor, people with mental illness and other disabilities, and immigrants—more than others.

Health care is a resource that is rationed. The United States is the only developed country in the world that does not have a government-funded universal or national program of health insurance. As a result, Americans with greater incomes and assets are more likely than low-income families to have health insurance and have greater access to health care services. It is for this reason that the 2010 health care reform legislation is heralded by some as groundbreaking. Supporters of this legislation anticipate that as previously uninsured people obtain insurance, access will be greatly improved.

Nicholas D. Kristof reiterates in "Access, Access, Access" (*New York Times*, March 17, 2010) the relationship between access to medical care and health status. He observes that U.S. life expectancy increased during the 1940s, largely because the nation's preparations—both military and civilian—for World War II (1939–1945) improved access to medical care. Kristof also observes

that "there is one group of Americans who do fine in international comparisons—and that's the 65-plus crowd. They have Medicare."

Various groups and organizations support the idea that health care is a fundamental human right, rather than a privilege. These organizations include Physicians for a National Health Program, the American Association of Retired Persons, National Health Care for the Homeless, Inc., and the Friends Committee on National Legislation, a Quaker public interest lobby.

Others disagree with the notion that access to health care is a fundamental right. For example, in "Healthcare Reform Passes" (March 22, 2010, http://www.campaignforliberty.com/article.php?view=713), Ron Paul (1935–; R-TX) decries government involvement in health care. Paul asserts that "citizens have a responsibility over their own life, but they also have the liberty to choose how they will live and protect their lives." He opposes the 2010 health care reform legislation, contending that "healthcare choices are a part of liberty, another part that is being stripped away. Government interference in healthcare has already infringed on choices available to people, but rather than getting out of the way, it is entrenching itself, and its corporatist cronies, even more deeply."

Jake Towne echoes Paul's sentiment in "Health Care Is NOT a Right" (December 23, 2009, http://www.campaignforliberty.com/article.php?view=466). He believes that because people pay for health care, as they do for other goods and services, it is a privilege. Towne opines that "to alleviate the pain of the starving and those without adequate medical care, we must turn not to the federal government but instead to ourselves."

CHAPTER 2

HEALTH CARE PRACTITIONERS

The art of medicine consists of amusing the patient while nature cures the disease.

—Voltaire

One of the first duties of the physician is to educate the masses not to take medicine.

—William Osler, *Sir William Osler: Aphorisms, from His Bedside Teachings and Writings* (1950)

PHYSICIANS

Physicians routinely perform medical examinations, provide preventive medicine services, diagnose illness, treat patients suffering from injury or disease, and offer counsel about how to achieve and maintain good health. There are two types of physicians trained in traditional Western medicine: the Doctor of Medicine (MD) is schooled in allopathic medicine and the Doctor of Osteopathy (DO) learns osteopathy. Allopathy is the philosophy and system of curing disease by producing conditions that are incompatible with disease, such as prescribing antibiotics to combat bacterial infection. The philosophy of osteopathy is different; it is based on recognition of the body's capacity for self-healing, and it emphasizes structural and manipulative therapies such as postural education, manual treatment of the musculoskeletal system (osteopathic physicians are trained in hands-on diagnosis and treatment), and preventive medicine. Osteopathy is also considered a holistic practice because it considers the whole person, rather than simply the diseased organ or system.

In modern medical practice, the philosophical differences may not be obvious to most health care consumers because MDs and DOs use many comparable methods of treatment, including prescribing medication and performing surgery. In fact, the American Osteopathic Association (2010, http://www.osteopathic.org/index.cfm?PageID=aoa_main), the national medical professional society that represents more than 67,000

DOs, admits that many people who seek care from osteopathic physicians may be entirely unaware of their physician's training, which emphasizes holistic interventions or special skills such as manipulative techniques. Like MDs, DOs complete four years of medical school and postgraduate residency training; may specialize in areas such as surgery, psychiatry, or obstetrics; and must pass state licensing examinations to practice.

Medical School, Postgraduate Training, and Qualifications

Modern medicine requires considerable skill and extensive training. The road to gaining admission to medical school and becoming a physician is long, difficult, and intensely competitive. Medical school applicants must earn excellent college grades, achieve high scores on entrance exams, and demonstrate emotional maturity and motivation to be admitted to medical school. Once admitted, medical students spend the first two years primarily in laboratories and classrooms learning basic medical sciences such as anatomy (detailed understanding of body structure), physiology (biological processes and vital functions), and biochemistry. They also learn how to take medical histories, perform complete physical examinations, and recognize symptoms of diseases. During their third and fourth years, the medical students work under supervision at teaching hospitals and clinics. By completing clerkships—spending time in different specialties such as internal medicine, obstetrics and gynecology, pediatrics, psychiatry, and surgery—they acquire the necessary skills and gain experience to diagnose and treat a wide variety of illnesses.

Following medical school, new physicians must complete a year of internship, also referred to as postgraduate year one, that emphasizes either general medical practice or one specific specialty and provides clinical experience in various hospital services (e.g., inpatient care, outpatient clinics, emergency departments, and operating rooms). In the past, many physicians entered practice after this first year of postgraduate training. However, in the present era of specialization most physicians choose to continue in residency training, which lasts an additional three to six years, depending on the specialty. Those who choose a subspecialty such as cardiology, infectious diseases, oncology, or plastic surgery must spend additional years in residency and may then choose to complete fellowship training. Immediately after residency, they are eligible to take an examination to earn board certification in their chosen specialty. Fellowship training involves a year or two of laboratory and clinical research work as well as opportunities to gain additional clinical and patient care expertise.

Medical School Applicants

According to the Association of American Medical Colleges (AAMC), in the press release "Medical School Enrollment Continues to Rise to Meet Physician Need" (October 20, 2009, http://www.aamc.org/newsroom/pressrel/2009/091020.htm), the number of students entering medical school for the 2008–09 academic year rose to 18,400, which was a 2% increase from the previous academic year. The students were selected from a pool of 42,269 applicants. Applications from African-Americans rose by 4% from the previous academic year, but applications from Hispanics fell by 1% and from Native Americans by 5%.

Conventional and Newer Medical Specialties

Rapid advances in science and medicine and changing needs have resulted in a variety of new medical and surgical specialties, subspecialties, and concentrations. For example, geriatrics, the medical subspecialty concerned with the prevention and treatment of diseases in older adults, has developed in response to growth in this population. The term *geriatrics* is derived from the Greek *geras* (old age) and *iatrikos* (physician). Geriatricians are physicians trained in primary care, such as internal medicine or family practice, who receive further training and become eligible for certification as specialists in the medical care of older adults. The American Geriatrics Society (AGS) indicates that the United States needs more geriatricians to care for its growing population of older adults. In "Fact Sheet: The American Geriatrics Society" (2010, http://www.americangeriatrics.org/about_us/who_we_are/faq_fact_sheet/), the AGS estimates that "a shortage of geriatricians exists in the United States and is projected to worsen over the next 20 years. Currently, there is one geriatrician for every 5,000 adults age 65 and older. In 2030, it is estimated that there will only be one geriatrician for every 7,665 older adults, representing a 50% decline over the next 25 years."

FIGURE 2.1

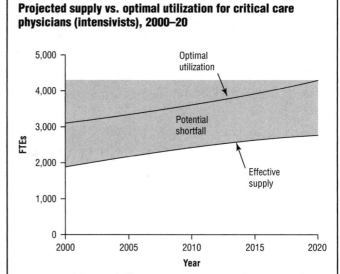

Projected supply vs. optimal utilization for critical care physicians (intensivists), 2000–20

FTE = Full-time equivalent

SOURCE: Elizabeth M. Duke, "Exhibit 15. Projected Supply vs. Optimal Utilization for Intensivists, 2000–2020," in *Report to Congress: The Critical Care Workforce: A Study of the Supply and Demand for Critical Care Physicians*, U.S. Department of Health and Human Services, Health Resources and Services Administration, May 2006, ftp://ftp.hrsa.gov/bhpr/nationalcenter/criticalcare.pdf (accessed May 7, 2010)

Another relatively new medical specialty has resulted in physician intensivists. Intensivists, as the name indicates, are trained to staff hospital intensive care units (ICUs, which are sometimes known as critical care units), where the most critically ill patients are cared for using a comprehensive array of state-of-the-art technology and equipment. This specialty arose in response to both the increasing complexity of care provided in ICUs and the demonstrated benefits of immediate availability of highly trained physicians to care for critically ill patients. The Health Resources and Services Administration (HRSA) notes in *The Critical Care Workforce: A Study of the Supply and Demand for Critical Care Physicians* (May 2006, ftp://ftp.hrsa.gov/bhpr/nationalcenter/criticalcare.pdf) that "demand for intensivists will continue to exceed available supply through the year 2020 if current supply and demand trends continue." Assuming optimal utilization, the HRSA predicts a shortfall of 1,500 intensivists in 2020. (See Figure 2.1.) According to Ognjen Gajic and Bekele Afessa of the Mayo Clinic in Rochester, Minnesota, in "Physician Staffing Models and Patient Safety in the ICU" (*Chest*, vol. 135, no. 4, April 2009), intensivists provide care only to a minority of ICU patients in the United States even though many studies demonstrate that the level of intensivist staffing is directly related to how well patients fare in the ICU—in that there is a positive association between intensivist staffing and good patient outcome. The researchers suggest that because the intensivist shortage is expected to increase, telemedicine (the use of telecommunications technology [e.g., telephone and videoconferencing] within the health care industry) may be a strategy to increase access to intensivists for critically ill patients and the physicians who care for them.

The fastest-growing new specialty is hospitalists—physicians who are hospital based as opposed to office based and who provide a variety of services from caring for hospitalized patients who do not have personal physicians to explaining complex medical procedures to patients and families and coordinating many aspects of inpatient care. Michael Heisler of the Sanford School of Medicine reports in "Hospitalists and Intensivists: Partners in Caring for the Critically Ill—The Time Has Come" (*Journal of Hospital Medicine*, vol. 5, no. 1, January 2010) that there were 28,000 hospitalists in the United States in 2009 and that their ranks are expected to grow in coming years. Heisler opines "that hospitalists are soon likely to care for the majority of elderly hospitalized patients in America."

More traditional medical specialties include:

- Anesthesiologist—administers anesthesia (partial or complete loss of sensation) and monitors patients in surgery
- Cardiologist—diagnoses and treats diseases of the heart and blood vessels
- Dermatologist—trained to diagnose and treat diseases of the skin, hair, and nails
- Family practitioner—delivers primary care to people of all ages and, when necessary, refers patients to other physician specialists
- Gastroenterologist—specializes in digestive system disorders
- Internist—provides diagnosis and nonsurgical treatment of a broad array of illnesses affecting adults
- Neurologist—specializes in the nervous system and provides diagnosis and treatment of brain, spinal cord, and nerve disorders
- Obstetrician-gynecologist—provides health care for women and their reproductive systems, as well as care for mothers and babies before, during, and immediately following delivery
- Oncologist—dedicated to the diagnosis and treatment of cancer
- Otolaryngologist—skilled in the medical and surgical treatment of ear, nose, and throat disorders and related structures of the face, head, and neck
- Pathologist—uses skills in microscopic chemical analysis and diagnostics to detect disease in body tissues and fluids

- Psychiatrist—specializes in the prevention, diagnosis, and treatment of mental health and emotional disorders
- Pulmonologist—specializes in diseases of the lungs and respiratory system
- Urologist—provides diagnosis as well as medical and surgical treatment of the urinary tract in both men and women as well as male reproductive health services

HIGH COSTS, LONG HOURS, AND LOW WAGES. According to the AAMC (2010, https://services.aamc.org/tsfreports/report_median.cfm?year_of_study=2010), the tuition and fees for the 2009–10 academic year at public medical schools were $25,209 for in-state residents and $45,858 for nonresidents. The tuition and fees at private medical schools were $42,906 for in-state residents and $43,431 for nonresidents. The AAMC reports that public medical school tuition and fees increased by an average of 6.8% for in-state residents and by 5% for nonresidents from the previous academic year. Similarly, private medical school tuition and fees increased by 4% for in-state residents and by 4.2% for nonresidents.

The AAMC indicates in "Medical Student Education: Costs, Debt, and Loan Repayment Facts" (October 2010, https://www.aamc.org/download/152968/data/10/debtfactcard.pdf) that the average 2010 medical school graduate had an educational debt of $157,944. Even though a physician's earning power is considerable, and many students are able to repay their debts during their first years of practice, some observers believe the extent of medical students' indebtedness may unduly influence their career choices. They may train for higher-paying specialties and subspecialties rather than follow their natural interests or opt to practice in underrepresented specialties or underserved geographic areas. The high cost of medical education is also believed to limit the number of minority applicants to medical school.

Historically, medical training has been difficult and involved long hours. Working long hours without adequate rest has been found to increase the occurrence of preventable medical errors and thereby adversely affect patient safety. In "The Response of the APPD, CoPS, and AAP to the Institute of Medicine Report on Resident Duty Hours" (*Pediatrics*, vol. 125, no. 4, April 2010), Susan Guralnick et al. note that the Institute of Medicine (IOM) published in December 2008 new recommendations about the hours and supervision of residents' training in the United States. The key IOM recommendations were:

- A maximum duration of 30 hours per shift, consisting of admitting patients for 16 hours plus a five-hour rest period between 10 p.m. and 8 a.m. and the remaining hours for education and transition of patient care

- 10 hours off after a day shift, 12 hours off after a night shift, and 14 hours off after an extended duty period of 30 hours

- Four-night maximum of night shifts; 48 hours off after three or four nights of consecutive duty

- Five days off per month

Representatives of professional societies including the American Academy of Pediatrics, the Association of Pediatric Program Directors (APPD), and the Council of Pediatric Specialties oppose many of the specific stipulations of the IOM recommendations. For example, the APPD opposes the IOM recommendation of a 30-hour day that consists of admitting patients for up to 16 hours, plus a five-hour sleep period between 10 p.m. and 8 a.m. with the remaining hours for transition and educational activities. The APPD proposes 24 hours of patient care and educational time plus three hours of transition time. These professional societies ask "that legislators, educational leaders, and organizations focus on patient safety, supervision, clinical outcomes, and educational outcomes rather than narrowly on the number of hours a resident physician works in training."

The Number of Physicians in Practice Is Increasing

In 2007, of the 941,304 physicians in the United States, 303,749 were primary care physicians. (See Table 2.1.) Primary care physicians are the front line of the health care system—the first health professionals most people see for medical problems or routine care. Family practitioners, internists, pediatricians, obstetrician/gynecologists, and general practitioners are considered to be primary care physicians. Primary care physicians tend to see the same patients regularly and develop relationships with patients over time as they offer preventive services, scheduled visits, follow-up, and urgent medical care. When necessary, they refer patients for consultation with, and care from, physician specialists.

In 2007, 562,897 physicians maintained office-based practices; 169,337 were in hospital-based practices and

TABLE 2.1

Medical doctors in primary care, by specialty, selected years 1949–2007

[Data are based on reporting by physicians]

Specialty	1949[a]	1960[a]	1970	1980	1990	1995	2000	2002	2006	2007
					Number					
Total doctors of medicine[b]	201,277	260,484	334,028	467,679	615,421	720,325	813,770	853,187	921,904	941,304
Active doctors of medicine[c]	191,577	247,257	310,845	414,916	547,310	625,443	692,368	719,431	766,836	776,554
General primary care specialists	113,222	125,359	134,354	170,705	213,514	241,329	274,653	286,294	300,907	303,749
General practice/family medicine	95,980	88,023	57,948	60,049	70,480	75,976	86,312	89,357	92,371	93,416
Internal medicine	12,453	26,209	39,924	58,462	76,295	88,240	101,353	106,499	113,340	114,449
Obstetrics/gynecology	—	—	18,532	24,612	30,220	33,519	35,922	36,810	37,996	38,186
Pediatrics	4,789	11,127	17,950	27,582	36,519	43,594	51,066	53,628	57,200	57,698
Primary care subspecialists	—	—	3,161	16,642	30,911	39,659	52,294	57,929	67,519	69,858
Family medicine	—	—	—	—	—	236	483	627	938	1,043
Internal medicine	—	—	1,948	13,069	22,054	26,928	34,831	38,821	44,914	46,403
Obstetrics/gynecology	—	—	344	1,693	3,477	4,133	4,319	4,228	4,337	4,408
Pediatrics	—	—	869	1,880	5,380	8,362	12,661	14,253	17,330	18,004
					Percent of active doctors of medicine					
General primary care specialists	59.1	50.7	43.2	41.1	39.0	38.6	39.7	39.8	39.2	39.1
General practice/family medicine	50.1	35.6	18.6	14.5	12.9	12.1	12.5	12.4	12.0	12.0
Internal medicine	6.5	10.6	12.8	14.1	13.9	14.1	14.6	14.8	14.8	14.7
Obstetrics/gynecology	—	—	6.0	5.9	5.5	5.4	5.2	5.1	5.0	4.9
Pediatrics	2.5	4.5	5.8	6.6	6.7	7.0	7.4	7.5	7.5	7.4
Primary care subspecialists	—	—	1.0	4.0	5.6	6.3	7.6	8.1	8.8	9.0
Family medicine	—	—	0.0	0.0	0.0	0.0	0.1	0.1	0.1	0.1
Internal medicine	—	—	0.6	3.1	4.0	4.3	5.0	5.4	5.9	6.0
Obstetrics/gynecology	—	—	0.1	0.4	0.6	0.7	0.6	0.6	0.6	0.6
Pediatrics	—	—	0.3	0.5	1.0	1.3	1.8	2.0	2.3	2.3

0.0 = Percent greater than zero but less than 0.05.
—Data not available.

[a]Active doctors of medicine (MDs) include those with address unknown and primary specialty not classified.
[b]Includes medical doctors engaged in federal and nonfederal patient care (office-based or hospital-based) and other professional activities.
[c]Starting with 1970 data, MDs who are inactive, have unknown address, or primary specialty not classified are excluded.
Notes: Data are as of December 31 except for 1990–1994 data, which are as of January 1, and 1949 data, which are as of midyear. Outlying areas include Puerto Rico, the U.S. Virgin Islands, and the Pacific islands of Canton, Caroline, Guam, Mariana, Marshall, American Samoa, and Wake.

SOURCE: "Table 109. Doctors of Medicine in Primary Care, by Specialty: United States and Outlying U.S. Areas, Selected Years 1949–2007," in *Health, United States, 2009: With Special Feature on Medical Technology*, U.S. Department of Health and Human Services, Centers for Disease Control and Prevention, National Center for Health Statistics, 2010, http://www.cdc.gov/nchs/data/hus/hus09.pdf#listtables (accessed May 7, 2010). Data from the American Medical Association (AMA).

TABLE 2.2

Medical doctors by activity and place of medical education, selected years 1975–2007

[Data are based on reporting by physicians]

Place of medical education and activity	1975	1985	1995	2000	2004	2005	2006	2007
				Number of doctors of medicine				
Total doctors of medicine	**393,742**	**552,716**	**720,325**	**813,770**	**884,974**	**902,053**	**921,904**	**941,304**
Active doctors of medicine[a]	340,280	497,140	625,443	692,368	744,143	762,438	766,836	776,554
Place of medical education:								
U.S. medical graduates	—	392,007	481,137	527,931	563,118	571,798	574,315	580,336
International medical graduates[b]	—	105,133	144,306	164,437	181,025	190,640	192,521	196,218
Activity:								
Patient care[c, d]	287,837	431,527	564,074	631,431	700,287	718,473	723,118	732,234
Office-based practice	213,334	329,041	427,275	490,398	538,538	563,225	560,411	562,897
General and family practice	46,347	53,862	59,932	67,534	73,234	74,999	74,900	75,952
Cardiovascular diseases	5,046	9,054	13,739	16,300	17,252	17,519	17,480	17,504
Dermatology	3,442	5,325	6,959	7,969	8,651	8,795	8,920	9,036
Gastroenterology	1,696	4,135	7,300	8,515	9,430	9,742	9,881	10,042
Internal medicine	28,188	52,712	72,612	88,699	101,776	107,028	107,284	108,552
Pediatrics	12,687	22,392	33,890	42,215	49,356	51,854	51,815	52,095
Pulmonary diseases	1,166	3,035	4,964	6,095	7,072	7,321	7,377	7,490
General surgery	19,710	24,708	24,086	24,475	25,229	26,079	25,592	25,434
Obstetrics and gynecology	15,613	23,525	29,111	31,726	33,811	34,659	34,225	34,405
Ophthalmology	8,795	12,212	14,596	15,598	16,304	16,580	15,765	15,852
Orthopedic surgery	8,148	13,033	17,136	17,367	18,632	19,115	19,220	19,299
Otolaryngology	4,297	5,751	7,139	7,581	8,160	8,206	8,199	8,177
Plastic surgery	1,706	3,299	4,612	5,308	5,845	6,011	6,016	6,100
Urological surgery	5,025	7,081	7,991	8,460	8,793	8,955	8,850	8,796
Anesthesiology	8,970	15,285	23,770	27,624	29,984	31,887	31,746	31,617
Diagnostic radiology	1,978	7,735	12,751	14,622	16,828	17,618	17,577	17,327
Emergency medicine	—	—	11,700	14,541	18,961	20,173	20,055	20,036
Neurology	1,862	4,691	7,623	8,559	9,632	10,400	10,423	10,476
Pathology, anatomical/clinical	4,195	6,877	9,031	10,267	10,653	11,747	11,465	11,191
Psychiatry	12,173	18,521	23,334	24,955	25,998	27,638	27,387	27,492
Radiology	6,970	7,355	5,994	6,674	6,900	7,049	6,954	6,913
Other specialty	15,320	28,453	29,005	35,314	36,037	39,850	39,280	39,111
Hospital-based practice	74,503	102,486	136,799	141,033	161,749	155,248	162,707	169,337
Residents and interns[e]	53,527	72,159	93,650	95,125	102,563	95,391	97,102	98,688
Full-time hospital staff	20,976	30,327	43,149	45,908	59,186	59,857	65,605	70,649
Other professional activity[f]	24,252	44,046	40,290	41,556	43,856	43,965	43,718	44,320
Inactive	21,449	38,646	72,326	75,168	92,323	99,823	108,344	111,551
Not classified	26,145	13,950	20,579	45,136	48,011	39,304	46,252	52,740
Unknown address	5,868	2,980	1,977	1,098	497	488	472	459

—Data not available.

[a]Doctors of medicine who are inactive, have unknown address, or primary specialty not classified are excluded.

[b]International medical graduates received their medical education in schools outside the United States and Canada.

[c]Specialty information is based on the physician's self-designated primary area of practice. Categories include generalists and specialists.

[d]Starting with 2003 data, estimates include federal and nonfederal doctors of medicine. Prior to 2003, estimates were for nonfederal doctors of medicine only.

[e]Starting with 1990 data, clinical fellows are included in this category. In prior years, clinical fellows were included in the other professional activity category.

[f]Includes medical teaching, administration, research, and other. Prior to 1990, this category also included clinical fellows.

Notes: Data for doctors of medicine are as of December 31, except for 1990–1994 data, which are as of January 1. Outlying areas include Puerto Rico, the U.S. Virgin Islands, and the Pacific islands of Canton, Caroline, Guam, Mariana, Marshall, American Samoa, and Wake.

SOURCE: "Table 108. Doctors of Medicine, by Place of Medical Education and Activity: United States and Outlying U.S. Areas, Selected Years 1975–2007," in *Health, United States, 2009: With Special Feature on Medical Technology,* U.S. Department of Health and Human Services, Centers for Disease Control and Prevention, National Center for Health Statistics, 2010, http://www.cdc.gov/nchs/data/hus/hus09.pdf#listtables (accessed May 7, 2010). Data from the American Medical Association (AMA).

98,688 were residents and interns. (See Table 2.2.) Besides the growing number of graduates of U.S. medical schools, the ranks of international medical graduates grew by 31,781, from 164,437 in 2000 to 196,218 in 2007.

The number of active physicians devoted to patient care, as opposed to research, administration, or other roles, varied by geographic region and by state, from a high of 39.1 physicians per 10,000 civilian population in Massachusetts in 2007 to a low of 17 physicians per 10,000 people in Idaho. (See Table 2.3.)

Physician Working Conditions and Earnings

Many physicians work long, irregular hours. The Bureau of Labor Statistics (BLS; December 17, 2009, http://www.bls.gov/oco/ocos074.htm) reports that in 2008, 43% of full-time physicians worked 50 hours or more per week performing patient care and administrative duties such as office management. Physicians and surgeons worked at 661,400 jobs in 2008, and 12% were self-employed. About 53% of physicians held salaried positions, and 19% were employed by private hospitals. Physicians in salaried positions, such as those employed

TABLE 2.3

Active physicians in patient care, by state, selected years 1975–2007

[Data are based on reporting by physicians]

State	Active physicians[a,b]					Physicians in patient care[a,b,c]				
	1975	1985	1995	2002	2007	1975	1985	1995	2002	2007
					Number per 10,000 civilian population					
United States	15.3	20.7	24.2	25.4	27.4	13.5	18.0	21.3	22.5	25.3
Alabama	9.2	14.2	18.4	19.9	21.6	8.6	13.1	17.0	18.3	20.5
Alaska	8.4	13.0	15.7	20.0	24.2	7.8	12.1	14.2	17.7	22.6
Arizona	16.7	20.2	21.4	18.9	22.3	14.1	17.1	18.2	17.6	20.6
Arkansas	9.1	13.8	17.3	19.2	20.4	8.5	12.8	16.0	17.8	19.3
California	18.8	23.7	23.7	24.0	26.1	17.3	21.5	21.7	21.8	24.2
Colorado	17.3	20.7	23.7	24.0	26.6	15.0	17.7	20.6	21.2	24.7
Connecticut	19.8	27.6	32.8	34.4	36.1	17.7	24.3	29.5	30.9	33.0
Delaware	14.3	19.7	23.4	25.2	26.2	12.7	17.1	19.7	21.5	24.4
District of Columbia	39.6	55.3	63.6	61.8	73.2	34.6	45.6	53.6	53.9	63.8
Florida	15.2	20.2	22.9	24.1	25.5	13.4	17.8	20.3	21.4	23.9
Georgia	11.5	16.2	19.7	20.4	21.4	10.6	14.7	18.0	18.8	20.0
Hawaii	16.2	21.5	24.8	27.7	31.7	14.7	19.8	22.8	25.2	29.4
Idaho	9.5	12.1	13.9	16.6	17.9	8.9	11.4	13.1	15.2	17.0
Illinois	14.5	20.5	24.8	26.0	27.7	13.1	18.2	22.1	23.1	25.7
Indiana	10.6	14.7	18.4	20.9	22.1	9.6	13.2	16.6	18.9	20.8
Iowa	11.4	15.6	19.2	19.9	21.4	9.4	12.4	15.1	15.7	19.2
Kansas	12.8	17.3	20.8	21.7	23.6	11.2	15.1	18.0	18.8	22.0
Kentucky	10.9	15.1	19.2	21.3	23.0	10.1	13.9	18.0	19.8	21.6
Louisiana	11.4	17.3	21.7	24.4	25.5	10.5	16.1	20.3	23.0	24.4
Maine	12.8	18.7	22.3	27.1	31.5	10.7	15.6	18.2	22.6	28.5
Maryland	18.6	30.4	34.1	35.3	40.0	16.5	24.9	29.9	31.2	35.1
Massachusetts	20.8	30.2	37.5	39.2	43.2	18.3	25.4	33.2	35.1	39.1
Michigan	15.4	20.8	24.8	25.8	28.1	12.0	16.0	19.0	20.1	25.1
Minnesota	14.9	20.5	23.4	25.3	28.4	13.7	18.5	21.5	23.3	26.6
Mississippi	8.4	11.8	13.9	17.1	18.1	8.0	11.1	13.0	15.6	17.1
Missouri	15.0	20.5	23.9	24.8	26.2	11.6	16.3	19.7	20.6	24.0
Montana	10.6	14.0	18.4	21.9	22.9	10.1	13.2	17.1	20.3	21.9
Nebraska	12.1	15.7	19.8	22.6	24.1	10.9	14.4	18.3	20.8	22.5
Nevada	11.9	16.0	16.7	17.9	19.6	10.9	14.5	14.6	16.1	18.5
New Hampshire	14.3	18.1	21.5	25.2	27.7	13.1	16.7	19.8	23.0	26.0
New Jersey	16.2	23.4	29.3	31.4	33.0	14.0	19.8	24.9	26.8	30.1
New Mexico	12.2	17.0	20.2	22.0	23.8	10.1	14.7	18.0	19.0	22.2
New York	22.7	29.0	35.3	36.5	38.2	20.2	25.2	31.6	32.6	35.1
North Carolina	11.7	16.9	21.1	23.3	24.7	10.6	15.0	19.4	21.4	23.1
North Dakota	9.7	15.8	20.5	22.5	24.5	9.2	14.9	18.9	20.8	23.4
Ohio	14.1	19.9	23.8	26.0	28.0	12.2	16.8	20.0	22.0	25.6
Oklahoma	11.6	16.1	18.8	19.2	20.7	9.4	12.9	14.7	14.8	18.7
Oregon	15.6	19.7	21.6	24.1	27.3	13.8	17.6	19.5	21.7	25.6
Pennsylvania	16.6	23.6	30.1	31.5	32.9	13.9	19.2	24.6	25.5	29.3
Rhode Island	17.8	23.3	30.4	33.4	36.8	16.1	20.2	26.7	29.7	34.0
South Carolina	10.0	14.7	18.9	21.5	22.9	9.3	13.6	17.6	19.9	21.7
South Dakota	8.2	13.4	16.7	20.1	22.4	7.7	12.3	15.7	18.6	21.3
Tennessee	12.4	17.7	22.5	24.2	25.9	11.3	16.2	20.8	22.5	24.4
Texas	12.5	16.8	19.4	20.3	21.4	11.0	14.7	17.3	18.1	20.0
Utah	14.1	17.2	19.2	19.8	20.9	13.0	15.5	17.6	17.9	19.5
Vermont	18.2	23.8	26.9	33.7	36.0	15.5	20.3	24.2	30.6	33.2
Virginia	12.9	19.5	22.5	24.5	26.9	11.9	17.8	20.8	22.5	25.1
Washington	15.3	20.2	22.5	24.7	26.8	13.6	17.9	20.2	22.3	24.8
West Virginia	11.0	16.3	21.0	23.7	25.5	10.0	14.6	17.9	19.8	23.1
Wisconsin	12.5	17.7	21.5	24.1	26.1	11.4	15.9	19.6	22.0	24.5
Wyoming	9.5	12.9	15.3	18.2	19.5	8.9	12.0	13.9	16.6	18.4

[a]Includes active doctors of medicine (MDs) and active doctors of osteopathy (DOs).
[b]Starting with 2003 data, federal and nonfederal physicians are included. Data prior to 2003 include nonfederal physicians only.
[c]Prior to 2006, excludes DOs. Excludes physicians in medical teaching, administration, research, and other nonpatient care activities. Includes residents.
Notes: Data for MDs are as of December 31. Data for DOs are as of May 31.

SOURCE: "Table 107. Active Physicians and Physicians in Patient Care, by State: United States, Selected Years 1975–2007," in *Health, United States, 2009: With Special Feature on Medical Technology*, U.S. Department of Health and Human Services, Centers for Disease Control and Prevention, National Center for Health Statistics, 2010, http://www.cdc.gov/nchs/data/hus/hus09.pdf#listtables (accessed May 7, 2010). Data from the American Medical Association (AMA), American Osteopathic Association, and American Association of Colleges of Osteopathic Medicine.

by health maintenance organizations, usually have shorter and more regular hours and enjoy more flexible work schedules than those in private practice. Instead of working as solo practitioners, growing numbers of physicians work in clinics or are partners in group practices or other integrated health care systems. Medical group practices allow physicians to have more flexible schedules, to realize purchasing economies of scale, to pool their money to finance expensive medical equipment, and to be better able to adapt to changes in health care delivery, financing, and reimbursement.

Physicians' earnings are among the highest of any profession. The BLS notes that the median annual total compensation (the point at which half earn more and half earn less) for primary care physicians in 2008 was $186,044 and for specialists it was $339,738. The range of salaries varies widely and is often based on a physician's specialty, the number of years in practice, the hours worked, and the geographic location. The Medical Group Management Association notes in *Physician Compensation*

and Production Survey: 2009 Report Based on 2008 Data (October 2009) that even though physician compensation rose slightly in 2008, most of the increases were outpaced by inflation.

Physician Visits

In 2007 Americans made 994.3 million office visits to physicians. (See Table 2.4.) Women aged 18 to 44 years visited physicians twice as often as men, and, as expected, people 75 years and older of both genders saw doctors more than twice as often as most younger people.

TABLE 2.4

Visits to physician offices by sex, age, and race, selected years 1995–2007

[Data are based on reporting by a sample of office-based physicians, hospital outpatient departments, and hospital emergency departments]

Age, sex, and race	All places[a]				Physician offices			
	1995	2000	2006	2007	1995	2000	2006	2007
	Number of visits in thousands							
Total	**860,859**	**1,014,848**	**1,123,354**	**1,200,017**	**697,082**	**823,542**	**901,954**	**994,321**
Under 18 years	194,644	212,165	231,535	240,813	150,351	163,459	181,560	194,959
18–44 years	285,184	315,774	317,502	335,440	219,065	243,011	234,063	257,257
45–64 years	188,320	255,894	310,667	334,088	159,531	216,783	256,494	283,890
45–54 years	104,891	142,233	164,692	170,514	88,266	119,474	133,402	141,478
55–64 years	83,429	113,661	145,975	163,574	71,264	97,309	123,092	142,412
65 years and over	192,712	231,014	263,649	289,675	168,135	200,289	229,837	258,214
65–74 years	102,605	116,505	124,089	142,528	90,544	102,447	108,063	127,805
75 years and over	90,106	114,510	139,560	147,147	77,591	97,842	121,774	130,409
	Number of visits per 100 persons							
Total, age-adjusted[b]	**334**	**374**	**380**	**402**	**271**	**304**	**305**	**332**
Total, crude	**329**	**370**	**382**	**405**	**266**	**300**	**307**	**336**
Under 18 years	275	293	315	327	213	226	247	264
18–44 years	264	291	287	304	203	224	212	233
45–64 years	364	422	418	439	309	358	345	373
45–54 years	339	385	384	392	286	323	311	325
55–64 years	401	481	465	503	343	412	392	438
65 years and over	612	706	740	799	534	612	645	712
65–74 years	560	656	665	746	494	577	579	669
75 years and over	683	766	824	859	588	654	719	761
Sex and age								
Male, age-adjusted[b]	290	325	328	351	232	261	262	290
Male, crude	277	314	322	345	220	251	256	285
Under 18 years	273	302	309	331	209	231	242	268
18–44 years	190	203	197	205	139	148	139	151
45–54 years	275	316	328	321	229	260	260	262
55–64 years	351	428	410	452	300	367	344	396
65–74 years	508	614	631	732	445	539	554	661
75 years and over	711	771	810	888	616	670	709	801
Female, age-adjusted[b]	377	420	431	452	309	345	346	374
Female, crude	378	424	440	462	310	348	355	384
Under 18 years	277	285	321	321	217	221	252	261
18–44 years	336	377	377	402	265	298	284	315
45–54 years	400	451	437	460	339	384	359	386
55–64 years	446	529	515	550	382	453	436	477
65–74 years	603	692	693	758	534	609	600	676
75 years and over	666	763	832	840	571	645	725	735
Race and age[c]								
White, age-adjusted[2]	339	380	384	398	282	315	317	335
White, crude	338	381	391	407	281	316	324	345
Under 18 years	295	306	325	330	237	243	263	273
18–44 years	267	301	292	298	211	239	225	235
45–54 years	334	386	379	381	286	330	317	324
55–64 years	397	480	465	498	345	416	402	442
65–74 years	557	641	672	735	496	568	593	666
75 years and over	689	764	820	856	598	658	721	765

TABLE 2.4

Visits to physician offices by sex, age, and race, selected years 1995–2007 [CONTINUED]

[Data are based on reporting by a sample of office-based physicians, hospital outpatient departments, and hospital emergency departments]

Age, sex, and race	All places[a]				Physician offices			
	1995	2000	2006	2007	1995	2000	2006	2007
Black or African American, age-adjusted	309	353	397	475	204	239	251	339
Black or African American, crude	281	324	379	450	178	214	235	317
Under 18 years	193	264	299	351	100	167	*188	247
18–44 years	260	257	331	380	158	149	180	241
45–54 years	387	383	438	490	281	269	272	341
55–64 years	414	495	515	592	294	373	347	444
65–74 years	553	656	615	900	429	512	458	748
75 years and over	534	745	744	966	395	568	569	769

*Estimates are considered unreliable.
[a]All places includes visits to physician offices and hospital outpatient and emergency departments.
[b]Estimates are age-adjusted to the year 2000 standard population using six age groups: under 18 years, 18–44 years, 45–54 years, 55–64 years, 65–74 years, and 75 years and over.
[c]Estimates by racial group should be used with caution because information on race was collected from medical records. In 2007, race data were missing and imputed for 29% of ambulatory care visits, including 32% of visits to physician offices, 16% of visits to hospital outpatient departments, and 15% of visits to hospital emergency departments. Information on the race imputation process used in each data year is available in the public use file documentation. Starting with 1999 data, the instruction for the race item on the patient record form was changed so that more than one race could be recorded. In previous years only one race could be checked. Estimates for race in this table are for visits where only one race was recorded. Because of the small number of responses with more than one racial group checked, estimates for visits with multiple races checked are unreliable and are not presented.
Notes: Rates for 1995–2000 were computed using 1990-based postcensal estimates of the civilian noninstitutionalized population as of July 1 adjusted for net underenumeration using the 1990 National Population Adjustment Matrix from the U.S. Census Bureau. Starting with 2001 data, rates were computed using 2000-based postcensal estimates of the civilian noninstitutionalized population as of July 1. The difference between rates for 2000 computed using 1990-based postcensal estimates and 2000 census counts is minimal. Rates will be overestimated to the extent that visits by institutionalized persons are counted in the numerator (for example, hospital emergency department visits by nursing home residents) and institutionalized persons are omitted from the denominator (the civilian noninstitutionalized population).

SOURCE: Adapted from "Table 91. Visits to Physician Offices, Hospital Outpatient Departments, and Hospital Emergency Departments, by Selected Characteristics: United States, Selected Years 1995–2007," in *Health, United States, 2009: With Special Feature on Medical Technology*, U.S. Department of Health and Human Services, Centers for Disease Control and Prevention, National Center for Health Statistics, 2010, http://www.cdc.gov/nchs/data/hus/hus09 .pdf#listtables (accessed May 7, 2010)

Physician Satisfaction

Changes in the health care delivery system—particularly the shift from traditional fee-for-service practice (paid for each visit, procedure, or treatment that is delivered) to managed care, with its efforts to standardize medical practice, which reduces physicians' ability to manage their time, schedules, and professional relationships—have been named as factors contributing to physicians' dissatisfaction with their choice of career. Other changes, including decreasing reimbursement and an ever-increasing emphasis on documentation to satisfy government and private payers, as well as administrative requirements that infringe on the time physicians would rather spend caring for patients, have also increased physician dissatisfaction.

Eric S. Williams et al. explain in "Understanding Physicians' Intentions to Withdraw from Practice: The Role of Job Satisfaction, Job Stress, Mental and Physical Health" (*Health Care Management Review*, vol. 35, no. 2, April–June 2010) that job satisfaction is strongly related to physicians' intentions to decrease the hours they work, change specialty, leave direct patient care, or quit medicine altogether.

Williams et al. reviewed the available literature describing the relationship of satisfaction or dissatisfaction to a variety of variables including stress, mental health, and physical health, as well as intentions to decrease hours worked, change specialty, or leave direct patient care. The researchers indicate that one of the most frequently mentioned workplace concerns of physicians is increasing workload and time pressure and that there is a strong association between dissatisfaction with workload and intentions to leave. Williams et al. then surveyed a sample of 5,704 of the more than 171,000 clinically active civilian physicians working primarily in patient care in office or hospital settings as family physicians and generalist internists.

As might be expected, the researchers find that higher perceived stress is associated with lower satisfaction levels that are related to greater intentions to quit, decrease work hours, change specialty, or leave direct patient care. They also discover that physicians experiencing burnout, anxiety, and depression appeared to attempt to cope with these feelings by leaving patient care in some way, rather than by quitting their job, decreasing work hours, or changing specialty. Some physicians planned to retire early. Others were able to assume administrative roles within their organization.

Williams et al. assert that when "primary care clinicians are recognized as patient advocates and encouraged to provide appropriate, effective, and timely access to specialty services for their patients," both physician satisfaction and the quality of care will improve.

REGISTERED NURSES

Registered nurses (RNs) are licensed by the state to care for the sick and to promote health. RNs supervise hospital care, administer medication and treatment as prescribed by physicians, monitor the progress of patients, and provide health education. Nurses work in a variety of settings, including hospitals, nursing homes, physicians' offices, clinics, and schools.

Education for Nurses

There are three types of education for RNs: associate's degrees (two-year community college programs), baccalaureate programs (four years of college), and post-graduate (master's degree and doctorate) programs. The baccalaureate degree provides more knowledge of community health services, as well as the psychological and social aspects of caring for patients, than does the associate's degree. Those who complete the four-year baccalaureate degree and the other advanced degrees are generally better prepared to eventually attain administrative or management positions and may have greater opportunities for upward mobility in related disciplines such as research, teaching, and public health.

The number of RNs grew from 2.2 million in 1999 to nearly 2.5 million in 2007. (See Table 2.5.) In *The Registered Nurse Population: Initial Findings from the 2008 National Sample Survey of Registered Nurses* (March 2010, http://bhpr.hrsa.gov/healthworkforce/rnsurvey/

TABLE 2.5

Health personnel by occupation, selected years 1999–2007

[Data are based on a semiannual mail survey of nonfarm establishments]

Occupation title	1999	2002	2005	2007	1999–2007 AAPC[b]	1999	2002	2005	2007	1999–2007 AAPC[b]
		Number of employees[a]					Mean hourly wage[c]			
Health care practitioner and technical occupations										
Audiologists	12,950	10,180	10,030	11,360	−1.6	$21.96	$24.92	$27.72	$30.61	4.2
Cardiovascular technologists and technicians	41,490	42,870	43,560	46,980	1 6	16.00	18.12	19.99	22.37	4.3
Dental hygienists	90,050	148,530	161,140	168,600	8.2	23.15	27.78	29.15	31.21	3.8
Diagnostic medical sonographers	29,280	36,530	43,590	46,770	6.0	21.04	23.90	26.65	29.13	4.2
Dietetic technicians	29,190	28,910	23,780	24,540	−2.1	10.09	11.59	12.20	12.83	3.0
Dietitians and nutritionists	41,320	45,150	48,850	52,800	3.1	17.96	20.16	22.09	24.05	3.7
Emergency medical technicians and paramedics	172,360	178,700	196,880	201,200	2.0	11.19	12.78	13.68	14.84	3.6
Licensed practical and licensed vocational nurses	688,510	692,290	710,020	719,240	0.5	13.95	15.53	17.41	18.72	3.7
Nuclear medicine technologists	17,880	17,090	18,280	20,410	1.7	20.40	25.13	29.10	31.43	5.6
Occupational therapists	78,950	78,580	87,430	91,920	1.9	24.96	25.50	28.41	31.51	3.0
Opticians, dispensing	58,860	61,790	70,090	62,420	0.7	12.11	13.38	14.80	16.10	3.6
Pharmacists	226,300	219,390	229,740	253,110	1.4	30.31	36.13	42.62	47.58	5.8
Pharmacy technicians	196,430	207,380	266,790	301,950	5.5	9.64	11.15	12.19	13.25	4.1
Physical therapists	131,050	130,290	151,280	161,850	2.7	28.05	28.93	31.42	34.39	2.6
Physician assistants	56,750	61,910	63,350	67,160	2.1	24.35	30.53	34.17	37.41	5.5
Psychiatric technicians	54,560	58,600	62,040	60,690	1.3	11.30	13.49	14.04	15.21	3.8
Radiation therapists	12,340	13,510	14,120	14,620	2.1	20.84	28.90	30.59	34.61	6.5
Radiologic technologists and technicians	177,850	173,540	184,580	200,370	1.5	17.07	19.30	22.60	24.59	4.7
Recreational therapists	30,190	26,130	23,260	23,240	−3.2	14.08	15.23	16.90	18.43	3.4
Registered nurses	2,205,430	2,239,530	2,368,070	2,468,340	1.4	21.38	23.96	27.35	30.04	4.3
Respiratory therapists	80,230	85,350	95,320	101,180	2.9	17.72	19.57	22.24	24.49	4.1
Respiratory therapy technicians	33,990	26,220	22,060	17,610	−7.9	16.07	16.79	18.57	20.00	2.8
Speech-language pathologists	85,920	87,030	94,660	103,810	2.4	22.99	24.75	27.89	30.64	3.7
Health care support occupations										
Dental assistants	175,160	268,220	270,720	283,680	6.2	11.60	13.42	14.41	15.52	3.7
Home health aides	577,530	569,670	663,280	834,580	4.7	9.04	9.16	9.34	10.03	1.3
Massage therapists	21,910	27,160	37,670	45,920	9.7	13.82	16.21	19.33	19.39	4.3
Medical assistants	281,480	361,960	382,720	434,540	5.6	10.89	11.93	12.58	13.59	2.8
Medical equipment preparers	29,070	35,490	41,790	43,790	5.3	10.20	11.50	12.42	13.43	3.5
Medical transcriptionists	97,260	99,160	90,380	86,990	−1.4	11.86	13.33	14.36	15.44	3.4
Nursing aides, orderlies, and attendants	1,308,740	1,329,310	1,391,430	1,390,260	0.8	8.59	9.87	10.67	11.50	3.7
Occupational therapist aides	9,250	8,040	6,220	7,640	−2.4	10.92	11.78	13.20	13.91	3.1
Occupational therapist assistants	17,290	17,970	22,160	25,130	4.8	15.97	17.76	19.13	21.72	3.9
Pharmacy aides	48,270	58,020	46,610	49,630	0.3	9.14	9.47	9.76	10.15	1.3
Physical therapist aides	44,340	37,330	41,930	43,350	−0.3	9.69	10.63	11.01	11.58	2.3
Physical therapist assistants	48,600	50,430	58,670	59,120	2.5	16.20	17.48	18.98	21.32	3.5
Psychiatric aides	51,100	56,260	56,150	58,310	1.7	10.76	11.42	11.47	12.54	1.9

[a]Estimates do not include self-employed workers and were rounded to the nearest 10.
[b]AAPC is average annual percent change.
[c]The mean hourly wage rate for an occupation is the total wages that all workers in the occupation earn in an hour divided by the total employment of the occupation.
Notes: This table excludes occupations such as dentists, physicians, and chiropractors, which have a large percentage of workers who are self-employed and/or not employed by establishments.

SOURCE: "Table 111. Employees and Wages, by Selected Healthcare Occupations: United States, Selected Years 1999–2007," in *Health, United States, 2009: With Special Feature on Medical Technology*, U.S. Department of Health and Human Services, Centers for Disease Control and Prevention, National Center for Health Statistics, 2010, http://www.cdc.gov/nchs/data/hus/hus09.pdf#listtables (accessed May 7, 2010)

FIGURE 2.2

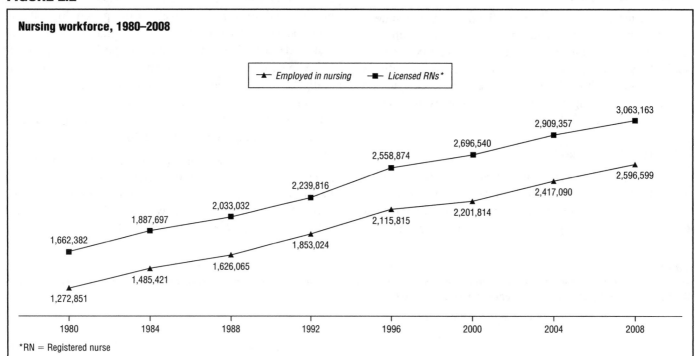

Nursing workforce, 1980–2008

*RN = Registered nurse

SOURCE: "Chart 1. U.S. Nursing Workforce, 1980–2008," in *The Registered Nurse Population: Initial Findings from the 2008 National Sample Survey of Registered Nurses*, U.S. Department of Health and Human Services, Health Resources and Services Administration, March 2010, http://bhpr.hrsa.gov/healthworkforce/rnsurvey/initialfindings2008.pdf (accessed May 10, 2010)

initialfindings2008.pdf), the HRSA reports that as of 2008 there were nearly 3.1 million RNs working in the United States. (See Figure 2.2.) This number represents a 5.3% increase from 2004, and the percentage of nurses working full time in the field rose from 58.4% to 63.2% during the same period. The largest percentage of increases occurred among those holding baccalaureate, master's, and doctorate degrees. Figure 2.3 shows the trend from 1980 to 2008 of increasing numbers of RNs entering the profession with bachelor's, master's, and doctorate degrees.

NEED FOR NURSES EXCEEDS SUPPLY. Even though the number of RNs holding baccalaureate degrees increased sharply during the 1990s, there is still a shortage of nurses that is predicted to persist until 2020. Some health care experts believe the shortage is intensifying because more lucrative fields are now open to women, the traditional nursing population. In health occupations alone, the percentage of female students entering traditionally male professions continues to increase. For example, during the 1980–81 academic year women accounted for just 19.8% of first-year dentistry students, compared with 43.2% of the class entering the 2006–07 academic year. (See Table 2.6.) Similarly, increasing percentages of women are attending medical school and training to become optometrists, pharmacists, podiatrists, and public health care workers. Meanwhile, the American Association of Colleges of Nursing indicates in the press release "Student Enrollment Expands at U.S. Nursing Colleges and Universities for the 9th Year

Despite Financial Challenges and Capacity Restraints" (December 2, 2009, http://www.aacn.nche.edu/Media/NewsReleases/2009/StudentEnrollment.html) that nursing school enrollment increased by just 3.5% from 2008 to 2009. According to the association, faculty shortages, budget cuts, and too few clinical training sites continue to hamper growth in nursing schools.

Industry observers believe this shortage results from a combination of factors including an aging population, a sicker population of hospitalized patients requiring more labor-intensive care, and a public perception that nursing is a thankless, unglamorous job that requires grueling physical labor, long hours, and low pay. In "The 50 Best Careers of 2010" (*U.S. News and World Report*, December 28, 2009), Liz Wolgemuth deems nursing a "good career," with salaries ranging from $43,400 to $92,200 per year and with excellent job security. Observers also note that the public, particularly high school students considering careers in health care, are unaware of the many new opportunities in nursing, such as advanced practice nursing, which offers additional independence and increased earning potential, and the technology-driven field of applied informatics (computer management of information).

ADVANCED PRACTICE NURSES AND PHYSICIAN ASSISTANTS

Much of the preventive medical care and treatment usually delivered by physicians may also be provided by

FIGURE 2.3

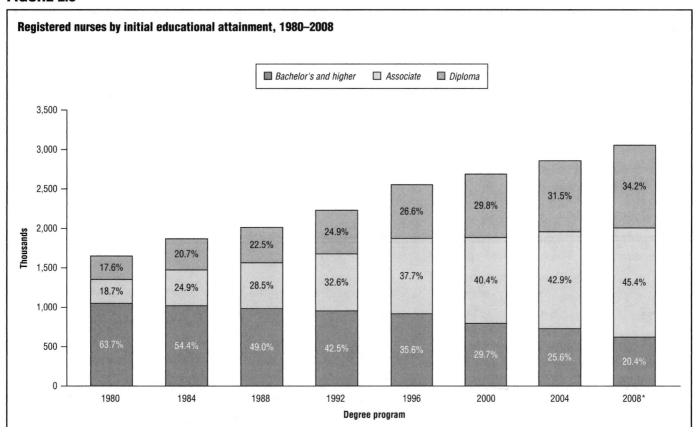

Registered nurses by initial educational attainment, 1980–2008

Legend: Bachelor's and higher | Associate | Diploma

Y-axis: Thousands

Year	Diploma	Associate	Bachelor's and higher
1980	17.6%	18.7%	63.7%
1984	20.7%	24.9%	54.4%
1988	22.5%	28.5%	49.0%
1992	24.9%	32.6%	42.5%
1996	26.6%	37.7%	35.6%
2000	29.8%	40.4%	29.7%
2004	31.5%	42.9%	25.6%
2008*	34.2%	45.4%	20.4%

Degree program

Note: The counts for all initial degrees may not add to the total registered nurse (RN) estimates for each survey due to incomplete information provided by respondents and the effect of rounding. Only those who provided educational preparation information are included in the calculations used for this chart.
*For 2008 initial education, there were 13,325 RNs with masters degrees (0.4%) and 954 RNs with doctoral degrees (0.03%).

SOURCE: "Chart 3. Distribution of the Registered Nurses according to Initial Nursing Education, 1980–2008," in *The Registered Nurse Population: Initial Findings from the 2008 National Sample Survey of Registered Nurses*, U.S. Department of Health and Human Services, Health Resources and Services Administration, March 2010, http://bhpr.hrsa.gov/healthworkforce/rnsurvey/initialfindings2008.pdf (accessed May 10, 2010)

midlevel practitioners—health professionals with less formal education and training than physicians. Advanced practice nurses make up a group that includes certified nurse midwives, nurse practitioners (NPs; RNs with advanced academic and clinical experience), and clinical nurse specialists (RNs with advanced nursing degrees who specialize in areas such as mental health, gerontology, cardiac or cancer care, or community or neonatal health). Physician assistants (PAs) are midlevel practitioners who work under the auspices, supervision, or direction of physicians. They conduct physical examinations, order and interpret laboratory and radiological studies, and prescribe medication. They even perform procedures (e.g., flexible sigmoidoscopy, biopsy, suturing, casting, and administering anesthesia) that were once performed exclusively by physicians.

The origins of each profession are key to understanding the differences between them. Nursing has the longer history, and nurses are recognized members of the health care team. For this reason, NPs were easily integrated into many practice settings.

PA is the newer of the two disciplines. PAs have been practicing in the United States since the early 1970s. The career originated as civilian employment for returning Vietnam War (1954–1975) veterans who had worked as medics. The veterans needed immediate employment and few had the educational prerequisites, time, or resources to pursue the training necessary to become physicians. At the same time, the United States was projecting a dire shortage of primary care physicians, especially in rural and inner-city practices. The use of PAs and NPs was seen as an ideal rapid response to the demand for additional medical services. They could be deployed quickly to serve remote communities or underserved populations for a fraction of the costs associated with physicians.

The numbers of PAs and NPs have increased dramatically since the beginning of the 1990s. The HRSA estimates in *Registered Nurse Population* that in 2008 there were 250,527 advanced practice nurses—158,348 NPs, 59,242 clinical nurse specialists, 34,821 certified RN anesthetists, and 19,134 certified nurse midwives. According to the American Academy of Physician Assistants (AAPA; http://aapa.org/about-pas/faq-about-pas), as of May 2010 there were 88,771 PAs eligible to practice.

TABLE 2.6

First-year and total enrollment of women in schools for selected health occupations, selected academic years 1980–81 through 2006–07

[Data are based on reporting by health professions associations]

Enrollment and occupation	Both sexes				Women			
	1980–1981	1990–1991[a]	2000–2001	2006–2007[b]	1980–1981	1990–1991[a]	2000–2001	2006–2007[b]
First-year enrollment	Number of students				Percent of students			
Dentistry	6,030	4,001	4,327	4,733	19.8	38.0	39.8	43.2
Medicine (allopathic)[c]	17,186	16,876	16,699	17,826	28.9	38.8	45.9	48.7
Medicine (osteopathic)	1,496	1,950	2,927	4,055	22.0	34.2	42.4	49.9
Nurses[d]	—	—	—	—	—	—	—	—
Optometry[b]	1,258	1,239	1,384	1,434	25.3	50.6	57.2	64.9
Pharmacy[c, e]	7,377	8,267	8,382	10,992	48.4	—	66.4	62.9
Podiatry	695	561	475	647	—	28.0	40.6	44.0
Public health[c]	3,348	4,289	5,840	7,382	—	62.1	69.8	69.8
Total enrollment								
Dentistry	22,842	15,951	17,349	19,038	17.0	34.4	38.7	44.3
Medicine (allopathic)[c]	65,189	65,163	69,414	73,100	26.5	37.3	44.6	48.5
Medicine (osteopathic)	4,940	6,792	10,817	14,409	19.7	32.7	41.1	50.3
Nurses[d]	—	—	—	177,822	—	—	—	90.1
Optometry[c]	4,641	4,760	5,428	5,488	—	47.3	55.5	64.2
Pharmacy[c, e]	26,617	29,797	34,481	48,592	47.4	62.4	65.9	64.2
Podiatry	2,577	2,154	1,968	1,879	11.9	28.9	36.4	45.7
Public health[c]	8,486	11,386	16,019	20,907	55.2	62.5	68.0	70.0

—Data not available.

[a]Percentage of women podiatry students is for 1991–1992.

[b]Starting with 2003–2004 data, osteopathic medicine data include the students of the Edward Via Virginia College of Osteopathic Medicine.

[c]Includes data from schools in Puerto Rico.

[d]Data are for generic (entry-level) or registered nurses seeking the baccalaureate degree. Gender data for first-year enrollment are not available.

[e]First-year enrollment data for pharmacy schools are for students in the first year of the final three years of pharmacy education. Prior to 2000–2001, pharmacy total enrollment data were for students in the final three years of pharmacy education. Starting in 2000–2001, pharmacy total enrollment data are for all students. In 2006, one pharmacy school did not report enrollment data.

Note: Total enrollment data are collected at the beginning of the academic year while first-year enrollment data are collected during the academic year.

SOURCE: "Table 114. First-Year and Total Enrollment of Women in Schools for Selected Health Occupations: United States, Selected Academic Years 1980–81 through 2006–07," in *Health, United States, 2009: With Special Feature on Medical Technology*, U.S. Department of Health and Human Services, Centers for Disease Control and Prevention, National Center for Health Statistics, 2010, http://www.cdc.gov/nchs/data/hus/hus09.pdf#listtables (accessed May 10, 2010). Non-government data from the American Dental Association, Association of American Medical Colleges, American Association of Colleges of Osteopathic Medicine, American Association of Colleges of Nursing, American Association of Colleges of Pharmacy, American Association of Colleges of Podiatric Medicine, and Association of Schools of Public Health.

Training, Certification, and Practice

Advanced practice nurses usually have considerable clinical nursing experience before completing certificate or master's degree NP programs. Key components of NP programs are instruction in nursing theory and practice and a period of direct supervision by a physician or NP. The American College of Nurse Practitioners (2010, http://www.acnpweb.org/i4a/pages/index.cfm?pageid=3465) explains that NPs are a scope of practice that varies from state to state, with "some states having independent practice for NPs (not requiring any physician involvement), [and] some with collaborative agreement required with a physician."

The Commission on Accreditation of Allied Health Education Programs accredits PA training programs. In "Becoming a Physician Assistant" (2010, http://www.aapa.org/about-pas/becoming-a-physician-assistant), the AAPA notes that most students have an undergraduate degree and health care experience before they enter a PA training program, which lasts an average of 26.5 months. Graduates sit for a national certifying examination and, once certified, must earn 100 hours of continuing medical education every two years and pass a recertification exam every six years.

PA practice is always delegated by the physician and conducted with physician supervision. The extent and nature of physician supervision varies from state to state. For example, Connecticut permits a physician to supervise up to six PAs, whereas California limits a supervising physician to two. Even though PAs work interdependently with physicians, supervision is not necessarily direct and onsite; some PAs working in remote communities are supervised primarily by telephone.

In *Vital Statistics* (March 2010, http://saaapa.aapa.org/images/stories/news/vitalstatssheet2010-final.pdf), the AAPA notes that in 2009 the mean (average) annual income of PAs who were employed full time was $93,105.

Distinctions between Midlevel Practitioners Blurring

Pohla Smith reports in "Doing Doctors' Work" (*Pittsburgh Post-Gazette*, March 12, 2008) that even though their training may be different, in terms of their day-to-day job responsibilities, NPs and PAs are becoming essentially interchangeable. Both types of practitioners diagnose and treat illness, take medical histories, and perform physical examinations. They can order diagnostic tests, prescribe medication, and assist in operating rooms and emergency departments.

In "Doctor Shortage? 28 States May Expand Nurses' Role" (Associated Press, April 13, 2010), Carla K. Johnson indicates that 28 states are considering expanding NPs' scopes of practice. In some states, such as Montana, NPs can practice without supervision from a physician, and in Massachusetts NPs are recognized as primary care practitioners on a par with physicians; however, other states still require NPs to work with physicians in practice. Even though NPs' roles have been gradually expanding over time, the Patient Protection and Affordable Care Act of 2010 may accelerate broadening the responsibilities of NPs, because it will extend health insurance coverage to millions of previously uninsured Americans, which will create demand for services that cannot be met by physicians alone.

Several provisions of the 2010 health care reform legislation expand the role of nurses by encouraging training and increasing compensation. These include:

- $50 million to clinics managed by nurses that provide care to low-income patients

- $50 million annually from 2012 to 2015 for hospitals to train nurses with advanced degrees to care for Medicare patients

- 10 percent bonuses from Medicare from 2011 to 2016 to primary care providers, including NPs, who work in physician-shortage areas

- An increase in Medicare reimbursement for certified nurse midwives, giving them the same compensation as physicians

DENTISTS

Dentists diagnose and treat problems of the teeth, gums, and mouth, take x-rays, apply protective plastic sealant to children's teeth, fill cavities, straighten teeth, and treat gum disease. The BLS (December 17, 2009, http://www.bls.gov/oco/ocos072.htm) reports that dentists worked at 141,900 jobs in 2008.

Fluoridation of community water supplies and improved dental hygiene have dramatically improved the dental health of Americans. Dental caries (cavities) among all age groups have declined significantly. As a result, many dental services are shifting focus from young people to adults. In the 21st century many adults are choosing to have orthodontic services, such as straightening their teeth. In addition, the growing older adult population

generally requires more complex dental procedures, such as endodontic (root canal) services, bridges, and dentures.

The overwhelming majority of dentists own solo dental practices, where only one dentist operates in each office. The BLS reports that in 2008 about 28% of dentists were self-employed, nearly all were in private practice, and nearly 15% of dentists belonged to a partnership. On average, dentists work between 35 and 40 hours per week and supervise staffers, such as dental assistants and hygienists. The BLS notes that self-employed dentists in general practice had mean annual wages of $142,870 in May 2008.

Dental Specialists

The ADA identifies nine recognized specialties in "Dentistry Definitions" (2010, http://www.ada.org/495.aspx). The BLS notes that in 2008 about 15% of dentists were specialists. Orthodontists, who straighten teeth, make up the largest group of specialists. The next largest group, oral and maxillofacial surgeons, operates on the mouth and jaws. The balance of the specialists concentrates in pediatric dentistry (dentistry for children), periodontics (treating the gums), prosthodontics (making dentures and artificial teeth), endodontics (root canals), public health dentistry (community dental health), and oral pathology (diseases of the mouth).

Training to Become a Dentist

Entry into dental schools requires two to four years of college-level predental education—most dental students have earned excellent grades and have at least a bachelor's degree when they enter dental school. Dentists should have good visual memory, excellent judgment about space and shape, a high degree of manual dexterity, and scientific ability. Development and maintenance of a successful private practice requires business acumen, the ability to manage and organize people and materials, and strong interpersonal skills.

Dental schools require applicants to take the Dental Admissions Test (DAT). During the admission process, schools consider scores earned on the DAT, applicants' grade-point averages, and information gleaned from recommendations and interviews. Dental school usually lasts four academic years. A student begins by studying the basic sciences, including anatomy, microbiology, biochemistry, and physiology. During the last two years students receive practical experience by treating patients, usually in dental clinics that are supervised by licensed dentists.

Visiting a Dentist

In 2007, 65.3% of Americans aged two years and older had visited a dentist at least once in the past year. (See Table 2.7.) Children aged two to 17 years (76.7%)

TABLE 2.7

Dental visits in the past year by selected characteristics, 1997, 2006, and 2007

[Data are based on household interviews of a sample of the civilian noninstitutionalized population]

Characteristic	2 years and over			2–17 years			18–64 years			65 years and over[a]		
	1997	2006	2007	1997	2006	2007	1997	2006	2007	1997	2006	2007
	Percent of persons with a dental visit in the past year[b]											
Total[c]	**65.1**	**64.9**	**65.3**	**72.7**	**75.7**	**76.7**	**64.1**	**62.4**	**62.7**	**54.8**	**58.0**	**57.7**
Sex												
Male	62.9	61.5	62.8	72.3	75.0	76.5	60.4	57.5	58.8	55.4	55.3	56.4
Female	67.1	68.2	67.7	73.0	76.5	76.9	67.7	67.1	66.5	54.4	60.0	58.7
Race[d]												
White only	66.4	65.7	66.4	74.0	76.4	77.2	65.7	63.3	64.2	56.8	59.5	59.7
Black or African American only	58.9	59.0	59.3	68.8	72.4	75.0	57.0	55.6	55.0	35.4	40.7	40.1
American Indian or Alaska Native only	55.1	55.4	57.8	66.8	72.0	85.4	49.9	51.0	45.6	*	*	41.2
Asian only	62.5	69.8	64.3	69.9	75.5	70.7	60.3	68.7	63.7	53.9	66.0	55.3
Native Hawaiian or other Pacific Islander only	—	*	*	—	*	*	—	*	*	—	*	*
2 or more races	—	65.8	62.7	—	78.1	75.3	—	54.9	55.2	—	62.9	41.6
Black or African American; white	—	72.3	70.7	—	79.5	76.6	—	59.5	57.7	—	*	70.8
American Indian or Alaska Native; white	—	55.7	55.6	—	69.6	75.9	—	48.5	51.0	—	62.9	35.7
Hispanic origin and race[d]												
Hispanic or Latino	54.0	53.0	55.8	61.0	66.3	71.2	50.8	47.2	48.9	47.8	44.2	48.0
Not Hispanic or Latino	66.4	66.9	67.0	74.7	78.1	78.1	65.7	64.9	65.1	55.2	58.9	58.4
White only	68.0	68.2	68.7	76.4	79.6	79.5	67.5	66.5	67.3	57.2	60.6	60.7
Black or African American only	58.8	59.0	59.3	68.8	72.4	75.0	56.9	55.5	55.1	35.3	40.9	39.6
Percent of poverty level[e]												
Below 100%	50.5	51.5	51.7	62.0	67.5	67.3	46.9	44.8	46.7	31.5	36.9	32.8
100%–less than 200%	50.8	52.0	52.8	62.5	68.4	70.2	48.3	46.8	47.0	40.8	44.5	43.3
200% or more	72.5	71.7	71.5	80.1	81.5	82.0	71.2	69.6	69.3	65.9	67.3	66.9
Hispanic origin and race and percent of poverty level[d, e]												
Hispanic or Latino:												
Below 100%	45.7	46.6	47.6	55.9	63.1	66.8	39.2	36.7	35.0	33.6	29.7	36.9
100%–less than 200%	47.2	47.5	51.0	53.8	62.2	69.4	43.5	40.7	40.6	47.9	36.5	48.1
200% or more	65.1	60.5	63.2	73.7	72.9	76.5	62.3	56.1	59.3	58.8	59.5	53.1
Not Hispanic or Latino:												
White only:												
Below 100%	51.7	55.1	53.9	64.4	71.6	65.1	50.6	50.6	54.8	32.0	41.4	32.5
100%–less than 200%	52.4	53.2	53.1	66.1	71.5	70.0	50.4	48.6	49.3	42.2	46.7	44.4
200% or more	73.8	73.4	73.6	81.3	83.3	83.5	72.7	71.7	71.7	67.0	68.1	69.0
Black or African American only:												
Below 100%	52.8	49.3	51.0	66.1	67.1	70.1	46.2	39.9	40.7	27.7	27.8	28.6
100%–less than 200%	48.7	52.8	53.8	61.2	70.1	72.1	46.3	48.7	48.6	26.9	28.6	28.7
200% or more	67.7	67.7	66.1	77.1	79.2	81.9	66.1	65.1	63.4	49.8	58.3	51.0

*Estimates are considered unreliable.

—Data not available.

[a]Based on the 1997–2007 National Health Interview Surveys, about 25%–30% of persons 65 years and over were edentulous (having lost all their natural teeth). In 1997–2007 about 68%–70% of older dentate persons compared with 16%–21% of older edentate persons had a dental visit in the past year.

[b]Respondents were asked "About how long has it been since you last saw or talked to a dentist?"

[c]Includes all other races not shown separately.

[d]The race groups, white, black, American Indian or Alaska Native, Asian, Native Hawaiian or other Pacific Islander, and 2 or more races, include persons of Hispanic and non-Hispanic origin. Persons of Hispanic origin may be of any race. Starting with 1999 data, race-specific estimates are tabulated according to the 1997 Revisions to the Standards for the Classification of Federal Data on Race and Ethnicity and are not strictly comparable with estimates for earlier years. The five single-race categories plus multiple-race categories shown in the table conform to the 1997 standards. Starting with 1999 data, race-specific estimates are for persons who reported only one racial group; the category 2 or more races includes persons who reported more than one racial group. Prior to 1999, data were tabulated according to the 1977 standards with four racial groups, and the Asian only category included Native Hawaiian or other Pacific Islander. Estimates for single-race categories prior to 1999 included persons who reported one race or, if they reported more than one race, identified one race as best representing their race. Starting with 2003 data, race responses of other race and unspecified multiple race were treated as missing, and then race was imputed if these were the only race responses. Almost all persons with a race response of other race were of Hispanic origin.

[e]Percent of poverty level is based on family income and family size and composition using U.S. Census Bureau poverty thresholds. Missing family income data were imputed for 25%–29% of persons 2 years of age and over in 1997–1998 and 31%–34% in 1999–2007.

Note: In 1997 the National Health Interview Survey questionnaire was redesigned.

SOURCE: Adapted from "Table 93. Dental Visits in the Past Year, by Selected Characteristics: United States, 1997, 2006, and 2007," in *Health, United States, 2009: With Special Feature on Medical Technology*, U.S. Department of Health and Human Services, Centers for Disease Control and Prevention, National Center for Health Statistics, 2010, http://www.cdc.gov/nchs/data/hus/hus09.pdf#listtables (accessed May 11, 2010)

were more likely to have visited a dentist than any other age group, and women aged 65 years and older (58.7%) were somewhat more likely to see a dentist than were men (56.4%). Among adults aged 18 to 64 years, the proportion of non-Hispanic whites (67.3%) visiting a dentist was considerably higher than the proportions of non-Hispanic African-Americans (55.1%) and Hispanics (48.9%). People who were poor or near poor were much less likely to visit a dentist annually than those who were not poor. For example, among adults aged 18 to 64 years,

46.7% of people who were 100% below the poverty level had visited a dentist in the past year, compared with 69.3% of people who were 200% or more above the poverty level.

SEVERE SHORTAGES OF DENTISTS IN SOME AREAS. The United States boasts the highest concentration of dentists of any country in the world. Nonetheless, health care planners caution that dentists' ranks will begin to decline in 2014, according to Roger Collier, in "United States Faces Dental Shortage" (October 21, 2009, http://www.cmaj.ca/earlyreleases/21oct09_dentist_shortage.dtl). Collier cites several factors that will exacerbate the existing shortage of general dentists. First, many dentists are choosing specialties such as orthodontics and are reluctant to practice in rural areas, where dentists are in short supply. Second, there have been dental school closures and the size of graduating classes are getting smaller. Third, female dentists tend to work fewer hours than male dentists. Finally, many practicing dentists are poised to retire.

ALLIED HEALTH CARE PROVIDERS

Many health care services are provided by an interdisciplinary team of health professionals. The complete health care team may include physicians, nurses, mid-level practitioners, and dentists; physical and occupational therapists; audiologists and speech-language pathologists; licensed practical nurses, nurses' aides, and home health aides; and pharmacists, optometrists, podiatrists, dental hygienists, social workers, registered dieticians, and others. Table 2.8 describes some of these allied heath professions. Specific health care teams are assembled to meet the varying needs of patients. For example, the team involved in stroke rehabilitation might include a physician, a nurse, a speech-language pathologist, a social worker, and physical and occupational therapists.

Because California is one of the most populous states in the country and among the top-10 economies of the world, trends in the health care workforce in California are often forerunners of the challenges and opportunities that other states may experience. According to the California Hospital Association (CHA), in *Allied Health: The Hidden Health Care Workforce—Addressing the Long Term Need for Qualified, Culturally Competent Allied Health Professionals* (July 2009, http://www.oshpd.ca.gov/rhpc/jobs/HiddenHealthCareWorkforceReport_09_V7.pdf), California faces a future shortage of allied health care professionals. Besides an unmet need for hospital nurses and pharmacists, the CHA describes a shortage of clinical laboratory scientists and medical laboratory technicians as "one of the most pressing workforce issues currently facing hospitals." The CHA lists several obstacles to growing the allied health care workforce, including an insufficient number of accredited educational programs, too few spaces in these programs, faculty shortages, and an insufficient number of clinical training sites where students gain experience.

TABLE 2.8

Allied health care providers

Dental hygienists provide services for maintaining oral health. Their primary duty is to clean teeth.
Emergency medical technicians (EMTs) provide immediate care to critically ill or injured people in emergency situations.
Home health aides provide nursing, household, and personal care services to patients who are homebound or disabled.
Licensed practical nurse (LPNs) are trained and licensed to provide basic nursing care under the supervision of registered nurses and doctors.
Medical records personnel analyze patient records and keep them up-to-date, complete, accurate, and confidential.
Medical technologists perform laboratory tests to help diagnose diseases and to aid in identifying their causes and extent.
Nurses' aides, orderlies, and attendants help nurses in hospitals, nursing homes, and other facilities.
Occupational therapists help disabled persons adapt to their disabilities. This may include helping a patient relearn basic living skills or modifying the environment.
Optometrists measure vision for corrective lenses and prescribe glasses.
Pharmacists are trained and licensed to make up and dispense drugs in accordance with a physician's prescription.
Physician assistants (PAs) work under a doctor's supervision. Their duties include performing routine physical exams, prescribing certain drugs, and providing medical counseling.
Physical therapists work with disabled patients to help restore function, strength and mobility. PTs use exercise, heat, cold, water, and electricity to relieve pain and restore function.
Podiatrists diagnose and treat diseases, injuries, and abnormalities of the feet. They may use drugs and surgery to treat foot problems.
Psychologists are trained in human behavior and provide counseling and testing services related to mental health.
Radiation technicians take and develop x-ray photographs for medical purposes.
Registered dietitians (RDs) are licensed to use dietary principles to maintain health and treat disease.
Respiratory therapists treat breathing problems under a doctor's supervision and help in respiratory rehabilitation.
Social workers help patients to handle social problems such as finances, housing, and social and family problems that arise out of illness or disability.
Speech pathologists diagnose and treat disorders of speech and communication.

SOURCE: "Allied Health Care Providers," U.S. Department of Commerce, Washington, DC

Physical and Occupational Therapists

Physical therapists (PTs) are licensed practitioners who work with patients to preserve and restore function, improve capabilities and mobility, and regain independence following an illness or injury. They also aim to prevent or limit disability and slow the progress of debilitating diseases. Treatment involves exercise to improve range of motion, balance, coordination, flexibility, strength, and endurance. PTs may also use electrical stimulation to promote healing, hot and cold packs to relieve pain and inflammation (swelling), and therapeutic massage.

According to the BLS (December 17, 2009, http://www.bls.gov/oco/ocos080.htm), PTs worked at 185,500 jobs in 2008, but some were part-time jobs and some PTs had two or more jobs at the same time. About 60% of practicing PTs worked in hospitals and physicians' offices; the remaining PTs were employed in outpatient rehabilitation clinics, nursing homes, and home health agencies. Even though most work in rehabilitation, PTs may specialize in areas such as sports medicine, pediatrics, or neurology. PTs often work as members of a health care team and may supervise PT assistants or aides. The BLS notes that the median annual wages for PTs were $72,790 in May 2008.

The BLS indicates that PTs are required to earn a master's or doctorate degree from an accredited physical therapy program. To practice physical therapy, PTs must obtain state licensure, and even though the requirements vary by state, licensure generally requires graduation from an accredited physical therapy education program and passing a national examination. Many states also require continuing education as a condition of maintaining licensure.

Occupational therapists (OTs) focus on helping people relearn and improve their abilities to perform the "activities of daily living," meaning the tasks they perform during the course of their work and home life. Examples of activities of daily living that OTs help patients regain are dressing, bathing, and meal preparation. For people with long-term or permanent disabilities, OTs may assist them to find new ways to accomplish their responsibilities on the job, sometimes by using adaptive equipment or by asking employers to accommodate workers with special needs such as people in wheelchairs. OTs use computer programs and simulations to help patients restore fine motor skills and practice reasoning, decision making, and problem solving.

A master's degree or higher in occupational therapy is the minimum educational requirement. The American Occupational Therapy Association states in "FAQ about the Entry-Level Master's and Doctoral Degrees for Occupational Therapist" (April 6, 2010, http://www.aota.org/Students/FAQDegrees.aspx) that "an entry-level degree for occupational therapists is the degree required to enter the profession and to be eligible to sit for the Occupational Therapist Registered ... examination administered by the National Board for Certification in Occupational Therapy.... Occupational therapy requires that the entry-level degree be a postbaccalaureate degree." The BLS (December 17, 2009, http://www.bls.gov/oco/ocos078.htm) reports that in 2008 OTs filled 104,500 jobs and that their median annual wages were $66,780.

The demand for PTs and OTs is expected to exceed the available supply through 2018. Besides hospital and rehabilitation center jobs, it is anticipated that PTs and OTs will increasingly be involved in school program efforts to meet the needs of disabled and special education students.

Pharmacists

Pharmacists are involved in many more aspects of patient care than simply compounding and dispensing medication from behind the drugstore counter. According to the American Pharmacists Association, pharmacists provide pharmaceutical care that both improves patient adherence to prescribed drug treatment and reduces the frequency of drug therapy mishaps, which can have serious and even life-threatening consequences.

Studies citing the value of pharmacists in patient care describe pharmacists improving the rates of immunization against disease (pharmacists can provide immunization in all 50 states, the District of Columbia, and Puerto Rico), assisting patients to better control chronic diseases such as asthma and diabetes, reducing the frequency and severity of drug interactions and adverse reactions, and helping patients effectively manage pain and symptoms of disease, especially at the end of life. Pharmacists also offer public health education programs about prescription medication safety, prevention of poisoning, appropriate use of nonprescription (over-the-counter) drugs, and medical self-care.

Pharmacists must obtain a doctoral degree, called a Pharm.D., from an accredited school of pharmacy. Training leading to the Pharm.D. generally takes four years to complete and some Pharm.D. graduates obtain additional training. All states require a license to practice pharmacy and 44 states and the District of Columbia also require the Multistate Pharmacy Jurisprudence Exam (MPJE), which tests pharmacy law. Some states also require additional exams and all require a stipulated number of hours of experience in a practice setting as a prerequisite for licensure.

The BLS (December 17, 2009, http://www.bls.gov/oco/ocos079.htm) reports that pharmacists worked at 269,900 jobs in 2008. About 65% worked in community pharmacies—either independently owned or part of a drugstore chain, grocery store, department store, or mass merchandiser. Most full-time salaried pharmacists worked about 40 hours per week, and many self-employed pharmacists worked more than 50 hours per week. About 22% worked in hospitals in 2008. The median annual wages of pharmacists in May 2008 was $106,410.

MENTAL HEALTH PROFESSIONALS

The mental health sector includes a range of professionals—psychiatrists, psychologists, psychiatric nurses, clinical social workers, and counselors—whose training, orientation, philosophy, and practice styles differ, even within a single discipline. For example, clinical psychologists may endorse and offer dramatically different forms of therapy—ranging from long-term psychoanalytic psychotherapy to short-term cognitive-behavioral therapy.

Psychiatrists

Psychiatrists are physicians who have completed residency training in the prevention, diagnosis, and treatment of mental illness, mental retardation, and substance abuse disorders. Because they are trained physicians, they are especially well equipped to care for people who have coexisting medical diseases and mental health problems and can prescribe medication including psychoactive drugs. Psychiatrists may also obtain additional training that prepares them to treat certain populations such as children and adolescents or older adults (this subspecialty is called geriatric psychiatry or geropsychiatry), or they may specialize in a specific treatment modality.

Psychologists

Research psychologists investigate the physical, cognitive, emotional, or social aspects of human behavior. They work in academic and private research centers and in business, nonprofit, and governmental organizations.

Clinical psychologists help mentally and emotionally disturbed clients better manage their symptoms and behaviors. Some work in rehabilitation, treating patients with spinal cord injuries, chronic pain or illness, stroke, arthritis, and neurologic conditions. Others help people cope during times of personal crisis, such as divorce or the death of a loved one. Psychologists are also called on to help communities recover from the trauma of natural or human-made disasters by working with, for example, people who have lost their homes to earthquakes, fires, or floods, or students who have witnessed school violence.

Clinical psychologists may specialize in health psychology, neuropsychology, or geropsychology. Health psychologists promote healthy lifestyles and behaviors and provide counseling such as smoking cessation, weight reduction, and stress management to assist people to reduce their health risks. Neuropsychologists often work in stroke rehabilitation and head injury programs, and geropsychologists work with older adults in institutional and community settings.

School psychologists identify, diagnose, and address students' learning and behavior problems. They work with teachers and school personnel to improve classroom management strategies and to design educational programs for students with disabilities or gifted and talented students. They also work with parents to help improve parenting skills.

Industrial-organizational psychologists aim to improve productivity and the quality of life in the workplace. They screen prospective employees and conduct training and development, counseling, and organizational development and analysis. Industrial-organizational psychologists examine aspects of work life. They work in organizational consultation, market research, systems design, or other applied psychology fields. For example, industrial-organizational psychologists may be involved in efforts to understand and influence consumer-purchasing behaviors.

Social psychologists consider interpersonal relationships and interactions with the social environment and social experience. Many social psychologists specialize in particular aspects of social psychology, such as group behavior, leadership, aggression, attitudinal change, or social perception.

EDUCATION, TRAINING, LICENSURE, AND EARNINGS. Most psychologists hold a doctorate degree in psychology, which requires between five and seven years of graduate study. Clinical psychologists must usually have earned a Doctor of Philosophy or a Doctor of Psychology degree and completed an internship of at least a one-year duration. An educational specialist degree qualifies an individual to work as a school psychologist; most school psychologists, however, complete a master's degree followed by a one-year internship. People with a master's degree in psychology may work as industrial-organizational psychologists or as psychological assistants, under the supervision of doctoral-level psychologists, and conduct research or psychological evaluations. Vocational and guidance counselors usually need two years of graduate education in counseling and one year of counseling experience. A master's degree in psychology requires at least two years of full-time graduate study. People with undergraduate degrees in psychology assist psychologists and other professionals in community mental health centers, vocational rehabilitation offices, and correctional programs.

Psychologists in clinical practice must be certified or licensed in all states and the District of Columbia. According to the BLS (December 17, 2009, http://www.bls.gov/oco/ocos056.htm), the median annual wages for clinical, counseling, and school psychologists was $64,140 in May 2008.

Psychiatric Nurses

Psychiatric nurses have earned a degree in nursing, are licensed as RNs, and have obtained additional experience in psychiatry. Advanced practice psychiatric nurses (RNs prepared at the master's level) may prescribe psychotropic medications and conduct individual, group, and family psychotherapy as well as perform crisis intervention and case management functions. Along with primary care physicians, they are often the first points of contact for people seeking mental health help.

The American Psychiatric Nurses Association (APNA) is the professional society that represents psychiatric nurses and examines the changing profile of the profession. According to the APNA, in "About Psychiatric-Mental Health Nurses (PMHNs)" (2010, http://www.apna.org/i4a/pages/index.cfm?pageid=3292), basic-level nurses usually start at an annual salary of $35,000 to $40,000, depending on the geographic location. Advanced practice nurses' salaries start at $60,000. Nurse executives can make $100,000 or more per year. Meanwhile, faculty members average about $65,000 per year, depending on the amount of education and experience.

Clinical Social Workers

Clinical social workers are the largest group of professionally trained mental health care providers in the United States. Clinical social workers offer psychotherapy or counseling and a range of diagnostic services in public agencies, clinics, and private practice. They assist people to improve their interpersonal relationships, solve personal and family problems, and advise them about how to function effectively in their communities.

According to the BLS (December 17, 2009, http://www.bls.gov/oco/ocos060.htm), social workers held 642,000 positions in the United States in 2008. Of this total, 292,600 were child, family, and school social workers, 138,700 were medical and public health social workers, and 137,300 were mental health and substance abuse social workers. The median annual wages of child, family, and school social workers were $39,530 in May 2008. Medical and public health social workers earned $46,650, and mental health and substance abuse social workers earned $37,210.

EDUCATION, CERTIFICATION, AND LICENSURE. A bachelor's degree in social work is usually the minimum requirement for employment as a social worker, and an advanced degree has become the standard for many positions. A master's degree in social work is necessary for positions in health and mental health settings and is typically required for certification for clinical work. Licensed clinical social workers hold a master's degree in social work along with additional clinical training. Supervisory, administrative, and staff training positions usually require an advanced degree, and university teaching positions and research appointments normally require a doctorate in social work.

All the states and the District of Columbia have licensing, certification, or registration requirements that delineate the scope of social work practice and the use of professional titles; however, standards for licensing vary by state. The National Association of Social Workers (2010, https://www.socialworkers.org/nasw/default.asp) represents 150,000 professional social workers and "works to enhance the professional growth and development of its members, to create and maintain professional standards, and to advance sound social policies."

Counselors

Counselors assist people with personal, family, educational, mental health, and job-related challenges and problems. Their roles and responsibilities depend on the clients they serve and on the settings in which they work. According to the BLS (December 17, 2009, http://www.bls.gov/oco/ocos067.htm), a master's degree is required to become a licensed counselor. In 2008, 49 states and the District of Columbia had some form of counselor credentialing, licensure, certification, or registry legislation governing

counselors who practice outside schools; however, requirements vary from state to state. The American Counseling Association (ACA; 2010, http://www.counseling.org/AboutUs/), which is the world's largest association for professional counselors, represents nearly 45,000 professional counselors in various practice settings. The ACA has taken an active role in advocating for certification, licensure, and registry of counselors.

The BLS notes that of the 665,500 counselors employed in the United States in 2008, 275,800 were educational, vocational, and school counselors, 129,500 were rehabilitation counselors, 113,300 were mental health counselors, 86,100 were substance abuse and behavioral disorder counselors, and 27,300 were marriage and family therapists.

Working in elementary, secondary, and postsecondary schools, educational, vocational, and school counselors work with people with disabilities and help them overcome the personal, social, and vocational effects of their disabilities. They advise people with disabilities that resulted from birth defects, illness or disease, accidents, or the stress of daily life.

Rehabilitation counselors help people with personal, social, and vocational challenges that result from birth defects, illness, disease, accidents, or the stress of daily life to gain independence and employment. They help design and coordinate activities for people in rehabilitation treatment facilities and perform client evaluations. Rehabilitation counselors plan and implement rehabilitation programs that may include personal and vocational counseling, training, and job placement.

Mental health counselors work in prevention programs to promote optimum mental health and provide a wide range of counseling services. They work closely with other mental health professionals, including psychiatrists, psychologists, clinical social workers, psychiatric nurses, and school counselors.

Substance abuse and behavioral disorder counselors help people overcome addictions to alcohol, drugs, gambling, and eating disorders. They counsel individuals, families, and groups in clinics, hospital-based outpatient treatment programs, community mental health centers, and inpatient chemical dependency treatment programs.

Marriage and family therapists use various techniques to intervene with individuals, families, and couples or to help them resolve emotional conflicts. They aim to modify perceptions and behavior, enhance communication and understanding among family members, and prevent family and individual crises. Individual marriage and family therapists may also offer psychotherapy to individuals, couples, and families to improve their interpersonal relationships.

Pastoral counselors offer a type of psychotherapy that combines spiritual resources with psychological understanding for healing and growth. According to the American Association of Pastoral Counselors (AAPC; 2009, http://aapc.org/content/what-pastoral-counseling), this therapeutic modality is more than simply the comfort, support, and encouragement a religious community can offer; instead, it provides "psychologically sound therapy that weaves in the religious and spiritual dimension." Typically, an AAPC-certified counselor has obtained a bachelor's degree from a college or university, a three-year professional degree from a seminary, and a specialized master's or doctorate degree in the mental health field.

The AAPC asserts that demand for spiritually based counseling is on the rise, in part because interest in spirituality is on the rise in the United States. The organization also believes that despite increased interest in psychotherapy and increasing numbers of therapists, managed mental health care has reduced the availability of, and payment for, counseling services for many people. As a result, more people are turning to clergy for help with personal, marital, and family issues as well as with faith issues. For many working poor Americans without health insurance benefits, free or low-cost counseling from pastoral counselors is the most accessible, available, affordable, and acceptable form of mental health care.

PRACTITIONERS OF COMPLEMENTARY AND ALTERNATIVE MEDICINE

The field of complementary and alternative medicine (CAM) is attracting a growing number of professionals. The National Center for Complementary and Alternative Medicine (NCCAM; April 2010, http://nccam.nih.gov/health/whatiscam/) defines alternative medicine as "a group of diverse medical and health care systems, practices, and products that are not generally considered part of conventional medicine." Even though there is some overlap between them, the NCCAM further distinguishes complementary, alternative, and integrative medicine in the following manner:

- Alternative medicine is therapy or treatment that is used instead of conventional medical treatment.

- Complementary medicine is nonstandard therapy or treatment that is used along with conventional medicine, not in place of it. Complementary medicine appears to offer health benefits, but there is less scientific evidence to support its utility than is generally available for conventional and integrative therapies.

- Integrative medicine is the combination of conventional medical treatment and CAM therapies that have been scientifically researched and have demonstrated evidence that they are both safe and effective.

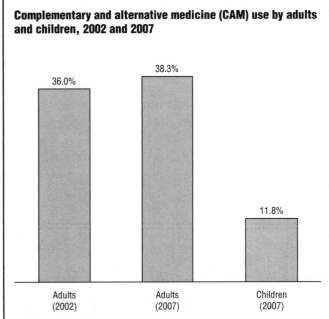

FIGURE 2.4

Complementary and alternative medicine (CAM) use by adults and children, 2002 and 2007

SOURCE: "Figure 1. CAM Use by U.S. Adults and Children," in *The Use of Complementary and Alternative Medicine in the United States*, National Institutes of Health, National Center for Complementary and Alternative Medicine, 2010, http://nccam.nih.gov/news/camstats/2007/72_dpi_CHARTS/chart1.htm (accessed May 12, 2010)

In general terms, alternative therapies are often entirely untested and unproven, whereas complementary and integrative practices that are used in conjunction with mainstream medicine have substantial scientific basis of demonstrated safety and efficacy (the ability of an intervention to produce the intended diagnostic or therapeutic effect in optimal circumstances).

There is considerable enthusiasm for and use of CAM approaches and practices. According to Patricia M. Barnes, Barbara Bloom, and Richard L. Nahin, in "Complementary and Alternative Medicine Use among Adults and Children: United States, 2007" (*National Health Statistics Reports*, no. 12, December 10, 2008), the 2007 National Health Interview Survey reveals that in 2007, 38.3% of American adults aged 18 years and older and 11.8% of children under the age of 18 used some form of CAM therapy within the 12 months preceding the survey. (See Figure 2.4.)

Figure 2.5 shows the 10 most frequently used CAM therapies in 2007:

- Natural products such as herbs, other botanicals, and enzymes (17.7%)

- Deep breathing (12.7%)

- Meditation (9.4%)

- Chiropractic and osteopathic care (8.6%)

- Massage (8.3%)

FIGURE 2.5

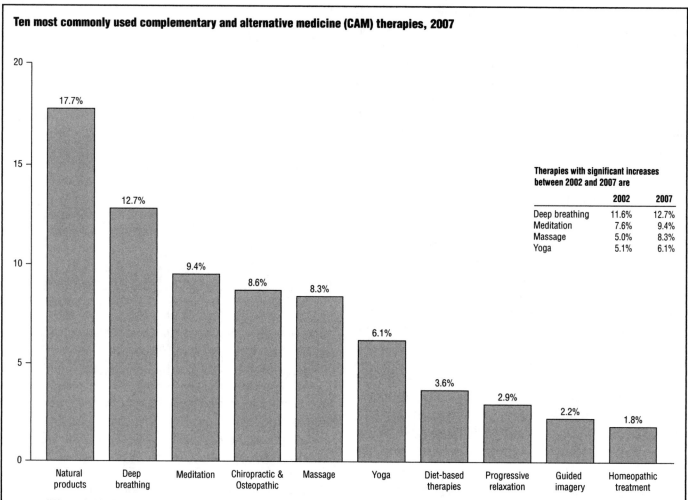

Ten most commonly used complementary and alternative medicine (CAM) therapies, 2007

Therapies with significant increases between 2002 and 2007 are

	2002	2007
Deep breathing	11.6%	12.7%
Meditation	7.6%	9.4%
Massage	5.0%	8.3%
Yoga	5.1%	6.1%

SOURCE: "Figure 4. 10 Most Common CAM Therapies among Adults—2007," in *The Use of Complementary and Alternative Medicine in the United States*, National Institutes of Health, National Center for Complementary and Alternative Medicine, 2010, http://nccam.nih.gov/news/camstats/2007/72_dpi_CHARTS/chart4.htm (accessed May 12, 2010)

- Yoga (6.1%)
- Diet-based therapies (3.6%)
- Progressive relaxation (2.9%)
- Guided imagery (2.2%)
- Homeopathic treatment (1.8%)

Homeopathic Medicine

Homeopathic medicine (also called homeopathy) is based on the belief that "like cures like" and uses very diluted amounts of natural substances to encourage the body's own self-healing mechanisms. Homeopathy was developed by the German physician Samuel Hahnemann (1755–1843) in the 1790s. Hahnemann found that he could produce symptoms of particular diseases by injecting small doses of various herbal substances. This discovery inspired him to administer to sick people extremely diluted formulations of substances that would produce the same symptoms they suffered from in an effort to stimulate natural recovery and regeneration.

According to Edzard Ernst of the University of Exeter, in "Homeopathy: What Does the 'Best' Evidence Tell Us?" (*Medical Journal of Australia*, vol. 192, no. 8, April 19, 2010), a rigorous review of studies evaluating homeopathy finds that homeopathic medicines have no effects beyond those of placebo. (A placebo is an inactive compound. The placebo effect is a health benefit, such as pain relief, that arises from the patient's expectation that the placebo will provide relief, rather than from the placebo itself.)

However, Bruno Van Brandt of Heel Inc. observes in "New Research in Physics Supports Homoeopathy: Is Avogadro's Number a Dogma?" (*Alternative Therapies in Health and Medicine*, vol. 16, no. 2, March–April 2010) that despite widespread condemnation, homeopathy continues to be employed by thousands of conventionally trained physicians. Brandt also asserts that recent research, such as the groundbreaking work in human immunodeficiency virus (HIV) research for which the French virologist Luc Montagnier (1932–) was awarded the 2008 Nobel Prize in Physiology or Medicine, supports the premise that exceedingly diluted homeopathic preparations can exert an effect.

Naturopathic Medicine

As its name suggests, naturopathic medicine (also called naturopathy) uses naturally occurring substances to prevent, diagnose, and treat disease. Even though it is now considered an alternative medicine system, it is one of the oldest medicine systems and has its origins in Native American culture and even draws from Greek, Chinese, and East Indian ideas about health and illness.

The guiding principles of modern naturopathic medicine are "first, do no harm" and "nature has the power to heal." Naturopathy seeks to treat the whole person, because disease is seen as arising from many causes rather than from a single cause. Naturopathic physicians are taught that "prevention is as important as cure" and to view creating and maintaining health as equally important as curing disease. They are instructed to identify and treat the causes of diseases rather than to act only to relieve symptoms.

Naturopathic treatment methods include nutritional counseling; use of dietary supplements, herbs, and vitamins; hydrotherapy (water-based therapies, usually involving whirlpool or other baths); exercise; manipulation; massage; heat therapy; and electrical stimulation. Because naturopathy draws on Chinese and Indian medical techniques, naturopathic physicians often use Chinese herbs, acupuncture, and East Indian medicines to treat disease.

In "Naturopathy and the Primary Care Practice" (*Primary Care: Clinics in Office Practice*, vol. 37, no. 1, March 2010), Sara A. Fleming and Nancy C. Gutknecht of the University of Wisconsin, Madison, describe naturopathy as "a distinct type of primary care medicine that blends age-old healing traditions with scientific advances and current research. Naturopathy is guided by a unique set of principles that recognize the body's innate healing capacity, emphasize disease prevention, and encourage individual responsibility to obtain optimal health." The researchers explain that "naturopathic physicians (NDs) are trained as primary care physicians in 4-year, accredited doctoral-level naturopathic medical schools." In 2010 there were 15 states and two U.S. territories that licensed and recognized naturopathic physicians.

Traditional Chinese Medicine

Traditional Chinese medicine (TCM) uses nutrition, acupuncture, massage, herbal medicine, and Qi Gong (exercises to improve the flow of vital energy through the body) to help people achieve balance and unity of their mind, body, and spirit. Practiced for more than 3,000 years by about a quarter of the world's population, TCM has been adopted by naturopathic physicians, chiropractors, and other CAM practitioners in the United States.

TCM views balancing *qi* (pronounced "chee"), the vital life force that flows over the surface of the body and through internal organs, as central to health, wellness, disease prevention, and treatment. This vital force or energy is thought to flow through the human body in meridians (channels). TCM practitioners believe that pain and disease develop when there is any sort of disturbance in the natural flow. TCM also seeks to balance the feminine and masculine qualities of yin and yang by using other techniques such as moxibustion, which is the stimulation of acupuncture points with heat, and cupping, in which the practitioner increases circulation by putting a heated jar on the skin of a body part. Herbal medicine is the most commonly prescribed treatment.

Acupuncture

Acupuncture is a Chinese practice that dates back more than 5,000 years. Chinese medicine describes acupuncture—the insertion of extremely thin, sterile needles to any of 360 specific points on the body—as a way to balance *qi*. When an acupuncturist determines that there is an imbalance in the flow of energy, needles are inserted at specific points along the meridians. Each point controls a different part of the body. Once the needles are in place, they are rotated gently or are briefly charged with a small electric current.

Traditional Western medicine explains the acknowledged effectiveness of acupuncture as the result of triggering the release of neurotransmitters and neuropeptides that influence brain chemistry and of pain-relieving substances called endorphins that occur naturally in the body. Besides providing lasting pain relief, acupuncture has demonstrated success in helping people with substance abuse problems, relieving nausea, heightening immunity by increasing total white blood cells and T-cell production, and assisting patients to recover from stroke and other neurological impairments. Imaging techniques confirm that acupuncture acts to alter brain chemistry and function.

Chiropractic Physicians

Chiropractic physicians treat patients whose health problems are associated mainly with the body's structural and neurological systems, especially the spine. These practitioners believe that interference with these systems can impair normal functions and lower resistance to disease. Chiropractic medicine asserts that misalignment or compression of, for example, the spinal nerves can alter many important body functions. According to the American Chiropractic Association, in "What Is Chiropractic?" (2010, http://www.acatoday.org/level2_css.cfm?T1ID=13&T2ID=61&BT1ID=21&BT2ID=94), the term *chiropractic* can be defined as "a health care profession that focuses on disorders of the musculoskeletal system and the nervous system, and the effects of these disorders on general health. Chiropractic care is used most often to treat neuromusculoskeletal complaints, including but not limited to back pain, neck pain, pain in the joints of the arms or legs, and headaches." Doctors of chiropractic medicine do not use or prescribe pharmaceutical drugs or perform surgery. Instead, they rely on adjustment and manipulation of the musculoskeletal system, particularly the spinal column.

Many chiropractors use nutritional therapy and prescribe dietary supplements; some employ a technique known as applied kinesiology to diagnose and treat disease. Applied kinesiology is based on the belief that every organ problem is associated with weakness of a specific muscle. Chiropractors who use this technique claim they can accurately identify organ system dysfunction without any laboratory or other diagnostic tests.

Besides manipulation, chiropractors also use a variety of other therapies to support healing and relax muscles before they make manual adjustments. These treatments include:

- Heat and cold therapy to relieve pain, speed healing, and reduce swelling

- Hydrotherapy to relax muscles and stimulate blood circulation

- Immobilization such as casts, wraps, traction, and splints to protect injured areas

- Electrotherapy to deliver deep tissue massage and boost circulation

- Ultrasound to relieve muscle spasms and reduce swelling

All states and the District of Columbia license chiropractors who meet the educational and examination requirements established by the state. According to the BLS (December 17, 2009, http://www.bls.gov/oco/ocos071.htm), in 2008 chiropractors worked at 49,100 jobs, and most were self-employed and in solo practice. In May 2008 the median annual wages of salaried chiropractors were $66,490. Visits to chiropractors are most often for treatment of lower back pain, neck pain, and headaches.

INCREASE IN HEALTH CARE EMPLOYMENT

The number of people working in health care services increased from 12.2 million in 2000 to 15.1 million in 2008. (See Table 2.9.) Health care workers are employed in medical offices, in outpatient and nursing care centers, and in patients' homes. Even though hospitals still employ a larger proportion of health care workers than any other service location, more patients are now able to receive treatment in physicians' offices, clinics, and other outpatient settings.

Why Is Health Care Booming?

Three major factors appear to have influenced the escalation in health care employment: advances in technology, the increasing amounts of money spent on health care, and the aging of the U.S. population. In other sectors of the economy, technology often replaces humans in the labor force. However, health care technology has increased the demand for highly trained specialists to operate the sophisticated equipment. Because of technological advances, patients are likely to undergo more tests and diagnostic procedures, take more drugs, see more specialists, and be subjected to more aggressive treatments than ever before.

The second factor involves the amount of money the nation spends on keeping its citizens in good health. The Centers for Medicare and Medicaid Services forecasts in *National Health Expenditure Projections, 2009–2019* (January 2010, http://www1.cms.gov/NationalHealth ExpendData/downloads/proj2009.pdf) that national health expenditures will rise from an average of $7,348 per person in 2010 to $11,997 per person in 2019. For each year that the amount of money spent on health care continues to grow, employment in the field grows as well. Some health care industry observers believe that government and private financing for the health care industry, unlike most other fields, is virtually unlimited.

The third factor contributing to the rise in the number of health care workers is the aging of the nation's population. There are greater numbers of older adults in the United States than ever before, and they are living longer. According to the U.S. Census Bureau, in the press release "Census Bureau Reports World's Older Population: Projected to Triple by 2050" (June 23, 2009, http://www.census.gov/newsroom/releases/archives/international _population/cb09-97.html), the U.S. population aged 65 years and older will more than double by 2050, rising from 39 million in 2010 to 89 million in 2050.

The increase in the number of older people is expected to boost the demand for home health care services, assisted living, and nursing home care. Many nursing homes now offer special care for stroke patients, people with Alzheimer's disease (a progressive cognitive impairment), and people who need a respirator to breathe. To care for such patients, nursing homes need more PTs, nurses' aides, and respiratory therapists—three of the fastest-growing occupations. In "Overview of the 2008–18 Projections" (December 17, 2009, http://www.bls.gov/oco/oco2003.htm), the BLS estimates that health care services will grow 24% between 2008 and 2018. The fastest-growing

TABLE 2.9

Persons employed in health service sites, by site and sex, 2000–08

[Data are based on household interviews of a sample of the civilian noninstitutionalized population]

Site	2000	2002	2003	2004	2005	2006	2007	2008
Both sexes				Number of persons in thousands				
All employed civilians[a]	136,891	136,485	137,736	139,252	141,730	144,427	146,047	145,362
All health service sites[b]	12,211	13,069	13,615	13,817	14,052	14,352	14,687	15,108
Offices and clinics of physicians	1,387	1,533	1,673	1,727	1,801	1,785	1,720	1,562
Offices and clinics of dentists	672	734	771	780	792	852	843	774
Offices and clinics of chiropractors	120	132	142	156	163	163	144	139
Offices and clinics of optometrists	95	113	92	93	98	98	114	110
Offices and clinics of other health practitioners[c]	143	149	250	274	275	292	299	195
Outpatient care centers	772	850	873	885	901	919	881	1,107
Home health care services	548	636	741	750	795	928	959	881
Other health care services[d]	1,027	1,188	943	976	1,045	1,096	1,334	1,647
Hospitals	5,202	5,330	5,652	5,700	5,719	5,712	5,955	6,241
Nursing care facilities	1,593	1,715	1,877	1,858	1,848	1,807	1,689	1,779
Residential care facilities, without nursing	652	689	601	618	615	700	749	673
Men								
All health service sites[b]	2,756	2,838	2,986	3,067	3,097	3,187	3,316	3,352
Offices and clinics of physicians	354	370	414	424	418	421	417	375
Offices and clinics of dentists	158	151	163	158	156	173	161	136
Offices and clinics of chiropractors	32	47	53	63	68	61	54	58
Offices and clinics of optometrists	26	29	29	24	27	29	26	24
Offices and clinics of other health practitioners[c]	38	42	63	69	80	80	71	52
Outpatient care centers	186	172	200	203	201	199	216	266
Home health care services	45	54	56	65	81	91	96	96
Other health care services[d]	304	362	297	314	311	344	399	470
Hospitals	1,241	1,195	1,263	1,333	1,347	1,337	1,464	1,451
Nursing care facilities	195	223	267	251	246	263	217	231
Residential care facilities, without nursing	177	193	181	164	162	189	195	193
Women								
All health service sites[b]	9,457	10,232	10,631	10,750	10,958	11,167	11,370	11,755
Offices and clinics of physicians	1,034	1,164	1,259	1,302	1,383	1,364	1,303	1,187
Offices and clinics of dentists	514	584	607	623	637	679	681	638
Offices and clinics of chiropractors	88	85	90	93	95	102	90	81
Offices and clinics of optometrists	69	84	64	69	71	69	88	86
Offices and clinics of other health practitioners[c]	106	106	186	204	195	213	228	143
Outpatient care centers	586	678	673	683	700	720	665	841
Home health care services	503	582	685	685	713	837	863	785
Other health care services[d]	723	826	646	662	734	752	935	1,176
Hospitals	3,961	4,135	4,390	4,366	4,372	4,376	4,491	4,790
Nursing care facilities	1,398	1,492	1,611	1,607	1,602	1,544	1,472	1,548
Residential care facilities, without nursing	475	496	420	454	453	511	554	480
Both sexes				Percent of employed civilians				
All health service sites	8.9	9.6	9.9	9.9	9.9	9.9	10.1	10.4
				Percent distribution				
All health service sites	100.0	100.0	100.0	100.0	100.0	100.0	100.0	100.0
Offices and clinics of physicians	11.4	11.7	12.3	12.5	12.8	12.4	11.7	10.3
Offices and clinics of dentists	5.5	5.6	5.7	5.6	5.6	5.9	5.7	5.1
Offices and clinics of chiropractors	1.0	1.0	1.0	1.1	1.2	1.1	1.0	0.9
Offices and clinics of optometrists	0.8	0.9	0.7	0.7	0.7	0.7	0.8	0.7
Offices and clinics of other health practitioners[c]	1.2	1.1	1.8	2.0	2.0	2.0	2.0	1.3
Outpatient care centers	6.3	6.5	6.4	6.4	6.4	6.4	6.0	7.3
Home health care services	4.5	4.9	5.4	5.4	5.7	6.5	6.5	5.8
Other health care services[d]	8.4	9.1	6.9	7.1	7.4	7.6	9.1	10.9
Hospitals	42.6	40.8	41.5	41.3	40.7	39.8	40.5	41.3
Nursing care facilities	13.0	13.1	13.8	13.4	13.2	12.6	11.5	11.8
Residential care facilities, without nursing	5.3	5.3	4.4	4.5	4.4	4.9	5.1	4.5

[a]Excludes workers under the age of 16 years.
[b]Data for health service sites for men and women may not sum to total for all health service sites for both sexes due to rounding.
[c]Includes health service sites such as psychologists' offices, nutritionists' offices, speech defect clinics, and other offices and clinics.
[d]Includes health service sites such as clinical laboratories, blood banks, CT-SCAN (computer tomography) centers, and other offices and clinics.
Notes: Annual data are based on data collected each month and averaged over the year. Health service sites are based on the North American Industry Classification System.

SOURCE: "Table 106. Persons Employed in Health Service Sites, by Site and Sex: United States, 2000–2008," in *Health, United States, 2009: With Special Feature on Medical Technology*, U.S. Department of Health and Human Services, Centers for Disease Control and Prevention, National Center for Health Statistics, 2010, http://www.cdc.gov/nchs/data/hus/hus09.pdf#listtables (accessed May 11, 2010)

TABLE 2.10

Occupations projected to grow fastest, 2008–18

Occupations	Percent change	Number of new jobs (in thousands)	Wages (May 2008 median)	Education/training category
Biomedical engineers	72	11.6	$77,400	Bachelor's degree
Network systems and data communications analysts	53	155.8	71,100	Bachelor's degree
Home health aides	50	460.9	20,460	Short-term on-the-job training
Personal and home care aides	46	375.8	19,180	Short-term on-the-job training
Financial examiners	41	11.1	70,930	Bachelor's degree
Medical scientists, except epidemiologists	40	44.2	72,590	Doctoral degree
Physician assistants	39	29.2	81,230	Master's degree
Skin care specialists	38	14.7	28,730	Postsecondary vocational award
Biochemists and biophysicists	37	8.7	82,840	Doctoral degree
Athletic trainers	37	6.0	39,640	Bachelor's degree
Physical therapist aides	36	16.7	23,760	Short-term on-the-job training
Dental hygienists	36	62.9	66,570	Associate degree
Veterinary technologists and technicians	36	28.5	28,900	Associate degree
Dental assistants	36	105.6	32,380	Moderate-term on-the-job training
Computer software engineers, applications	34	175.1	85,430	Bachelor's degree
Medical assistants	34	163.9	28,300	Moderate-term on-the-job training
Physical therapist assistants	33	21.2	46,140	Associate degree
Veterinarians	33	19.7	79,050	First professional degree
Self-enrichment education teachers	32	81.3	35,720	Work experience in a related occupation
Compliance officers, except agriculture, construction, health and safety, and transportation	31	80.8	48,890	Long-term on-the-job training

SOURCE: "Table 1. Occupations with the Fastest Growth," in *Occupational Outlook Handbook, 2010–11 Edition: Overview of the 2008–18 Projections*, U.S. Department of Labor, Bureau of Labor Statistics, 2009, http://www.bls.gov/oco/oco2003.htm#industry (accessed May 12, 2010)

health care occupations will be personal and home health aides, medical scientists, PAs, skin care specialists, PT assistants, and dental assistants. Table 2.10 shows some of the fastest-growing health care occupations as well as their educational requirements and median wages in May 2008.

Another factor that will likely further increase the demand for health care workers is the 2010 health care reform legislation. When the millions of previously uninsured Americans obtain coverage and enter the health care system, additional health care resources (i.e., workers and facilities) will be required. The legislation may also improve the way in which physicians and other health care workers deliver care. For example, previously uninsured Americans who may have used hospital emergency departments to obtain needed medical care will be able to access preventive services in physicians' offices and clinics. This group may also seek care when the symptoms of sickness first appear, when diseases and disorders are more amenable to treatment, rather than waiting until the situation requires emergency treatment.

However, health care professionals also see potential problems with some of the provisions of the new legislation. For example, in "Doctors Divided on How New Health-Care Law Will Affect Them" (*Washington Post*, March 27, 2010), Rachel Saslow reports that some hospital departments and clinics may have to reduce staff and hours because the legislation failed to overturn reductions in Medicare reimbursement.

CHAPTER 3
HEALTH CARE INSTITUTIONS

A hospital is no place to be sick.

—Samuel Goldwyn

HOSPITALS

The first hospitals in the United States were established more than 200 years ago. No records of hospitals in the early colonies exist, but almshouses, which sheltered the poor, also cared for those who were ill. The first almshouse opened in 1662 in the Massachusetts Bay Colony. In 1756 the Pennsylvania Hospital in Philadelphia became the first U.S. institution devoted entirely to care of the sick.

Until the late 1800s, U.S. hospitals had a bad reputation. The upper classes viewed hospitals as places for the poor who could not afford home care, and the poor saw hospitalization as a humiliating consequence of personal economic failure. People from all walks of life thought hospitals were places to go to die.

TYPES OF HOSPITALS

The American Hospital Association (AHA) notes in "Fast Facts on US Hospitals" (November 11, 2009, http://www.aha.org/aha/resource-center/Statistics-and-Studies/fast-facts.html) that in 2008 there were 5,815 hospitals in the United States that were described as short stay or long term, depending on the length of time a patient spends before being discharged. Short-stay facilities include community, teaching, and public hospitals. Sometimes short-stay hospitals are referred to as acute care facilities because the services provided within them focus on pressing problems or medical conditions, such as a heart attack, rather than on long-term chronic conditions, such as the need for rehabilitation following a head injury. Long-term hospitals are usually rehabilitation and psychiatric hospitals or facilities for the treatment of tuberculosis or other pulmonary (respiratory) diseases.

Hospitals are also distinguished by their ownership, scope of services, and whether they are teaching hospitals with academic affiliations. Hospitals may be operated as proprietary (for-profit) businesses—owned either by corporations or individuals such as the physicians on staff—or they may be voluntary—owned by not-for-profit corporations or religious organizations or operated by federal, state, or city governments. Voluntary, not-for-profit hospitals are usually governed by a board of trustees, who are selected from among community business and civic leaders and who serve without pay to oversee hospital operations.

Most community hospitals offer emergency services as well as a range of inpatient and outpatient medical and surgical services. There are more than 1,000 tertiary hospitals in the United States, which are hospitals that provide highly specialized services such as neonatal intensive care units (for care of sick newborns), trauma services, or cardiovascular surgery programs. A majority of tertiary hospitals serve as teaching hospitals.

Teaching hospitals are those community and tertiary hospitals affiliated with medical schools, nursing schools, or allied health professions training programs. Teaching hospitals are the primary sites for training new physicians, where interns and residents work under the supervision of experienced physicians. Nonteaching hospitals may also maintain affiliations with medical schools and some serve as sites for nursing and allied health professions students as well as for physicians-in-training.

Community Hospitals

The most common type of hospital in the United States is the community, or general, hospital. Community hospitals, where most people receive care, are typically small, with 50 to 500 beds. The AHA reports in "Fast Facts on US Hospitals" that in 2008 there were 5,010 community hospitals, with 808,069 staffed beds, in the

United States. These hospitals normally provide quality care for routine medical and surgical problems. Since the 1980s many smaller hospitals have closed down because they are no longer profitable. The larger ones, usually located in cities and adjacent suburbs, are often equipped with a full complement of medical and surgical personnel and state-of-the-art equipment.

Some community hospitals are not-for-profit corporations that are supported by local funding. These include hospitals supported by religious, cooperative, or osteopathic organizations. During the 1990s increasing numbers of not-for-profit community hospitals converted their ownership status, becoming proprietary hospitals that are owned and operated on a for-profit basis by corporations. These hospitals joined investor-owned corporations because they needed additional financial resources to maintain their existence in an increasingly competitive industry. Investor-owned corporations acquire not-for-profit hospitals to build market share, expand their provider networks, and penetrate new health care markets. According to the AHA, there were 2,923 not-for-profit community hospitals and 982 investor-owned, for-profit community hospitals in 2008.

Teaching Hospitals

Most teaching hospitals, which provide clinical training for medical students and other health care professionals, are affiliated with a medical school and have several hundred beds. Many of the physicians on staff at the hospital also hold teaching positions at the university that is affiliated with the hospital. These physicians may serve as classroom instructors in addition to teaching physicians-in-training at the bedsides of the patients. Patients in teaching hospitals understand that they may be examined by medical students and residents as well as by their primary attending physician.

One advantage of obtaining care at a university-affiliated teaching hospital is the opportunity to receive treatment from highly qualified physicians with access to the most advanced technology and equipment. A disadvantage is the inconvenience and invasion of privacy that may result from multiple examinations performed by residents and students. When compared with smaller community hospitals, some teaching hospitals have reputations for being impersonal; however, patients with complex, unusual, or difficult diagnoses usually benefit from the presence of acknowledged medical experts and more comprehensive resources that are available at these facilities.

Public Hospitals

Public hospitals are owned and operated by federal, state, or city governments. Many have a continuing tradition of caring for the poor. They are usually located in the inner cities and are often in precarious financial situations because many of their patients are unable to pay for services. These hospitals depend heavily on Medicaid payments that are supplied by federal and state agencies or on grants from local governments. Medicaid is a program run by both the federal and state governments for the provision of health care insurance to people younger than 65 years of age who cannot afford to pay for private health insurance. The federal government matches the states' contribution to provide a certain minimal level of available coverage, and the states may offer additional services at their own expense. In "Fast Facts on US Hospitals," the AHA indicates that there were 1,105 state and local government community hospitals and 213 federal government hospitals in 2008.

TREATING SOCIETY'S MOST VULNERABLE MEMBERS. Increasingly, public hospitals must bear the burden of the weaknesses in the nation's health care system. The major problems in U.S. society are readily apparent in the emergency departments and corridors of public hospitals: poverty, drug and alcohol abuse, crime-related and domestic violence, untreated or inadequately treated chronic conditions such as high blood pressure and diabetes, and infectious diseases such as acquired immunodeficiency syndrome (AIDS) and tuberculosis.

LOSING MONEY. The typical public hospital provides millions of dollars in health care and fails to recoup these costs from reimbursement by private insurance, Medicaid, and Medicare (a program run by the federal government through which people aged 65 years and older receive health care insurance). Jack Zwanzige, Nasreen Khan, and Anil Bamezai note in "The Relationship between Safety Net Activities and Hospital Financial Performance" (*BMC Health Services Research*, vol. 10, no. 1, January 14, 2010) that at the close of the 20th century all U.S. hospitals were forced to take steps to reduce health care costs and faced reduced Medicare and Medicaid reimbursement. However, these changes may have disproportionately affected the nation's public hospitals, which provide "safety net" services and serve vulnerable populations such as poor and uninsured patients. (According to the Institute of Medicine, in "America's Health Care Safety Net: Intact but Endangered" [June 2000, http://www.iom.edu/], safety net services are offered by providers "that deliver a significant level of health care to uninsured, Medicaid, and other vulnerable patients." The IOM also explains that "these providers have two distinguishing characteristics: (1) either by legal mandate or explicitly adopted mission, they offer care to patients regardless of their ability to pay for those services; and (2) a substantial share of their patient mix are uninsured, Medicaid, and other vulnerable patients.") In response to these fiscal pressures, some hospitals closed and others decreased the quantity or quality of services provided. Others responded by streamlining services and pursuing paying patients.

According to Jennifer Lubell, in "Don't Let the Numbers Fool You" (*Modern Healthcare*, vol. 38, no. 35, September 1, 2008), in 2007 the U.S. Census Bureau reported a 3.2% decline in the numbers of uninsured people—from 47 million or 15.8% of the population in 2006 to 45.7 million or 15.3% of the population in 2007. Lubbell observes that it appeared that the public health safety net (government entitlement programs, public hospitals, and clinics) was making up the difference in the uninsured numbers, in that there were fewer uninsured people and more people were covered by government health programs. The percentage of the population covered by government health programs increased from 27% in 2006 to 27.8% in 2007, with the number of people covered by these programs also increasing, from 80.3 million to 83 million during this same period. Lubell also notes that the number of people using Medicaid increased by 1.3 million from 2006 to 2007 and that Medicare numbers grew by 1 million.

PROVIDING NEEDED SERVICES. The National Association of Public Hospitals and Health Systems (NAPH; 2010, http://naph.org/Main-Menu-Category/About-NAPH/About-Our-Members.aspx) believes the mission of public hospitals is to respond to the needs of their communities. The NAPH represents 140 hospitals and health care systems that provide care to patients and serve as community resources. Many of the NAPH-member hospitals are also major academic centers, where they train medical and dental residents as well as nursing and allied health professionals.

In the press release "Numbers of Uninsured on Rise in Nation's Public Hospitals" (February 24, 2010, http://www.naph.org/Main-Menu-Category/Newsroom/2010-Press-Releases/Rise-in-Uninsured-Press-Release.aspx), the NAPH reports that since the start of the economic recession, safety net public hospitals have treated 23% more uninsured patients and have seen uncompensated care rise 10%. Larry S. Gage, the president of the NAPH, is quoted as saying, "Safety net public hospitals are treating record numbers of uninsured patients in the current economic crisis while also facing severe budget cuts in many states. ... America's public hospitals are in a precarious situation and Medicaid cuts at the state level will hinder their ability to continue serving as our nation's health care safety net. The impact will weaken the fragile viability of the nation's safety net and force public hospitals to close their doors due to inadequate financing."

Following the passage of the Patient Protection and Affordable Care Act of 2010, Gage issued the press release "NAPH Praises House of Representatives for Passing Historic Bill" (March 22, 2010, http://naph.org/Main-Menu-Category/Newsroom/2010-Press-Releases.aspx), in which he praised the legislation. He explained that "NAPH has worked since its inception nearly 30 years ago to achieve comprehensive health reform that expands coverage for the uninsured and underinsured. The 140 safety net hospitals and health systems that make up NAPH's membership know that the historic vote this weekend by the House of Representatives will save lives and improve access for tens of millions of Americans all across the nation."

Hospital Emergency Departments: More Than They Can Handle

For many Americans, the hospital emergency department has replaced the physician's office as the place to seek health care services. With no insurance and little money, many people go to the only place that will take them without question. Insurance companies and health care planners estimate that more than half of all emergency department visits are for nonemergency treatment.

Poor and near poor children up to 18 years of age of all races were more likely to visit emergency departments (28.6% and 23%, respectively) in 2007 than those who were not poor (17%). (See Table 3.1.) In 2007, 27.3% of children on Medicaid visited emergency departments at least once, as opposed to 17.1% of children who were privately insured and 17.7% of uninsured children. In the 18 years and older age group, 29.9% of poor people and 23.6% of the near poor made at least one visit to the emergency department in 2007. (See Table 3.2.) Of adults aged 18 to 64 years, 16.9% of people who were privately insured visited the emergency department at least once in 2007, as opposed to 37.9% of those who had Medicaid and 20.3% of those who were uninsured.

Even though any type of hospital can experience slow emergency department service, public hospitals are frequently underfunded and understaffed, and service can be exceedingly slow. All-day waits in the emergency department for initial treatment are not uncommon. The U.S. Government Accountability Office (GAO) observes in *Hospital Emergency Departments: Crowding Continues to Occur, and Some Patients Wait Longer Than Recommended Time Frames* (April 2009, http://www.gao.gov/new.items/d09347.pdf) that in 2006 wait times in the emergency department were longer than those reported in 2003 and that in some cases the wait times exceeded the time frames recommended by the National Center for Health Statistics (NCHS). For example, the average wait time to see a physician in 2006 was 37 minutes, even though the recommended time was one to 14 minutes. The GAO also finds that in 2006, 27.3% of emergency departments diverted emergency patients to other medical facilities, presumably because the emergency department was overcrowded and unable to accommodate additional patients.

TABLE 3.1

Emergency department visits within the past 12 months among children under 18, by selected characteristics, 1997, 2006, and 2007

[Data are based on household interviews of a sample of the civilian noninstitutionalized population]

Characteristic	Under 18 years			Under 6 years			6–17 years		
	1997	2006	2007	1997	2006	2007	1997	2006	2007
	Percent of children with one or more emergency department visits								
All children[a]	19.9	21.3	20.2	24.3	28.2	23.9	17.7	17.9	18.3
Race[b]									
White only	19.4	21.2	20.0	22.6	28.0	22.9	17.8	17.9	18.5
Black or African American only	24.0	25.0	23.1	33.1	33.6	30.7	19.4	21.0	19.2
American Indian or Alaska Native only	24.1	19.7	22.0	24.3	*	30.6	24.0	*	17.1
Asian only	12.6	13.4	11.4	20.8	19.6	16.8	8.6	10.2	8.1
Native Hawaiian or other Pacific Islander only	—	*	*	—	*	*	—	*	*
2 or more races	—	17.1	22.3	—	19.8	23.3	—	15.2	21.6
Hispanic origin and race[b]									
Hispanic or Latino	21.1	19.7	18.0	25.7	28.5	23.9	18.1	14.5	14.6
Not Hispanic or Latino	19.7	21.7	20.8	24.0	28.2	23.9	17.6	18.7	19.2
White only	19.2	21.5	20.5	22.2	27.6	22.4	17.7	18.7	19.6
Black or African American only	23.6	25.3	23.4	32.7	34.0	31.0	19.2	21.3	19.5
Percent of poverty level[c]									
Below 100%	25.1	25.8	28.1	29.5	32.6	34.3	22.2	21.6	24.0
100%–less than 200%	22.0	22.1	22.5	28.0	30.3	25.9	19.0	17.8	20.5
200% or more	17.3	19.3	16.7	20.5	25.3	18.6	15.8	16.7	15.9
Hispanic origin and race and percent of poverty level[b, c]									
Hispanic or Latino:									
Percent of poverty level:									
Below 100%	21.9	21.0	22.6	25.0	31.1	29.9	19.6	14.3	17.5
100%–less than 200%	20.8	20.5	16.2	28.8	27.3	21.6	15.6	16.3	12.8
200% or more	20.4	17.7	15.8	23.4	26.5	19.7	18.7	13.3	14.1
Not Hispanic or Latino:									
White only:									
Percent of poverty level:									
Below 100%	25.5	27.5	33.3	27.2	32.3	35.4	24.4	24.6	31.8
100%–less than 200%	22.3	22.9	26.7	25.8	33.3	28.0	20.7	18.2	26.0
200% or more	17.2	20.0	17.2	20.1	24.9	18.4	15.9	17.9	16.7
Black or African American only:									
Percent of poverty level:									
Below 100%	29.3	31.1	29.3	39.5	37.7	41.2	23.0	27.3	22.7
100%–less than 200%	22.5	24.8	23.3	31.7	32.9	26.8	18.5	21.1	21.2
200% or more	17.7	19.4	17.6	22.6	29.6	22.7	15.9	15.7	15.5
Health insurance status at the time of interview[d]									
Insured	19.8	21.9	20.5	24.4	28.5	24.2	17.5	18.5	18.5
Private	17.5	19.2	17.1	20.9	24.5	18.6	15.9	17.0	16.4
Medicaid	28.2	27.2	27.3	33.0	34.2	32.0	24.1	22.3	23.9
Uninsured	20.2	16.8	17.7	23.0	25.4	20.4	18.9	13.7	16.9
Health insurance status prior to interview[d]									
Insured continuously all 12 months	19.6	21.5	20.3	24.1	27.9	23.9	17.3	18.2	18.4
Uninsured for any period up to 12 months	24.0	26.0	23.8	27.1	36.2	28.5	21.9	21.1	21.8
Uninsured more than 12 months	18.4	12.8	15.1	19.3	17.6	*	18.1	11.5	13.6
Percent of poverty level and health insurance status prior to interview[c, d]									
Below 100%:									
Insured continuously all 12 months	26.3	26.5	28.6	30.9	31.7	34.8	22.8	23.1	24.1
Uninsured for any period up to 12 months	26.5	32.2	31.3	29.7	41.8	39.6	24.4	25.7	26.0
Uninsured more than 12 months	17.5	12.5	19.0	16.0	*	*	18.0	9.8	19.8
100%–less than 200%:									
Insured continuously all 12 months	21.8	22.4	23.0	28.0	30.8	25.2	18.6	17.6	21.5
Uninsured for any period up to 12 months	24.5	27.1	26.0	29.7	32.9	32.2	21.0	24.8	23.2
Uninsured more than 12 months	19.5	12.9	16.6	22.5	*	*	18.6	11.0	13.1

MAJORITY OF EMERGENCY DEPARTMENT PATIENTS HAVE HEALTH INSURANCE. Because people without health insurance or a usual source of care often resort to using hospital emergency departments, many industry observers assume that the crowding and long waits in the emergency department are at least in part caused by uninsured patients seeking care for routine problems such as colds, allergies, or back pain. In "Frequent Users of Emergency Departments: The Myths, the Data, and the Policy Implications" (*Annals of Emergency Medicine*,

TABLE 3.1

Emergency department visits within the past 12 months among children under 18, by selected characteristics, 1997, 2006, and 2007

[CONTINUED]

[Data are based on household interviews of a sample of the civilian noninstitutionalized population]

Characteristic	Under 18 years			Under 6 years			6–17 years		
	1997	2006	2007	1997	2006	2007	1997	2006	2007
200% or more:									
Insured continuously all 12 months	17.1	19.5	17.0	20.3	25.2	19.2	15.6	17.0	16.1
Uninsured for any period up to 12 months	20.7	20.0	16.9	21.3	34.4	*	20.4	13.6	18.4
Uninsured more than 12 months	17.9	13.3	9.3	19.2	*	*	17.3	14.5	*

*Estimates are considered unreliable.
—Data not available.
[a]Includes all other races not shown separately and unknown health insurance status.
[b]The race groups, white, black, American Indian or Alaska Native, Asian, Native Hawaiian or other Pacific Islander, and 2 or more races, include persons of Hispanic and non-Hispanic origin. Persons of Hispanic origin may be of any race. Starting with 1999 data, race-specific estimates are tabulated according to the 1997 Revisions to the Standards for the Classification of Federal Data on Race and Ethnicity and are not strictly comparable with estimates for earlier years. The five single-race categories plus multiple-race categories shown in the table conform to the 1997 Standards. Starting with 1999 data, race-specific estimates are for persons who reported only one racial group; the category 2 or more races includes persons who reported more than one racial group. Prior to 1999, data were tabulated according to the 1977 standards with four racial groups and the Asian only category included Native Hawaiian or other Pacific Islander. Estimates for single-race categories prior to 1999 included persons who reported one race or, if they reported more than one race, identified one race as best representing their race. Starting with 2003 data, race responses of other race and unspecified multiple race were treated as missing, and then race was imputed if these were the only race responses. Almost all persons with a race response of other race were of Hispanic origin.
[c]Percent of poverty level is based on family income and family size and composition using U.S. Census Bureau poverty thresholds. Missing family income data were imputed for 21%–25% of children in 1997–1998 and 27%–31% in 1999–2007.
[d]Health insurance categories are mutually exclusive. Persons who reported both Medicaid and private coverage are classified as having private coverage. Starting with 1997 data, state-sponsored health plan coverage is included as Medicaid coverage. Starting with 1999 data, coverage by the Children's Health Insurance Program (CHIP) is included with Medicaid coverage. In addition to private and Medicaid, the insured category also includes military, other government, and Medicare coverage. Persons not covered by private insurance, Medicaid, CHIP, state-sponsored or other government-sponsored health plans (starting in 1997), Medicare, or military plans are considered to have no health insurance coverage. Persons with only Indian Health Service coverage are considered to have no health insurance coverage.

SOURCE: Adapted from "Table 88. Emergency Department Visits within the Past 12 Months among Children under 18 Years of Age, by Selected Characteristics: United States, 1997, 2006, and 2007," in *Health, United States, 2009: With Special Feature on Medical Technology*, U.S. Department of Health and Human Services, Centers for Disease Control and Prevention, National Center for Health Statistics, 2010, http://www.cdc.gov/nchs/data/hus/hus09.pdf#listtables (accessed May 11, 2010)

vol. 56, no. 1, July 2010), Eduardo LaCalle and Elaine Rabin of the Mount Sinai School of Medicine refute this hypothesis and characterize frequent users of emergency medical care (adults who made four or more emergency department visits in one year) as people with insurance who also make frequent use of other health care services such as clinics and physicians' offices. The researchers conclude that "frequent ED users are a heterogeneous group along many dimensions and defy popular assumptions and many frequent users present with true medical needs, which may explain why existing attempts to address the phenomena have had mixed success at best."

HOSPITALS TRY TO EASE THE PAIN OF WAITING. In an effort to distinguish themselves from competitors and increase patient satisfaction with care, some hospitals are promising patients in the emergency department that they will not have to wait more than 30 minutes to be seen. Even though this guarantee does not apply when the emergency department has multiple critical patients or is so full that ambulances are being diverted to other hospitals, Tammie Smith notes in "Hospital Offering a Time Guarantee" (*Richmond Times-Dispatch*, March 20, 2006) that under typical circumstances participating hospitals are attempting to reduce the average waiting time to see a physician—46.5 minutes—to under half an hour. When the guarantees are not met and patients have to wait longer, they may be compensated with an apology

and movie tickets, prepaid gas cards, restaurant gift certificates, or even free medical care.

In "Emergency Department. Hospitals Aim to Help Patients Pick an ED by Posting Wait Times on the Web" (*Hospitals and Health Networks*, vol. 84, no. 2, February 2010), Denene Brox reports that some hospitals post "up-to-the-minute ED wait times on the Internet." By using these websites, health care consumers with urgent, but not life-threatening medical problems, can choose the area hospital with the shortest wait time. Participating hospitals hope that informing prospective patients about wait times will result in higher levels of patient satisfaction.

HOSPITALIZATION

Table 3.3 shows that the discharge rate increased among people aged 65 years and older from 1990 to 2004 and then stabilized from 2005 to 2006. The discharge rates for all other age groups steadily declined during this period until 2005. In 2006 the discharge rates increased slightly for people aged 18 to 44 years but declined or remained relatively stable for all other age groups.

In 2006 the hospital discharge rate was 1,153.1 per 10,000 population. (See Table 3.3.) The rate for females was 1,312.3 per 10,000 population, and for males it was 1,000.5 per 10,000 population. Male patients had longer average lengths of stay (ALOS) than female patients—5.2 days compared with 4.4 days. ALOS and

TABLE 3.2

Emergency department visits within the past 12 months among adults, by selected characteristics, selected years 1997–2007

[Data are based on household interviews of a sample of the civilian noninstitutionalized population]

Characteristic	One or more emergency department visits				Two or more emergency department visits			
	1997	2000	2006	2007	1997	2000	2006	2007
	Percent of adults with emergency department visits							
18 years and over, age-adjusted[a, b]	19.6	20.2	20.5	20.2	6.7	6.9	7.5	7.4
18 years and over, crude[a]	19.6	20.1	20.4	20.1	6.7	6.8	7.4	7.3
Age								
18–44 years	20 7	20.5	20.5	20.3	6.8	7.0	7.3	7.4
18–24 years	26.3	25.7	24.9	23.3	9.1	8.8	9.6	8.7
25–44 years	19.0	18.8	18.9	19.3	6.2	6.4	6.5	6.9
45–64 years	16.2	17.6	18.4	18.3	5.6	5.6	6.8	6.5
45–54 years	15.7	17.9	17.9	18.0	5.5	5.8	6.3	6.6
55–64 years	16.9	17.0	18.9	18.7	5.7	5.3	7.5	6.4
65 years and over	22.0	23.7	24.5	23.1	8.1	8.6	9.0	9.0
65–74 years	20.3	21.6	20.6	20.2	7.1	7.4	6.8	7.6
75 years and over	24.3	26.2	28.9	26.5	9.3	10.0	11.6	10.6
Sex[b]								
Male	19.1	18.7	19.0	18.4	5.9	5.7	6.0	6.2
Female	20.2	21.6	22.1	21.9	7.5	7.9	8.9	8.6
Race[b, c]								
White only	19.0	19.4	20.1	19.6	6.2	6.4	7.0	6.9
Black or African American only	25.9	26.5	25.6	26.3	11.1	10.8	11.3	11.3
American Indian or Alaska Native only	24.8	30.3	21.1	26.7	13.1	12.6	10.5	11.3
Asian only	11.6	13.6	13.6	11.9	2.9	3.8	3.8	4.5
Native Hawaiian or other Pacific Islander only	—	*	*	*	—	*	*	*
2 or more races	—	32.5	24.5	28.3	—	11.3	9.4	14.2
American Indian or Alaska Native; White	—	33.9	21.9	29.9	—	9.4	*	17.2
Hispanic origin and race[b, c]								
Hispanic or Latino	19.2	18.3	17.3	18.2	7.4	7.0	5.7	6.7
Mexican	17.8	17.4	15.4	16.1	6.4	7.1	4.8	5.6
Not Hispanic or Latino	19.7	20.6	21.1	20.6	6.7	6.9	7.7	7.5
White only	19.1	19.8	20.8	20.1	6.2	6.4	7.3	7.0
Black or African American only	25.9	26.5	25.8	26.2	11.0	10.8	11.3	11.4
Percent of poverty level[b, d]								
Below 100%	28.1	29.0	28.2	29.9	12.8	13.3	13.0	14.1
100%–less than 200%	23.8	23.9	24.0	23.6	9.3	9.6	10.6	10.2
200% or more	17.0	18.0	18.2	17.8	4.9	5.2	5.5	5.6
Hispanic origin and race and percent of poverty level[b, c, d]								
Hispanic or Latino:								
Below 100%	22.1	22.4	20.7	25.0	9.8	9.7	6.8	11.8
100%–less than 200%	19.2	18.1	16.0	17.0	8.1	6.7	5.9	6.2
200% or more	17.6	16.8	16.5	16.6	5.4	6.1	5.2	5.4
Not Hispanic or Latino:								
White only:								
Below 100%	29.5	30.1	31.7	32.6	13.0	13.9	15.2	14.9
100%–less than 200%	24.3	25.5	26.3	25.6	9.1	10.4	11.7	11.1
200% or more	16.8	17.7	18.3	17.7	4.8	5.0	5.3	5.4
Black or African American only:								
Below 100%	34.6	35.4	31.4	32.2	17.5	17.4	15.8	15.8
100%–less than 200%	29.2	28.5	30.3	28.6	12.8	12.2	13.6	13.4
200% or more	19.7	22.6	21.5	22.8	7.2	8.0	8.5	8.7
Health insurance status at the time of interview[e, f]								
18–64 years:								
Insured	18.8	19.5	19.9	19.4	6.1	6.4	7.2	7.0
Private	16.9	17.6	17.2	16.9	4.7	5.1	5.3	5.1
Medicaid	37.6	42.2	39.0	37.9	19.7	21.0	20.7	21.2
Uninsured	20.0	19.3	18.9	20.3	7.5	6.9	6.9	7.4

discharge rates varied by geography—ALOS ranged from 4.2 days in the Midwest to 5.2 days in the Northeast. Furthermore, the discharge rate per 10,000 population ranged from 964.1 in the West to 1,261.4 in the Northeast.

Organ Transplants

Organ transplants are a viable means of saving lives, and according to the United Network for Organ Sharing's (UNOS) Organ Procurement and Transplantation Network (OPTN; July 23, 2010, http://optn.transplant

TABLE 3.2

Emergency department visits within the past 12 months among adults, by selected characteristics, selected years 1997–2007 [CONTINUED]

[Data are based on household interviews of a sample of the civilian noninstitutionalized population]

*Estimates are considered unreliable.

—Data not available.

[a]Includes all other races not shown separately and unknown health insurance status.

[b]Estimates are for persons 18 years of age and over and are age-adjusted to the year 2000 standard population using five age groups: 18–44 years, 45–54 years, 55–64 years, 65–74 years, and 75 years and over.

[c]The race groups, white, black, American Indian or Alaska Native, Asian, Native Hawaiian or other Pacific Islander, and 2 or more races, include persons of Hispanic and non-Hispanic origin. Persons of Hispanic origin may be of any race. Starting with 1999 data, race-specific estimates are tabulated according to the 1997 Revisions to the Standards for the Classification of Federal Data on Race and Ethnicity and are not strictly comparable with estimates for earlier years. The five single-race categories shown in the table conform to the 1997 standards. Starting with 1999 data, race-specific estimates are for persons who reported only one racial group; the category 2 or more races includes persons who reported more than one racial group. Prior to 1999, data were tabulated according to the 1977 standards with four racial groups, and the Asian only category included Native Hawaiian or other Pacific Islander. Estimates for single-race categories prior to 1999 included persons who reported one race or, if they reported more than one race, identified one race as best representing their race. Starting with 2003 data, race responses of other race and unspecified multiple race were treated as missing, and then race was imputed if these were the only race responses. Almost all persons with a race response of other race were of Hispanic origin.

[d]Percent of poverty level is based on family income and family size and composition using U.S. Census Bureau poverty thresholds. Missing family income data were imputed for 26%–30% of persons 18 years of age and over in 1997–1998 and 32%–35% in 1999–2007.

[e]Estimates for persons 18–64 years of age are age-adjusted to the year 2000 standard population using three age groups: 18–44 years, 45–54 years, and 55–64 years of age.

[f]Health insurance categories are mutually exclusive. Persons who reported both Medicaid and private coverage are classified as having private coverage. Starting with 1997 data, state-sponsored health plan coverage is included as Medicaid coverage. Starting with 1999 data, coverage by the Children's Health Insurance Program (CHIP) is included with Medicaid coverage. In addition to private and Medicaid, the insured category also includes military plans, other government-sponsored health plans, and Medicare, not shown separately. Persons not covered by private insurance, Medicaid, CHIP, state-sponsored or other government-sponsored health plans (starting in 1997), Medicare, or military plans are considered to have no health insurance coverage. Persons with only Indian Health Service coverage are considered to have no health insurance coverage.

SOURCE: Adapted from "Table 89. Emergency Department Visits within the Past 12 Months among Adults 18 Years of Age and over, by Selected Characteristics: United States, Selected Years 1997–2007," in *Health, United States, 2009: With Special Feature on Medical Technology*, U.S. Department of Health and Human Services, Centers for Disease Control and Prevention, National Center for Health Statistics, 2010, http://www.cdc.gov/nchs/data/hus/hus09.pdf#listtables (accessed May 11, 2010)

.hrsa.gov/), 28,463 transplants were performed in 2009. The UNOS compiles data on organ transplants, distributes organ donor cards, and maintains a registry of patients waiting for organ transplants. It reports that as of July 30, 2010, 107,810 Americans were waiting for a transplant. The UNOS/OPTN (October 2009, http://www.ustransplant.org/annual_reports/current/Chapter_I_AR_CD.htm#1) also states that at the close of 2006 there were 173,339 people living with functioning organ transplants. Nonetheless, many patients died waiting for an organ transplant because demand for organs continued to outpace supply.

In February 2004 the UNOS/OPTN revised and strengthened its policies to guard against potential medical errors in transplant candidate and donor matching. The policy revisions were developed in response to a systematic review of a medical error in February 2003, when a teenager named Jesica Santillan (1985–2003) died after receiving a heart-lung transplant from a blood-type incompatible donor at Duke University Medical Center. News of this tragic error immediately prompted transplant centers throughout the United States to perform internal audits of their protocols and procedures to ensure appropriate donor-recipient matching.

The key policy revisions included stipulations that:

- The blood type of each transplant candidate and donor must be independently verified by two staff members at the institution involved at the time blood type is entered into the national database.

- Each transplant program and organ procurement organization (OPO) must establish a protocol to ensure blood-type data for transplant candidates, and donors are accurately entered into the national database and communicated to transplant teams. The UNOS will verify the existence and effective use of these protocols during routine audits of OPOs and transplant programs.

- Organs must only be offered to candidates specifically identified on the computer-generated list of medically suitable transplant candidates for a given organ offer. If the organ offer is not accepted for any candidate on a given match run, an OPO may give transplant programs the opportunity to update transplant candidate data and rerun a match to see if any additional candidates are identified.

The UNOS resolved to continuously review national policies and procedures for organ placement and to recommend policy and procedure enhancements to maximize the efficiency of organ placement and the safety of transplant candidates and recipients. As of July 2010, there had been no further reported occurrences of unintentional blood-type incompatible transplants.

The risks associated with organ transplant were, however, publicized once again in 2005 and 2006, when two transplant recipients from the same organ donor contracted West Nile virus, a potentially serious illness that is transmitted by mosquitoes. Even though 28,116 transplants were performed in the United States in 2005, according to the OPTN (July 23, 2010, http://optn.transplant.hrsa.gov/), and these two recipients were the only ones reported to have become ill from

TABLE 3.3

Hospital discharges, days of care, and average length of stay by selected characteristics, selected years 1980–2006

[Data are based on a sample of hospital records]

Characteristic	1980[a]	1985[a]	1990	1995	2000	2004	2005	2006
	Discharges per 10,000 population							
Total, age-adjusted[b]	**1,744.5**	**1,522.3**	**1,252.4**	**1,180.2**	**1,132.8**	**1,184.3**	**1,162.4**	**1,153.1**
Total, crude	**1,676.8**	**1,484.1**	**1,222.7**	**1,157.4**	**1,128.3**	**1,192.3**	**1,174.4**	**1,168.7**
Age								
Under 18 years	756.5	614.0	463.5	423.7	402.6	430.2	411.0	393.9
Under 1 year	2,317.6	2,137.9	1,915.3	1,977.6	2,027.6	2,065.3	1,949.3	1,818.4
1–4 years	864.6	650.2	466.9	457.1	458.0	458.9	429.7	418.8
5–17 years	609.3	477.4	334.1	290.2	268.6	296.2	286.5	276.0
18–44 years	1,578.8	1,301.2	1,026.6	914.3	849.4	910.8	898.0	906.7
18–24 years	1,570.3	1,297.8	1,065.3	928.9	854.1	863.5	862.4	870.4
25–44 years	1,582.8	1,302.5	1,013.8	909.9	847.9	927.2	910.3	919.3
25–34 years	1,682.9	1,416.9	1,140.3	1,015.0	942.5	1,021.8	1,007.8	1,011.2
35–44 years	1,438.3	1,153.1	868.8	808.0	764.8	841.8	821.5	834.6
45–64 years	1,947.6	1,707.8	1,354.5	1,185.4	1,114.2	1,177.9	1,147.0	1,161.2
45–54 years	1,750.2	1,470.7	1,123.9	984.7	920.8	997.2	964.3	970.5
55–64 years	2,153.6	1,948.0	1,632.6	1,483.4	1,415.0	1,436.3	1,402.4	1,422.1
65 years and over	3,836.9	3,698.0	3,341.2	3,477.4	3,533.6	3,628.9	3,595.6	3,507.9
65–74 years	3,158.4	2,972.6	2,616.3	2,600.0	2,546.0	2,592.3	2,628.9	2,533.6
75 years and over	4,893.0	4,756.1	4,340.3	4,590.7	4,619.6	4,702.2	4,588.4	4,512.6
75–84 years	4,638.6	4,464.2	3,957.0	4,155.7	4,124.4	4,269.7	4,131.7	4,025.9
85 years and over	5,764.6	5,728.9	5,606.3	5,925.1	6,050.9	5,856.7	5,758.1	5,711.4
Sex[b]								
Male	1,543.9	1,382.5	1,130.0	1,048.5	990.8	1,025.7	1,013.0	1,000.5
Female	1,951.9	1,675.6	1,389.5	1,317.3	1,277.3	1,349.0	1,319.6	1,312.3
Sex and age								
Male, all ages	1,390.4	1,240.2	1,002.2	941.7	910.6	964.9	959.0	954.9
Under 18 years	762.6	626.4	463.1	431.3	408.6	436.4	412.2	401.5
18–44 years	950.9	776.9	579.2	507.2	450.0	464.8	471.1	476.8
45–64 years	1,953.1	1,775.6	1,402.7	1,212.0	1,127.4	1,183.6	1,148.8	1,175.7
65–74 years	3,474.1	3,255.2	2,877.6	2,762.2	2,649.1	2,685.0	2,742.6	2,584.3
75–84 years	5,093.5	5,031.8	4,417.3	4,361.1	4,294.1	4,540.5	4,388.1	4,220.3
85 years and over	6,372.3	6,406.9	6,420.9	6,387.9	6,166.6	5,838.3	5,984.1	5,983.5
Female, all ages	1,944.0	1,712.2	1,431.7	1,362.9	1,336.6	1,411.3	1,382.2	1,375.3
Under 18 years	750.2	601.0	464.1	415.7	396.2	423.7	409.8	385.9
18–44 years	2,180.2	1,808.3	1,468.0	1,318.0	1,248.1	1,361.9	1,330.9	1,343.5
45–64 years	1,942.5	1,645.9	1,309.7	1,160.5	1,101.7	1,172.5	1,145.3	1,147.3
65–74 years	2,916.6	2,754.8	2,411.2	2,469.4	2,461.0	2,514.4	2,533.1	2,490.7
75–84 years	4,370.4	4,130.4	3,678.9	4,024.1	4,013.5	4,087.4	3,957.7	3,893.0
85 years and over	5,500.3	5,458.0	5,289.6	5,743.7	6,003.3	5,865.0	5,654.4	5,584.1
Geographic region[b]								
Northeast	1,622.9	1,428.7	1,332.2	1,335.3	1,274.8	1,287.9	1,245.9	1,261.4
Midwest	1,925.2	1,584.7	1,287.5	1,132.8	1,109.2	1,143.9	1,174.9	1,168.0
South	1,814.1	1,569.4	1,325.0	1,252.4	1,209.2	1,255.5	1,202.5	1,198.8
West	1,519.7	1,469.6	1,006.6	967.4	894.0	1,011.5	1,005.9	964.1
	Days of care per 10,000 population							
Total, age-adjusted[b]	**13,027.0**	**10,017.9**	**8,189.3**	**6,386.2**	**5,576.8**	**5,686.8**	**5,541.7**	**5,474.7**
Total, crude	**12,166.8**	**9,576.6**	**7,840.5**	**6,201.7**	**5,546.5**	**5,741.2**	**5,620.9**	**5,577.8**
Age								
Under 18 years	3,415.1	2,812.3	2,263.1	1,846.7	1,789.7	1,931.8	1,918.3	1,857.6
Under 1 year	13,213.9	14,141.2	11,484.7	10,834.5	11,524.0	12,434.5	12,131.6	11,624.2
1–4 years	3,333.5	2,280.4	1,700.1	1,525.6	1,482.2	1,416.8	1,355.3	1,405.4
5–17 years	2,698.5	2,049.8	1,633.2	1,240.3	1,172.1	1,281.8	1,300.9	1,239.1
18–44 years	8,323.6	6,294.7	4,676.7	3,517.2	3,093.8	3,349.3	3,305.0	3,360.6
18–24 years	7,174.6	5,287.2	4,015.9	2,987.4	2,679.5	2,817.3	2,819.9	2,889.4
25–44 years	8,861.4	6,685.2	4,895.5	3,676.4	3,225.5	3,532.5	3,472.8	3,524.5
25–34 years	8,497.5	6,688.9	4,939.7	3,536.1	3,161.7	3,427.4	3,434.3	3,462.2
35–44 years	9,386.6	6,680.4	4,844.8	3,812.3	3,281.5	3,627.4	3,507.9	3,581.9
45–64 years	15,969.5	12,015.9	9,139.3	6,574.5	5,515.4	5,915.8	5,717.3	5,793.0
45–54 years	13,167.2	9,692.8	6,996.6	5,162.0	4,374.2	4,911.4	4,711.2	4,667.4
55–64 years	18,895.4	14,369.5	11,722.6	8,671.6	7,290.8	7,352.0	7,124.0	7,333.6

West Nile virus, they suffered the worst possible outcome. Both developed encephalitis (a brain infection), fell into coma, and died. These cases catalyzed transplant physicians and public health officials to intensify organ safety protocols and procedures.

SURGICAL CENTERS AND URGENT CARE CENTERS

Ambulatory surgery centers (also called surgicenters) are equipped to perform routine surgical procedures that do not require an overnight hospital stay. A surgical

TABLE 3.3

Hospital discharges, days of care, and average length of stay by selected characteristics, selected years 1980–2006 [CONTINUED]

[Data are based on a sample of hospital records]

Characteristic	1980[a]	1985[a]	1990	1995	2000	2004	2005	2006
				Days of care per 10,000 population				
65 years and over	40,983.5	32,279.7	28,956.1	23,736.5	21,118.9	20,486.0	19,882.8	19,197.5
65–74 years	31,470.3	24,373.3	20,878.2	16,847.0	14,389.7	14,051.7	13,985.3	13,170.2
75 years and over	55,788.2	43,812.7	40,090.8	32,478.1	28,518.6	27,148.7	25,939.4	25,413.1
75–84 years	51,836.2	40,521.6	35,995.1	28,947.5	25,397.8	24,540.6	23,155.3	22,671.7
85 years and over	69,332.0	54,782.4	53,616.9	43,305.9	37,537.8	34,110.0	33,071.5	32,165.5
Sex[b]								
Male	12,475.8	9,792.1	8,057.8	6,239.0	5,358.8	5,411.5	5,301.3	5,208.8
Female	13,662.9	10,340.4	8,404.5	6,548.8	5,809.7	5,996.5	5,828.7	5,764.2
Sex and age								
Male, all ages	10,674.1	8,518.8	6,943.0	5,507.5	4,860.8	5,049.4	4,979.7	4,947.3
Under 18 years	3,473.1	2,942.7	2,335.7	1,998.0	1,955.7	2,015.2	2,006.2	1,968.0
18–44 years	6,102.4	4,746.6	3,517.4	2,729.7	2,175.0	2,255.6	2,282.7	2,375.6
45–64 years	15,894.9	12,290.1	9,434.2	6,822.7	5,704.4	6,123.8	5,773.5	6,004.3
65–74 years	33,697.6	26,220.5	22,515.5	17,697.4	14,897.4	14,423.4	14,502.6	13,262.1
75–84 years	54,723.3	44,087.4	38,257.8	29,642.6	26,616.7	26,458.3	25,106.9	23,972.7
85 years and over	77,013.1	58,609.5	60,347.3	45,263.6	37,765.3	34,025.9	35,179.0	32,604.0
Female, all ages	13,560.1	10,566.3	8,691.1	6,863.4	6,202.7	6,407.7	6,239.5	6,186.8
Under 18 years	3,354.5	2,675.5	2,186.8	1,687.9	1,615.1	1,844.4	1,826.1	1,741.8
18–44 years	10,450.7	7,792.0	5,820.3	4,297.9	4,010.8	4,455.4	4,341.8	4,361.5
45–64 years	16,037.1	11,765.5	8,865.1	6,341.7	5,336.4	5,718.2	5,663.9	5,592.2
65–74 years	29,764.7	22,949.2	19,592.7	16,162.0	13,971.3	13,739.5	13,549.0	13,092.4
75–84 years	50,133.3	38,424.7	34,628.3	28,502.5	24,601.0	23,249.9	21,830.1	21,782.1
85 years and over	65,990.5	53,253.6	51,000.5	42,538.6	37,444.4	34,147.9	32,103.5	31,960.3
Geographic region[b]								
Northeast	14,024.4	11,143.1	10,266.8	8,389.7	7,185.9	6,875.9	6,636.5	6,608.5
Midwest	14,871.9	10,803.6	8,306.5	5,908.8	5,005.3	4,987.1	4,954.3	4,893.5
South	12,713.5	9,642.6	8,204.1	6,659.9	5,925.1	6,141.7	5,830.4	5,844.8
West	9,635.2	8,300.7	5,755.1	4,510.6	4,082.0	4,575.1	4,690.3	4,451.6
				Average length of stay in days				
Total, age-adjusted[b]	**7.5**	**6.6**	**6.5**	**5.4**	**4.9**	**4.8**	**4.8**	**4.7**
Total, crude	**7.3**	**6.5**	**6.4**	**5.4**	**4.9**	**4.8**	**4.8**	**4.8**
Age								
Under 18 years	4.5	4.6	4.9	4.4	4.4	4.5	4.7	4.7
Under 1 year	5.7	6.6	6.0	5.5	5.7	6.0	6.2	6.4
1–4 years	3.9	3.5	3.6	3.3	3.2	3.1	3.2	3.4
5–17 years	4.4	4.3	4.9	4.3	4.4	4.3	4.5	4.5
18–44 years	5.3	4.8	4.6	3.8	3.6	3.7	3.7	3.7
18–24 years	4.6	4.1	3.8	3.2	3.1	3.3	3.3	3.3
25–44 years	5.6	5.1	4.8	4.0	3.8	3.8	3.8	3.8
25–34 years	5.0	4.7	4.3	3.5	3.4	3.4	3.4	3.4
35–44 years	6.5	5.8	5.6	4.7	4.3	4.3	4.3	4.3
45–64 years	8.2	7.0	6.7	5.5	5.0	5.0	5.0	5.0
45–54 years	7.5	6.6	6.2	5.2	4.8	4.9	4.9	4.8
55–64 years	8.8	7.4	7.2	5.8	5.2	5.1	5.1	5.2
65 years and over	10.7	8.7	8.7	6.8	6.0	5.6	5.5	5.5
65–74 years	10.0	8.2	8.0	6.5	5.7	5.4	5.3	5.2
75 years and over	11.4	9.2	9.2	7.1	6.2	5.8	5.7	5.6
75–84 years	11.2	9.1	9.1	7.0	6.2	5.7	5.6	5.6
85 years and over	12.0	9.6	9.6	7.3	6.2	5.8	5.7	5.6
Sex[b]								
Male	8.1	7.1	7.1	6.0	5.4	5.3	5.2	5.2
Female	7.0	6.2	6.0	5.0	4.5	4.4	4.4	4.4
Sex and age								
Male, all ages	7.7	6.9	6.9	5.8	5.3	5.2	5.2	5.2
Under 18 years	4.6	4.7	5.0	4.6	4.8	4.6	4.9	4.9
18–44 years	6.4	6.1	6.1	5.4	4.8	4.9	4.8	5.0
45–64 years	8.1	6.9	6.7	5.6	5.1	5.2	5.0	5.1
65–74 years	9.7	8.1	7.8	6.4	5.6	5.4	5.3	5.1
75–84 years	10.7	8.8	8.7	6.8	6.2	5.8	5.7	5.7
85 years and over	12.1	9.1	9.4	7.1	6.1	5.8	5.9	5.4

center requires less sophisticated and expensive equipment than a hospital operating room. Minor surgery, such as biopsies, abortions, hernia repair, and many cosmetic surgery procedures, are performed at outpatient surgical centers. Most procedures are done under local anesthesia, and patients go home the same day.

Most ambulatory surgery centers are freestanding, but some are located on hospital campuses or are next

TABLE 3.3

Hospital discharges, days of care, and average length of stay by selected characteristics, selected years 1980–2006 [CONTINUED]

[Data are based on a sample of hospital records]

Characteristic	1980[a]	1985[a]	1990	1995	2000	2004	2005	2006
				Average length of stay in days				
Female, all ages	7.0	6.2	6.1	5.0	4.6	4.5	4.5	4.5
Under 18 years	4.5	4.5	4.7	4.1	4.1	4.4	4.5	4.5
18–44 years	4.8	4.3	4.0	3.3	3.2	3.3	3.3	3.2
45–64 years	8.3	7.1	6.8	5.5	4.8	4.9	4.9	4.9
65–74 years	10.2	8.3	8.1	6.5	5.7	5.5	5.3	5.3
75–84 years	11.5	9.3	9.4	7.1	6.1	5.7	5.5	5.6
85 years and over	12.0	9.8	9.6	7.4	6.2	5.8	5.7	5.7
Geographic region[b]								
Northeast	8.6	7.8	7.7	6.3	5.6	5.3	5.3	5.2
Midwest	7.7	6.8	6.5	5.2	4.5	4.4	4.2	4.2
South	7.0	6.1	6.2	5.3	4.9	4.9	4.8	4.9
West	6.3	5.6	5.7	4.7	4.6	4.5	4.7	4.6

[a]Comparisons of data from 1980–1985 with data from subsequent years should be made with caution because estimates of change may reflect improvements in the survey design rather than true changes in hospital use.
[b]Estimates are age-adjusted to the year 2000 standard population using six age groups: under 18 years, 18–44 years, 45–54 years, 55–64 years, 65–74 years, and 75 years and over.
Notes: Excludes newborn infants. Rates are based on the civilian population as of July 1. Rates for 1990–1999 are not strictly comparable with rates for 2000 and beyond because population estimates for 1990–1999 have not been revised to reflect the 2000 census.

SOURCE: "Table 99. Discharges, Days of Care, and Average Length of Stay in Nonfederal Short-Stay Hospitals, by Selected Characteristics: United States, Selected Years 1980–2006," in *Health, United States, 2009: With Special Feature on Medical Technology*, U.S. Department of Health and Human Services, Centers for Disease Control and Prevention, National Center for Health Statistics, 2010, http://www.cdc.gov/nchs/data/hus/hus09.pdf#listtables (accessed May 12, 2010)

to physicians' offices or clinics. Facilities are licensed by their state and must be equipped with at least one operating room, an area for preparing patients for procedures, a patient recovery area, and x-ray and clinical laboratory services. Also, surgical centers must have a registered nurse on the premises when patients are in the facility.

Urgent care centers (also called urgicenters) are usually operated by private, for-profit organizations and provide up to 24-hour care on a walk-in basis. These centers fill several special needs in a community. They provide convenient, timely, and easily accessible care in an emergency when the nearest hospital is miles away. The centers are normally open during the hours when most physicians' offices are closed, and they are economical to operate because they do not provide hospital beds. They usually treat problems such as cuts that require sutures, sprains and bruises from accidents, and various infections. Many provide inexpensive immunizations, and some offer routine health care for people who do not have a regular source of medical care. Urgent care may be more expensive than a visit to the family physician, but an urgent care center visit is usually less expensive than treatment from a traditional hospital emergency department.

Clinics and Urgent Care Centers in Stores, Malls, and Chains

Pat Pollert, Darla Dobberstein, and Ronald Wiisanen observe in "Jumping into the Healthcare Retail Market: Our Experience" (*Frontiers of Health Services Management*, vol. 24, no. 3, Spring 2008) that retail-based clinics are being established throughout the United States in grocery stores, drug stores, shopping malls, and chains such as Target and Walmart. Pollert, Dobberstein, and Wiisanen describe their experience of operating a retail-based clinic in Fargo, North Dakota. Initially, their clinic was opposed by some area physicians, who were concerned that the clinic would undermine continuity and quality of care because clinic practitioners rarely see patients more than once and patients do not return for follow-up visits. However, customer feedback was overwhelmingly positive. Customers appreciated the convenience and described the clinic as "efficient, effective and friendly."

Retail-based clinics offer more than simply convenient locations. Many welcome walk-in patients and offer extended hours, flat fees for physician visits, low-cost immunizations, and comfortable surroundings. They also emphasize unscheduled care much more than do most primary care practices. Furthermore, many do not bill insurance companies; patients pay in cash or by credit card.

According to the drug store chain Walgreens, in the press release "Walgreens Named as One of Fast Company Magazine's Most Innovative Health Care Companies" (February 18, 2010, http://takecarehealth.com/about/press-release.aspx?id=02.18.10_1), in 2010 its Take Care Clinics were located in 357 locations in 19 states. The clinics accept many kinds of health insurance, are open seven days a week, and offer evening hours on weeknights.

LONG-TERM CARE FACILITIES

Families are still the major caretakers of older, dependent, and disabled members of American society. However, the number of people aged 65 years and older living in long-term care facilities such as nursing homes is rising because the population in this age group is increasing rapidly. Even though many older people now live longer, healthier lives, the increase in overall length of life has expanded the need for long-term care facilities.

Growth of the home health care industry in the early 1990s only slightly slowed the increase in the numbers of Americans entering nursing homes. Assisted living and continuing-care retirement communities offer other alternatives to nursing home care. When it is possible, many older adults prefer to remain in the community and receive health care in their home.

Types of Nursing Homes

Nursing homes fall into three broad categories: residential care facilities, intermediate care facilities, and skilled nursing facilities. Each provides a different range and intensity of services:

- A residential care facility (RCF) normally provides meals and housekeeping for its residents, plus some basic medical monitoring, such as administering medications. This type of home is for people who are fairly independent and do not need constant medical attention but need help with tasks such as laundry and cleaning. Many RCFs also provide social activities and recreational programs for their residents.

- An intermediate care facility (ICF) offers room and board and nursing care as necessary for people who can no longer live independently. As in the RCF, exercise and social programs are provided, and some ICFs also offer physical therapy and rehabilitation programs.

- A skilled nursing facility (SNF) provides around-the-clock nursing care, plus on-call physician coverage. The SNF is for patients who need intensive nursing care and services such as occupational therapy, physical therapy, respiratory therapy, and rehabilitation.

Number of Nursing Home Residents Is Rising

The National Nursing Home Survey (NNHS) is a continuing series of national sample surveys of nursing homes, their residents, and their staff. The surveys were conducted in 1973–74, 1977, 1985, 1995, 1997, 1999, and 2004. Even though each survey focused on different aspects of care, they all provide some common basic information about nursing homes, their residents, and their staff from two perspectives: the provider of services and the recipient. Data about the facilities include characteristics such as size, ownership, Medicare/Medicaid certification, occupancy rate, number of days of care provided, and expenses. The surveys gathered demographic data, health status, and services received by nursing home residents. The most recent NNHS for which data are available was conducted in 2004 and the results were published in *2004 National Nursing Home Survey* (2006, http://www.cdc.gov/nchs/data/nnhsd/nursinghomefacilities2006 .pdf). The nursing homes included in this survey had at least three beds and were either certified (by Medicare or Medicaid) or had a state license to operate as a nursing home.

The NNHS reports that in 2004 the nation's 16,100 certified nursing homes housed more than 1.7 million beds and had occupancy rates of 86.3%. Nursing homes averaged 107.6 beds per facility. In 2004, 61.5% of all nursing homes were privately owned, 54.2% were affiliated with a chain, 30.8% were operated by not-for-profit volunteer organizations, and only 7.7% were operated by governmental agencies.

Most residents of nursing homes are the "oldest old" (people aged 85 years and older). Out of the total 1.3 million nursing home residents aged 65 years and older in 2004, the so-called oldest old accounted for 674,500 (52%) of all nursing home residents. (See Table 3.4.)

In December 2008 the Centers for Medicare and Medicaid Services (CMS) began the Five-Star Quality Rating System (https://www.cms.gov/CertificationandComplianc/ 13_FSQRS.asp) for the nation's 16,100 certified nursing homes. The CMS also provides a nursing home checklist (http://www.medicare.gov/Nursing/Checklist.pdf) to help consumers assess and compare nursing homes. Furthermore, the CMS offers the website "Nursing Home Compare" (http://www.medicare.gov/NHCompare/Include/ DataSection/Questions/ProximitySearch.asp), which contains detailed information about every Medicare- and Medicaid-certified nursing home in the country.

Diversification of Nursing Homes

To remain competitive with home health care and the increasing array of alternative living arrangements for the elderly, many nursing homes offer alternative services and programs. These services include adult day care and visiting nurse services for people who still live at home. Other programs include respite plans that allow caregivers who need to travel for business or vacation to leave an elderly relative in the nursing home temporarily.

One of the most popular nontraditional services is subacute care, which is comprehensive inpatient treatment for people recovering from acute illnesses such as pneumonia, injuries such as a broken hip, and chronic diseases such as arthritis that do not require intensive, hospital-level treatment. This level of care also enables nursing homes to expand their markets by offering services to younger patients.

TABLE 3.4

Nursing home residents age 65 and older, by age, sex, and race, selected years 1973–2004

[Data are based on a sample of nursing home residents]

Age, sex, and race	Number of residents in hundreds					Residents per 1,000 population[a]				
	1973–1974	1985	1995	1999	2004	1973–1974	1985	1995	1999	2004
Age										
65 years and over, age-adjusted[b]	—	—	—	—	—	58.5	54.0	46.4	43.3	34.8
65 years and over, crude	9,615	13,183	14,229	14,695	13,173	44.7	46.2	42.8	42.9	36.3
65–74 years	1,631	2,121	1,897	1,948	1,741	12.3	12.5	10.2	10.8	9.4
75–84 years	3,849	509	5,096	5,176	4,687	57.7	57.7	46.1	43.0	36.1
85 years and over	4,136	5,973	7,235	7,571	6,745	257.3	220.3	200.9	182.5	138.8
Male										
65 years and over, age-adjusted[b]	—	—	—	—	—	42.5	38.8	33.0	30.6	24.1
65 years and over, crude	2,657	3,344	3,571	3,778	3,369	30.0	29.0	26.2	26.5	22.2
65–74 years	651	806	795	841	754	11.3	10.8	9.6	10.3	8.9
75–84 years	1,023	1,413	1,443	1,495	1,409	39.9	43.0	33.5	30.8	27.0
85 years and over	983	1,126	1,333	1,442	1,206	182.7	145.7	131.5	116.5	80.0
Female										
65 years and over, age-adjusted[b]	—	—	—	—	—	67.5	61.5	52.8	49.8	40.4
65 years and over, crude	6,958	9,839	10,658	10,917	9,804	54.9	57.9	54.3	54.6	46.4
65–74 years	980	1,315	1,103	1,107	988	13.1	13.8	10.7	11.2	9.8
75–84 years	2,826	3,677	3,654	3,681	3,278	68.9	66.4	54.3	51.2	42.3
85 years and over	3,153	4,847	5,902	6,129	5,539	294.9	250.1	228.1	210.5	165.2
White[c]										
65 years and over, age-adjusted[b]	—	—	—	—	—	61.2	55.5	45.8	41.9	34.0
65 years and over, crude	9,206	12,274	12,715	12,796	11,489	46.9	47.7	42.7	42.1	36.2
65–74 years	1,501	1,878	1,541	1,573	1,342	12.5	12.3	9.3	10.0	8.5
75–84 years	3,697	4,736	4,513	4,406	4,058	60.3	59.1	45.0	40.5	35.2
85 years and over	4,008	5,660	6,662	6,817	6,089	270.8	228.7	203.2	181.8	139.4
Black or African American[c]										
65 years and over, age-adjusted[b]	—	—	—	—	—	28.2	41.5	50.8	55.5	49.9
65 years and over, crude	377	820	1,229	1,459	1,454	22.0	35.0	45.5	51.0	47.7
65–74 years	122	225	296	303	345	11.1	15.4	18.5	18.2	20.2
75–84 years	134	306	475	587	546	26.7	45.3	57.8	66.5	55.5
85 years and over	121	290	458	569	563	105.7	141.5	168.2	182.8	160.7

—Category not applicable.

[a]Rates are calculated using estimates of the civilian population of the United States including institutionalized persons.

[b]Age-adjusted to the year 2000 population standard using the following three age groups: 65–74 years, 75–84 years, and 85 years and over.

[c]Starting with 1999 data, the instruction for the race item on the current resident questionnaire was changed so that more than one race could be recorded. In previous years, only one racial category could be checked. Estimates for racial groups presented in this table are for residents for whom only one race was recorded. Estimates for residents where multiple races were checked are unreliable due to small sample sizes and are not shown.

Notes: Residents are persons on the roster of the nursing home as of the night before the survey. Residents for whom beds are maintained even though they may be away on overnight leave or in a hospital are included. People residing in personal care or domiciliary care homes are excluded.

SOURCE: "Table 105. Nursing Home Residents 65 Years of Age and over, by Age, Sex, and Race: United States, Selected Years 1973–2004," in *Health, United States, 2009: With Special Feature on Medical Technology*, U.S. Department of Health and Human Services, Centers for Disease Control and Prevention, National Center for Health Statistics, 2010, http://www.cdc.gov/nchs/data/hus/hus09.pdf#listtables (accessed May 12, 2010)

Innovation Improves Quality of Nursing Home Care

Even though industry observers and the media frequently raise concerns about the care provided in nursing homes and publicize instances of elder abuse and other quality of care issues, several organizations have actively sought to develop models of health service delivery that improve the clinical care and quality of life for nursing home residents. In *Evaluation of the Wellspring Model for Improving Nursing Home Quality* (August 2002, http://www.cmwf.org/usr_doc/stone_wellspringevaluation.pdf), a report that examines one such model in eastern Wisconsin, Robyn Stone et al. evaluate the Wellspring model of nursing home quality improvement.

Wellspring is a group of not-for-profit nursing homes that are governed by a group called the Wellspring Alliance. Founded in 1994, the alliance aims to improve the clinical care delivered to its nursing home residents and the work environment for its employees. Based on the Wellspring philosophy that education and collaboration are paramount to success, the program began by equipping nursing home personnel with the skills needed to perform their jobs and by organizing employees in teams working toward shared goals. The Wellspring model of service delivery uses a multidisciplinary clinical team approach (nurse practitioners, social service professionals, food service personnel, nursing assistants, and facility and housekeeping personnel) to solve problems and develop approaches to better meet residents' needs. Each of these teams represents an important innovation because it allows health professionals and other workers to interact as peers and share resources, information, and decision making in a cooperative, supportive environment.

Stone et al. observe that there was more cooperation, responsibility, and accountability within the teams and the institutions than what was noted at other comparable facilities. Besides finding a strong organizational culture that seemed committed to quality patient care, the researchers document measurable improvements in specific areas including:

- Wellspring facilities had lower rates of staff turnover than comparable Wisconsin facilities during the same period, probably because Wellspring workers felt valued by management and experienced greater job satisfaction than other nursing home personnel

- The Wellspring model did not require additional resources to institute, and Wellspring facilities operated at lower costs than comparable facilities

- Wellspring facilities' performance, as measured by a federal survey, improved

- Wellspring personnel appeared more attentive to residents' needs and problems and sought to anticipate and promptly resolve problems

- An organizational commitment to training and shared decision making, along with improved quality of interactions and relationships among staff and between staff and residents, significantly contributed to enhanced quality of life for residents

James Fett describes in "Social Accountability: Building Bonds in Our Communities" (*BESTPractices*, July–August 2004) the ambitious social outreach programs of one of the charter Wellspring organizations, St. Paul Elder Services, which serves a community of 13,000 residents in Kaukauna, Wisconsin. St. Paul Elder Services provides several types of uncompensated care as well as programs and services to fulfill the unmet needs of older adults in the community. Examples of these services include free blood pressure screenings at senior housing complexes, adult day care for people suffering from dementia, warm-water exercise classes, diabetic menu planning classes, continence management programs, and foot, nail, and ear cleaning services. Fett explains that "our community is the source of our residents, volunteers, associates and philanthropy. . . . Social accountability . . . communicates our message of commitment, performance and excellence. Through this process, we have created and strengthened a level of trust and cooperation, improving the quality of life for everyone involved."

In *A Process Evaluation of the Implementation of the Lutheran Wellspring Alliance of the Carolinas* (August 2008, http://www.aahsa.org/uploadedFiles/IFAS/Publications _amp;_Products/Wellspring%20Report_final.pdf), a report that examines the evolution and implementation of the Wellspring model of nursing home quality improvement, Natasha Bryant, Janice Heineman, and Robyn Stone evaluate how adopting the Wellspring model changed the lives of residents, staff, and families in nine Lutheran Carolina nursing homes. The researchers assert, "The nursing home workers interviewed believed that the Wellspring program improved the quality of life and care for residents. The Wellspring program provided workers with best practices and tools that enabled them to better care for residents. The staff, therefore, has a better understanding of the overall care process for the resident and can provide better care." Bryant, Heineman, and Stone also observe that a higher percentage of family members rated the facilities as "excellent" or "good" after the Wellspring model was implemented.

MENTAL HEALTH FACILITIES

In earlier centuries mental illness was often considered a sign of possession by the devil or, at best, a moral weakness. A change in these attitudes began in the late 18th century, when mental illness was perceived to be a treatable condition. It was then that the concept of asylums was developed, not only to lock the mentally ill away but also to provide them with "relief" from the conditions they found troubling.

In the 21st century mental health care is provided in a variety of treatment settings by different types of organizations. The following mental health organizations offer diagnostic and therapeutic mental health services:

- A psychiatric hospital (public or private) provides 24-hour inpatient care to people with mental illnesses in a hospital setting. It may also offer 24-hour residential care and less than 24-hour care, but these are not requirements. Psychiatric hospitals are operated under state, county, private for-profit, and private not-for-profit auspices.

- General hospitals with separate psychiatric services, units, or designated beds are under government or nongovernmental auspices and maintain assigned staff for 24-hour inpatient care, 24-hour residential care, and less than 24-hour care (outpatient care or partial hospitalization) to provide mental health diagnosis, evaluation, and treatment.

- Veterans Administration (VA) hospitals are operated by the U.S. Department of Veterans Affairs and include VA general hospital psychiatric services and VA psychiatric outpatient clinics that exclusively serve people entitled to VA benefits.

- Outpatient mental health clinics that provide only ambulatory mental health services. Generally, a psychiatrist has overall medical responsibility for clients and establishes the philosophy and orientation of the mental health program.

- Community mental health centers were funded under the Federal Community Mental Health Centers Act of 1963 and subsequent amendments to the act. During the early 1980s, when the federal government reverted to funding mental health services through block grants to the states rather than by funding them directly, the federal government stopped tracking these mental health organizations individually, and statistical reports include them in the category "all other mental health organizations." This category also includes freestanding psychiatric outpatient clinics, freestanding partial care organizations, and multiservice mental health organizations such as residential treatment centers. These so-called community mental health centers have sliding scale fees and accept Medicaid, Medicare, private health insurance, and private fee-for-service (paid for each visit, procedure, or treatment that is delivered) payment. Mental health care is also available from not-for-profit mental health or counseling services offered by health and social service agencies, such as Catholic Social Services, family and children's service agencies, Jewish Family Services, and Lutheran Social Services, that are staffed by qualified mental health professionals to provide counseling services.

- Residential treatment centers for emotionally disturbed children serve children and youth primarily under the age of 18 years, provide 24-hour residential services, and offer a clinical program that is directed by a psychiatrist, psychologist, social worker, or psychiatric nurse who holds a master's or doctorate degree.

Where Are the Mentally Ill?

The chronically mentally ill reside either in mental hospitals or in community settings, such as with families, in boarding homes and shelters, in single-room-occupancy hotels (usually inexpensive hotels or boardinghouses), in prison, or even on the streets as part of the homeless population. The institutionalized mentally ill are those people with psychiatric diagnoses who have lived in mental hospitals for more than one year or those with diagnosed mental illness who are living in nursing homes.

Declining mental health expenditures have resulted in fewer available services for specific populations of the mentally ill, particularly those who could benefit from inpatient or residential care. Even for people without conditions requiring institutional care there are barriers to access. The U.S. surgeon general's landmark report *Mental Health: A Report of the Surgeon General, 1999* (1999, http://www.mentalhealth.samhsa.gov/features/surgeongeneralreport/home.asp) describes the U.S. mental health service system as largely uncoordinated and fragmented, in part because it involves so many different sectors—health and social welfare agencies, public and private hospitals, housing, criminal justice, and education—and because it is funded through many different sources. Finally, inequalities in insurance coverage for mental health, coupled with the stigma associated with mental illness and treatment, have also limited access to services.

The NCHS reveals in *Health, United States, 2009* (2010, http://www.cdc.gov/nchs/data/hus/hus09.pdf) that the number of mental health organizations for 24-hour inpatient treatment steadily declined from 3,942 in 1990 to 2,891 in 2004. (See Table 3.5.) Except for Department of Veterans Affairs medical centers, all other service sites and types of organizations diminished in capacity. The number of beds per 100,000 civilian population fell from 128.5 in 1990 to just 71.2 in 2004. This decline was not necessarily a result of better treatment for the mentally ill but a consequence of reduced funding for inpatient facilities. Many of the patients who were once housed in mental institutions (including some who had been lifelong residents in these facilities) were forced to fend for themselves on the streets or in prison.

Besides mental health units or beds in acute care medical/surgical hospitals and physicians' offices, mental health care and treatment is offered in the offices of other mental health clinicians such as psychologists, clinical social workers, and marriage and family therapists, as well as in other settings. Private psychiatric hospitals provide outpatient mental health evaluation and therapy in day programs as well as inpatient care. Like acute care hospitals, these facilities are accredited by the Joint Commission on Accreditation of Health Care Organizations and may offer outpatient services by way of referral to a local network of qualified mental health providers.

National Goals for Mental Health Service Delivery

Healthy People 2010 (November 2000, http://www.healthypeople.gov/document/tableofcontents.htm) is a set of health objectives for the United States to achieve during the first decade of the 21st century. Fourteen of the 467 health objectives enumerated in *Healthy People 2010* relate to mental health and mental disorders. Even though nearly all the objectives intend to reduce the incidence and prevalence of mental illness in the United States and improve access to care and treatment, several specifically address service delivery issues related to mental health professionals and treatment facilities.

As of July 2010, the objectives for *Healthy People 2020* were being established. Eleven of the proposed objectives were carried over from *Healthy People 2010* and three other proposed objectives were modified (October 30,

TABLE 3.5

Mental health organizations and beds for 24-hour hospital and residential treatment, by type of organization, selected years 1986–2004

[Data are based on inventories of mental health organizations]

Type of organization	1986	1990	1994	1998	2000	2002	2004
	\multicolumn{7}{c}{Number of mental health organizations}						
All organizations	3,512	3,942	3,853	3,741	3,211	3,044	2,891
State and county mental hospitals	285	278	270	237	229	227	237
Private psychiatric hospitals	314	464	432	347	271	255	264
Nonfederal general hospital psychiatric services	1,351	1,577	1,539	1,595	1,325	1,231	1,230
Department of Veterans Affairs (VA) medical centers[a]	139	131	136	124	134	132	—
Residential treatment centers for emotionally disturbed children	437	501	472	462	476	510	458
All other organizations[b]	986	991	1,004	976	776	689	702
	\multicolumn{7}{c}{Number of beds}						
All organizations	267,613	325,529	293,139	269,148	214,186	211,040	212,231
State and county mental hospitals	119,033	102,307	84,063	71,266	61,833	57,314	57,034
Private psychiatric hospitals	30,201	45,952	42,742	31,731	26,402	24,996	28,422
Nonfederal general hospital psychiatric services	45,808	53,576	53,455	54,775	40,410	40,520	41,403
Department of Veterans Affairs medical centers[a]	26,874	24,779	21,346	17,173	8,989	9,581	—
Residential treatment centers for emotionally disturbed children	24,547	35,170	32,691	32,040	33,508	39,407	33,835
All other organizations[b]	21,150	63,745	58,842	62,163	43,044	39,222	51,536
	\multicolumn{7}{c}{Beds per 100,000 civilian population[c]}						
All organizations	111.7	128.5	110.9	94.0	74.8	72.2	71.2
State and county mental hospitals	49.7	40.4	31.8	24.9	21.6	19.6	19.1
Private psychiatric hospitals	12.6	18.1	16.2	11.1	9.2	8.6	9.5
Nonfederal general hospital psychiatric services	19.1	21.2	20.2	19.1	14.1	13.9	13.9
Department of Veterans Affairs medical centers[a]	11.2	9.9	8.1	6.0	3.1	3.3	—
Residential treatment centers for emotionally disturbed children	10.3	13.9	12.4	11.2	11.7	13.5	11.4
All other organizations[b]	8.8	25.2	22.2	21.7	15.0	13.4	17.3

—Data not available.

[a]Department of Veterans Affairs medical centers (VA general hospital psychiatric services and VA psychiatric outpatient clinics) were dropped from the survey as of 2004.
[b]Includes freestanding psychiatric outpatient clinics, partial care organizations, and multiservice mental health organizations.
[c]Civilian population estimates for 2000 and beyond are based on the 2000 census as of July 1; population estimates for 1992–1998 are 1990 postcensal estimates.

SOURCE: "Table 116. Mental Health Organizations and Beds for 24-Hour Hospital and Residential Treatment, by Type of Organization: United States, Selected Years 1986–2004," in *Health, United States, 2009: With Special Feature on Medical Technology*, U.S. Department of Health and Human Services, Centers for Disease Control and Prevention, National Center for Health Statistics, 2010, http://www.cdc.gov/nchs/data/hus/hus09.pdf#listtables (accessed May 12, 2010)

2009, http://www.healthypeople.gov/hp2020/Objectives/TopicArea.aspx?id=34&TopicArea=Mental+Health+and+Mental+Disorders). The proposed objectives that were retained were:

- Reduce the suicide rate

- Reduce the rate of suicide attempts by adolescents

- Increase the proportion of homeless adults with mental health problems who receive mental health services

- Reduce the proportion of adolescents who engage in disordered eating behaviors in an attempt to control their weight

- Increase the proportion of primary care facilities that provide mental health treatment onsite or by paid referral

- Increase the proportion of children with mental health problems who receive treatment

- Increase the proportion of juvenile residential facilities that screen admissions for mental health problems

- Increase the proportion of counties served by community-based jail diversion programs and/or mental health courts for adults with mental health problems

- Increase the number of States and the District of Columbia that track consumers' satisfaction with the mental health services they receive

- Increase the number of States, Territories, and the District of Columbia with an operational mental health plan that addresses cultural competence

- Increase the number of States, Territories, and the District of Columbia with an operational mental health plan that addresses specialized mental health services for elderly persons

The proposed objectives that were modified were:

- Increase the proportion of persons with serious mental illness (SMI) who are employed

- Increase the proportion of adults with mental disorders who receive treatment

- Increase the proportion of persons with co-occurring substance abuse and mental disorders who receive treatment for both disorders

Also, there were two new proposed objectives for *Healthy People 2020*:

- Increase depression screening by primary care providers

- Decrease the annual prevalence of Major Depressive Episode (MDE).

MDE is a serious depression with symptoms such as despondency, feelings of worthlessness, and even suicidal thoughts.

HOME HEALTH CARE

The concept of home health care began as postacute care after hospitalization, an alternative to longer, costlier lengths of stay in regular hospitals. Home health care services have grown tremendously since the 1980s, when prospective payment (payments made before, rather than after, care is received) for Medicare patients sharply reduced hospital lengths of stay. During the mid-1980s Medicare began reimbursing hospitals using a rate scale based on diagnosis-related groups—hospitals received a fixed amount for providing services to Medicare patients based on their diagnoses. This form of payment gave hospitals powerful financial incentives to use fewer resources because they could keep the difference between the prospective payment and the amount they actually spent to provide care. Hospitals experienced losses when patients had longer lengths of stay and used more services than were covered by the standardized diagnosis-related group prospective payment.

According to the article "Home Health Care" (*Family Economics and Nutrition Review*, Spring 1996), home health care grew faster during the early 1990s than any other segment of health services. Its growth may be attributable to the observation that in many cases caring for patients at home is preferable to and more cost effec-

tive than care provided in a hospital, nursing home, or some other residential facility. Oftentimes, older adults are more comfortable and much happier living in their own home or with family members. Disabled people may also be able to function better at home with limited assistance than in a residential setting with full-time monitoring.

Home health care agencies provide a wide variety of services. Services range from helping with activities of daily living, such as bathing, doing light housekeeping, and making meals, to skilled nursing care, such as the nursing care needed by AIDS or cancer patients. The number of Medicare-certified home health agencies has varied in response to reimbursement, growing from 2,924 in 1980 to 8,437 in 1996, then declining to 6,928 in 2003. (See Table 3.6.) In 2007 the number of Medicare-certified home health agencies rose to 9,024, the highest it has ever been.

In 1972 Medicare extended home health care coverage to people under 65 years of age only if they were disabled or suffered from end-stage renal disease. Before 2000 Medicare coverage for home health care was limited to patients immediately following discharge from the hospital. By 2000 Medicare covered beneficiaries' home health care services with no requirement for previous hospitalization. There were also no limits to the number of professional visits or to the length of coverage. As long as the patient's condition warranted it, the following services were provided:

- Part-time or intermittent skilled nursing and home health aide services

- Speech-language pathology services

TABLE 3.6

Medicare-certified providers and suppliers, selected years 1975–2007

[Data are compiled from various Centers for Medicare and Medicaid Services data systems]

Providers or suppliers	1975	1980	1985	1990	1996	1999	2001	2003	2005	2007
					Number of providers or suppliers					
Skilled nursing facilities	—	5,052	6,451	8,937	—	14,913	14,841	14,838	15,006	15,054
Home health agencies	2,242	2,924	5,679	5,730	8,437	7,857	7,099	6,928	8,090	9,024
Clinical Laboratory Improvement Act facilities	—	—	—	—	159,907	171,018	168,333	176,947	196,296	206,065
End-stage renal disease facilities	—	999	1,393	1,937	2,876	3,787	3,991	4,309	4,755	5,095
Outpatient physical therapy	117	419	854	1,195	2,302	2,867	2,874	2,961	2,962	2,915
Portable x-ray	132	216	308	443	555	666	675	641	553	550
Rural health clinics	—	391	428	551	2,775	3,453	3,334	3,306	3,661	3,781
Comprehensive outpatient rehabilitation facilities	—	—	72	186	307	522	518	587	634	539
Ambulatory surgical centers	—	—	336	1,197	2,112	2,894	3,147	3,597	4,445	4,964
Hospices	—	—	164	825	1,927	2,326	2,267	2,323	2,872	3,255

—Data not available.

Notes: Data for 1975–1990 are as of July 1. Data for 1996–1999 and 2004–2007 are as of December 31. Data for 2001, 2002, and 2003 are as of December 2000, December 2001, and December 2002, respectively.

SOURCE: "Table 120. Medicare-Certified Providers and Suppliers: United States, Selected Years 1975–2007," in *Health, United States, 2009: With Special Feature on Medical Technology*, U.S. Department of Health and Human Services, Centers for Disease Control and Prevention, National Center for Health Statistics, 2010, http://www.cdc.gov/nchs/data/hus/hus09.pdf#listtables (accessed May 12, 2010)

- Physical and occupational therapy
- Medical social services
- Medical supplies
- Durable medical equipment (with a 20% co-payment)

Over time, the population receiving home health care services has changed. Since 2000 much of home health care is associated with rehabilitation from critical illnesses, and fewer users are long-term patients with chronic conditions. This changing pattern of utilization reflects a shift from longer-term care for chronic conditions to short-term, postacute care. Compared with postacute care users, the long-term patients are older, more functionally disabled, more likely to be incontinent, and more expensive to serve.

Medicare Limits Home Health Care Services

The Balanced Budget Act of 1997 cut approximately $16.2 billion from the federal government's home health care expenditures over a period of five years. The act sought to return home health care to its original concept of short-term care plus skilled nursing and therapy services. As a result of this shift away from personal care and "custodial care" services and toward short-term, skilled nursing services, some Medicare beneficiaries who received home health care lost coverage for certain personal care services, such as assistance with bathing, dressing, and eating.

The Balanced Budget Act sharply curtailed the growth in home health care spending, which affected health care providers. Nonetheless, the aging population and the financial imperative to prevent or minimize institutionalization (hospitalization or placement in a long-term care facility) combined to generate increasing expenditures for home health care services. Medicare expenditures for home health care rose from $4 billion in 2000 to $6.6 billion in 2008, which represented 2.8% of Medicare expenditures. (See Table 3.7.) In contrast, payments to skilled nursing facilities accounted for 10.3% ($24.2 billion) of expenditures in 2008, and inpatient hospital expenditures were 55.4% ($130.5 billion) of the total.

HOSPICE CARE

In medieval times hospices were refuges for the sick, the needy, and travelers. The modern hospice movement developed in response to the need to provide humane care to terminally ill patients, while at the same time offering support to their families. The British physician Cicely Saunders (1918–2005) pioneered the hospice concept in Britain during the late 1960s and helped introduce it in the United States during the 1970s. The care provided by hospice workers is called palliative care, and it aims to relieve patients' pain and the accompanying symptoms of terminal illness without seeking to cure the illness.

Hospice is a philosophy, an approach to care for the dying, and it is not necessarily a physical facility. Hospice may refer to a place—a freestanding facility or a designated floor in a hospital or nursing home—or to a program such as hospice home care, where a team of health professionals helps the dying patient and family at home. Hospice teams may involve physicians, nurses, social workers, pastoral counselors, and trained volunteers. The goal of hospice care is to provide support and care for people at the end of life, enabling them to remain as comfortable as possible.

Hospice workers consider the patient and family as the "unit of care" and focus their efforts on attending to emotional, psychological, and spiritual needs as well as to physical comfort and well-being. The programs provide respite care, which offers relief at any time for families who may be overwhelmed and exhausted by the demands of caregiving and may be neglecting their own needs for rest and relaxation. Finally, hospice programs work to prepare relatives and friends for the loss of their loved ones. Hospice offers bereavement support groups and counseling to help deal with grief and may even help with funeral arrangements.

The hospice concept is different from most other health care services because it focuses on care rather than on cure. Hospice workers try to minimize the two greatest fears associated with dying: fear of isolation and fear of pain. Potent, effective medications are offered to patients in pain, with the goal of controlling pain without impairing alertness so that patients may be as comfortable as possible.

Hospice care also emphasizes living life to its fullest. Patients are encouraged to stay active for as long as possible, to do things they enjoy, and to learn something new each day. Quality of life, rather than length of life, is the focus. In addition, whenever it is possible, family and friends are urged to be the primary caregivers in the home. Care at home helps both patients and family members enrich their lives and face death together.

Ira Byock, the former president of the American Academy of Hospice and Palliative Medicine, explains the concept of hospice care in *Dying Well: The Prospect for Growth at the End of Life* (1997): "Hospice care differs noticeably from the modern medical approach to dying. Typically, as a hospice patient nears death, the medical details become almost automatic and attention focuses on the personal nature of this final transition—what the patient and family are going through emotionally and spiritually. In the more established system, even as people die, medical procedures remain the first

TABLE 3.7

Medicare enrollees and expenditures by type of service, selected years 1970–2008

[Data are compiled from various sources by the Centers for Medicare and Medicaid Services]

Medicare program and type of service	1970	1980	1990	1995	2000	2003	2004	2005	2006	2007	2008[a]
Enrollees					Number in millions						
Total Medicare[b]	**20.4**	**28.4**	**34.3**	**37.6**	**39.7**	**41.2**	**41.9**	**42.6**	**43.4**	**44.3**	**45.2**
Hospital insurance	20.1	28.0	33.7	37.2	39.3	40.7	41.5	42.2	43.1	43.9	44.9
Supplementary medical insurance (SMI)[c]	19.5	27.3	32.6	35.6	37.3	38.6	—	—	—	—	—
Part B	19.5	27.3	32.6	35.6	37.3	38.6	39.1	39.8	40.4	41.1	41.7
Part D[d]	—	—	—	—	—	—	1.2	1.8	27.0	30.8	32.1
Expenditures					Amount in billions						
Total Medicare	**$ 7.5**	**$ 36.8**	**$ 111.0**	**$184.2**	**$221.8**	**$280.8**	**$308.9**	**$336.4**	**$408.3**	**$431.7**	**$468.1**
Total hospital insurance (HI)	**5.3**	**25.6**	**67.0**	**117.6**	**131.1**	**154.6**	**170.6**	**182.9**	**191.9**	**203.1**	**235.6**
HI payments to managed care organizations[e]	—	0.0	2.7	6.7	21.4	19.5	20.8	24.9	32.9	39.0	50.6
HI payments for fee-for-service utilization	5.1	25.0	63.4	109.5	105.1	134.5	146.5	156.6	159.6	163.4	172.8
Inpatient hospital	4.8	24.1	56.9	82.3	87.1	109.1	117.0	123.2	124.1	124.2	130.5
Skilled nursing facility	0.2	0.4	2.5	9.1	11.1	14.8	17.2	19.4	20.3	22.5	24.2
Home health agency	0.1	0.5	3.7	16.2	4.0	4.9	5.4	6.0	5.9	6.2	6.6
Hospice	—	—	0.3	1.9	2.9	5.7	6.8	8.0	9.3	10.5	11.7
Home health agency transfer[f]	—	—	—	—	1.7	−2.2	—	—	—	—	—
Medicare Advantage premiums[g]	—	—	—	—	—	—	—	—	0.0	0.1	0.9
Accounting error (calendar year 2005–2008)[h]	—	—	—	—	—	—	—	−1.9	−3.9	−2.7	8.5
Administrative expenses[i]	0.2	0.5	0.9	1.4	2.9	2.8	3.3	3.3	3.3	3.2	3.6
Total supplementary medical insurance (SMI)[e]	**2.2**	**11.2**	**44.0**	**66.6**	**90.7**	**126.1**	**138.3**	**153.5**	**216.4**	**228.6**	**232.6**
Total Part B	**2.2**	**11.2**	**44.0**	**66.6**	**90.7**	**126.1**	**137.9**	**152.4**	**169.0**	**178.9**	**183.3**
Part B payments to managed care organizations[e]	0.0	0.2	2.8	6.6	18.4	17.3	18.7	22.0	31.5	38.9	47.6
Part B payments for fee-for-service utilization[j]	1.9	10.4	39.6	58.4	72.2	104.3	116.2	125.0	130.2	134.6	141.0
Physician/supplies[k]	1.8	8.2	29.6	—	—	—	—	—	—	—	—
Outpatient hospital[l]	0.1	1.9	8.5	—	—	—	—	—	—	—	—
Independent laboratory[m]	0.0	0.1	1.5	—	—	—	—	—	—	—	—
Physician fee schedule	—	—	—	31.7	37.0	48.3	54.1	57.7	58.2	58.9	60.8
Durable medical equipment	—	—	—	3.7	4.7	7.5	7.7	8.0	8.3	8.1	8.9
Laboratory[n]	—	—	—	4.3	4.0	5.5	6.1	6.3	6.7	7.1	7.3
Other[o]	—	—	—	9.9	13.6	22.6	25.0	26.7	28.0	28.9	30.2
Hospital[p]	—	—	—	8.7	8.4	15.3	17.4	19.2	21.3	22.4	23.8
Home health agency	0.0	0.2	0.1	0.2	4.5	5.1	5.9	7.1	7.8	9.2	10.0
Home health agency transfer[f]	—	—	—	—	−1.7	2.2	—	—	—	—	—
Medicare Advantage premiums	—	—	—	—	—	—	—	—	0.0	0.1	0.1
Accounting error (calendar year 2005–2008)[h]	—	—	—	—	—	—	—	1.9	3.9	2.7	−8.5
Administrative expenses[i]	0.2	0.6	1.5	1.6	1.8	2.4	2.8	2.6	2.9	2.5	3.0
Part D start-up costs[q]	—	—	—	—	—	—	0.2	0.7	0.2	0.0	0.0
Total Part D[d]	**—**	**—**	**—**	**—**	**—**	**—**	**0.4**	**1.1**	**47.4**	**49.7**	**49.3**
				Percent distribution of expenditures							
Total hospital insurance (HI)	**100.0**	**100.0**	**100.0**	**100.0**	**100.0**	**100.0**	**100.0**	**100.0**	**100.0**	**100.0**	**100.0**
HI payments to managed care organizations[e]	—	0.0	4.0	5.7	16.3	12.6	12.2	13.6	17.2	19.2	21.5
HI payments for fee-for-service utilization	97.0	97.9	94.6	93.1	80.2	87.0	85.9	85.6	83.2	80.5	73.4
Inpatient hospital	91.4	94.3	85.0	70.0	66.4	70.6	68.6	67.4	64.6	61.2	55.4
Skilled nursing facility	4.7	1.5	3.7	7.8	8.5	9.6	10.1	10.6	10.6	11.1	10.3
Home health agency	1.0	2.1	5.5	13.8	3.1	3.1	3.2	3.3	3.1	3.1	2.8
Hospice	—	—	0.5	1.6	2.2	3.7	4.0	4.4	4.9	5.2	5.0

priority. With hospice, they move to the background as the personal comes to the fore."

According to the National Hospice and Palliative Care Organization (NHPCO), in *NHPCO Facts and Figures: Hospice Care in America* (2009, http://www.nhpco.org/files/public/Statistics_Research/NHPCO_facts_and_figures.pdf), the use of hospice care is increasing in the United States. The NHPCO estimates that in 2008, 1.5 million patients received hospice care and 963,000 patients died in hospice programs. In 2008 Medicare and Medicaid expenditures for hospice care totaled $11.7 billion and accounted for 4.9% of Medicare expenditures. (See Table 3.7.)

MANAGED CARE ORGANIZATIONS

Managed health care is the sector of the health insurance industry in which health care providers are not independent businesses run by, for example, private medical practitioners but are instead administrative firms that manage the allocation of health care benefits. In contrast to conventional indemnity insurers that do not govern the provision of medical care services and simply pay for them, managed care firms have a significant voice in how services are administered to enable them to exert better control over health care costs. (Indemnity insurance is traditional fee-for-service coverage in which providers are paid according to the service performed.)

TABLE 3.7

Medicare enrollees and expenditures by type of service, selected years 1970–2008 [CONTINUED]

[Data are compiled from various sources by the Centers for Medicare and Medicaid Services]

Medicare program and type of service	1970	1980	1990	1995	2000	2003	2004	2005	2006	2007	2008[a]
Home health agency transfer[f]	—	—	—	—	1.3	−1.4	—	—	—	—	—
Medicare Advantage premiums[g]	—	—	—	—	—	—	—	—	0.0	0.0	0.4
Accounting error (calendar year 2005–2008)[h]	—	—	—	—	—	—	—	−1.0	−2.0	−1.3	3.6
Administrative expenses[i]	3.0	2.1	1.4	1.2	2.2	1.8	2.0	1.8	1.7	1.6	1.5

—Category not applicable or data not available.

0.0 = Quantity greater than 0 but less than 0.05.

[a]Preliminary estimates.

[b]Average number enrolled in the hospital insurance (HI) and/or supplementary medical insurance (SMI) programs for the period.

[c]Starting with 2004 data, the SMI trust fund consists of two separate accounts: Part B (which pays for a portion of the costs of physicians' services, outpatient hospital services, and other related medical and health services for voluntarily enrolled individuals) and Part D (Medicare Prescription Drug Account, which pays private plans to provide prescription drug coverage).

[d]The Medicare Modernization Act, enacted on December 8, 2003, established within SMI two Part D accounts related to prescription drug benefits: the Medicare Prescription Drug Account and the Transitional Assistance Account. The Medicare Prescription Drug Account is used in conjunction with the broad, voluntary prescription drug benefits that began in 2006. The Transitional Assistance Account was used to provide transitional assistance benefits, beginning in 2004 and extending through 2005, for certain low-income beneficiaries prior to the start of the new prescription drug benefit. The amounts shown for Total Part D expenditures—and thus for total SMI expenditures and total Medicare expenditures—for 2006 and later years include estimated amounts for premiums paid directly from Part D beneficiaries to Part D prescription drug plans.

[e]Medicare-approved managed care organizations.

[f]For 1998 to 2003 data, reflects annual home health HI to SMI transfer amounts.

[g]When a beneficiary chooses a Medicare Advantage plan whose monthly premium exceeds the benchmark amount, the additional premiums (that is, amounts beyond those paid by Medicare to the plan) are the responsibility of the beneficiary. Beneficiaries subject to such premiums may choose to either reimburse the plans directly or have the additional premiums deducted from their Social Security checks. The amounts shown here are only those additional premiums deducted from Social Security checks. These amounts are transferred to the HI trust and SMI trust funds and then transferred from the trust funds to the plans.

[h]Represents misallocation of benefit payments between the HI trust fund and the Part B account of the SMI trust fund from May 2005 to September 2007, and the transfer made in June 2008 to correct the misallocation.

[i]Includes expenditures for research, experiments and demonstration projects, peer review activity (performed by Peer Review Organizations from 1983 to 2001 and by Quality Review Organizations from 2002 to present), and to combat and prevent fraud and abuse.

[j]Type-of-service reporting categories for fee-for-service reimbursement differ before and after 1991.

[k]Includes payment for physicians, practitioners, durable medical equipment, and all suppliers other than independent laboratory through 1990. Starting with 1991 data, physician services subject to the physician fee schedule are shown. Payments for laboratory services paid under the laboratory fee schedule and performed in a physician office are included under Laboratory beginning in 1991. Payments for durable medical equipment are shown separately beginning in 1991. The remaining services from the Physician/supplies category are included in Other.

[l]Includes payments for hospital outpatient department services, skilled nursing facility outpatient services, Part B services received as an inpatient in a hospital or skilled nursing facility setting, and other types of outpatient facilities. Starting with 1991 data, payments for hospital outpatient department services, except for laboratory services, are listed under Hospital. Hospital outpatient laboratory services are included in the Laboratory line.

[m]Starting with 1991 data, those independent laboratory services that were paid under the laboratory fee schedule (most of the independent lab category) are included in the Laboratory line; the remaining services are included in the Physician fee schedule and Other lines.

[n]Payments for laboratory services paid under the laboratory fee schedule performed in a physician office, independent lab, or in a hospital outpatient department.

[o]Includes payments for physician-administered drugs; freestanding ambulatory surgical center facility services; ambulance services; supplies; freestanding end-stage renal disease (ESRD) dialysis facility services; rural health clinics; outpatient rehabilitation facilities; psychiatric hospitals; and federally qualified health centers.

[p]Includes the hospital facility costs for Medicare Part B services that are predominantly in the outpatient department, with the exception of hospital outpatient laboratory services, which are included on the Laboratory line. Physician reimbursement is included on the Physician fee schedule line.

[q]Part D start-up costs were funded through the SMI Part B account in 2004–2008.

Notes: All data shown are estimates and are subject to revision. Percents may not sum to totals because of rounding. Estimates for Medicare-covered services furnished to Medicare enrollees residing in the United States, Puerto Rico, Virgin Islands, Guam, other outlying areas, foreign countries, and unknown residence.

SOURCE: Adapted from "Table 142. Medicare Enrollees and Expenditures and Percent Distribution, by Medicare Program and Type of Service: United States and Other Areas, Selected Years 1970–2008," in *Health, United States, 2009: With Special Feature on Medical Technology*, U.S. Department of Health and Human Services, Centers for Disease Control and Prevention, National Center for Health Statistics, 2010, http://www.cdc.gov/nchs/data/hus/hus09.pdf#listtables (accessed May 12, 2010)

Managed care, which has a primary purpose of controlling service utilization and costs, represents a rapidly growing segment of the health care industry. The beneficiaries of employer-funded health plans (people who receive health benefits from their employers), as well as Medicare and Medicaid recipients, often find themselves in this type of health care program. The term *managed care organization* covers several types of health care delivery systems, such as health maintenance organizations (HMOs), preferred provider organizations (PPOs), and utilization review groups that oversee diagnoses, recommend treatments, and manage costs for their beneficiaries.

Health Maintenance Organizations

HMOs began to grow during the 1970s as alternatives to traditional health insurance, which was becoming increasingly expensive. The HMO Act of 1973 was a federal law requiring employers with more than 24 employees to offer an alternative to conventional indemnity insurance in the form of a federally qualified HMO. The intent of the act was to stimulate HMO development, and the federal government has been promoting HMOs since the administration of President Richard M. Nixon (1913–1994), maintaining that groups of physicians following certain rules of practice can slow rising medical costs and improve health care quality.

HMOs are health insurance programs organized to provide complete coverage for subscribers' (also known as enrollees or members) health needs for negotiated, prepaid prices. The subscribers (and/or their employers) pay a fixed amount each month; in turn, the HMO group provides, at no extra charge or at a minimal charge, preventive care, such as routine checkups, screening, and immunizations, and care for any illness or accident. The monthly fee also covers inpatient hospitalization and referral services. HMO members benefit from reduced out-of-pocket costs (they do not pay deductibles), they do not have to file claims or fill out insurance forms, and they generally pay only nominal co-payments for each office visit. Members are usually locked into the plan for a specified period—usually one year. If the necessary service is available within the HMO, patients must normally use an HMO doctor. There are several types of HMOs:

- Staff model—the "purest" form of managed care. All primary care physicians are employees of the HMO and practice in a centralized location such as an outpatient clinic that may also house a laboratory, pharmacy, and facilities for other diagnostic testing. The staff model offers the HMO the greatest opportunities to manage both cost and quality of health care services.

- Group model—in which the HMO contracts with a group of primary care and multispecialty health providers. The group is paid a fixed amount per patient to provide specific services. The administration of the medical group determines how the HMO payments will be distributed among the physicians and other health care providers. Group model HMOs are usually located in hospitals or in clinic settings and have on-site pharmacies. Participating physicians usually do not have any fee-for-service patients.

- Network model—in which the HMO contracts with two or more groups of health providers that agree to provide health care at negotiated prices to all members enrolled in the HMO.

- Independent practice association (IPA) model—in which the HMO contracts with individual physicians or medical groups that then provide medical care to HMO members at their own offices. The individual physicians agree to follow the practices and procedures of the HMO when caring for the HMO members; however, they generally also maintain their own private practices and see fee-for-service patients as well as HMO members. IPA physicians are paid by capitation (literally, per head) for the HMO patients and by conventional methods for their fee-for-service patients. Physician members of the IPA guarantee that the care for each HMO member for which they are responsible will be delivered within a fixed budget. They guarantee this by allowing the HMO to withhold an amount of their payments (usually about 20% per year). If at year's end the physician's cost for providing care falls within the preset amount, then the physician receives all the monies withheld. If the physician's costs of care exceed the agreed-on amount, the HMO may retain any portion of the

monies it has withheld. This arrangement places physicians and other providers such as hospitals, laboratories, and imaging centers at risk for keeping down treatment costs, and this at-risk formula is the key to HMO cost-containment efforts.

Some HMOs offer an open-ended or point-of-service (POS) option that allows members to choose their own physicians and hospitals, either within or outside the HMO. However, a member who chooses an outside provider will generally have to pay a larger portion of the expenses. Physicians not contracting with the HMO but who see HMO patients are paid according to the services performed. POS members are given an incentive to seek care from contracted network physicians and other health care providers through comprehensive coverage offerings.

The Kaiser Family Foundation indicates in "Health Insurance & Managed Care" (http://statehealthfacts.org/comparecat.jsp?cat=7&rgn=6&rgn=1) that as of July 2008, 64.5 million HMO members were served by 577 HMOs operating in the United States. In *Health, United States, 2007* (2007, http://www.cdc.gov/nchs/data/hus/hus07.pdf), the NCHS notes that HMO enrollment grew during the 1990s and reached about 30% of the U.S. population in 2000. However, the Kaiser Family Foundation states that by July 2008 HMO enrollment had declined to just 21.4% of the U.S population.

HMO enrollment varies by geographic region, with the highest levels of enrollment in the New England states and the far West. According to the Kaiser Family Foundation, 52.9% of the populations in the District of Columbia, 47.7% in Hawaii, 42.9% in California, and 34.3% in Massachusetts were enrolled in HMOs as of July 2008. In contrast, 0.2% of the populations in Alaska and 1.5% in Mississippi were covered by HMOs.

HMOs Have Fans and Critics

HMOs have been the subject of considerable debate among physicians, payers, policy makers, and health care consumers. Many physicians feel HMOs interfere in the physician-patient relationship and effectively prevent them from practicing medicine the way they have traditionally practiced. These physicians claim they know their patients' conditions and are, therefore, in the best position to recommend treatment. The physicians resent being advised and overruled by insurance administrators. (Physicians can recommend the treatment they believe is best, but if the insurance company will not cover the costs, patients may be unwilling to undergo the recommended treatment.)

The HMO industry counters that its evidence-based determinations (judgments about the appropriateness of care that reflect scientific research) are based on the experiences of many thousands of physicians and, therefore, it knows which treatment is most likely to be successful. The industry maintains that, in the past, physician-chosen treatments were not scrutinized or even assessed for effectiveness, and as a result most physicians did not really know whether the treatment they prescribed was optimal for the specific medical condition.

Furthermore, the HMO industry cites the slower increase in health care expenses as another indicator of its management success. Industry spokespeople note that any major change in how the industry is run would lead to increasing costs. They claim that HMOs and other managed care programs are bringing a more rational approach to the health care industry while maintaining health care quality and controlling costs.

Still, many physicians resent that, with a few exceptions, HMOs are not financially liable for their decisions. When a physician chooses to forgo a certain procedure and negative consequences result, the physician may be held legally accountable. When an HMO informs a physician that it will not cover a recommended procedure and the HMO's decision is found to be wrong, it cannot be held directly liable. Many physicians assert that because HMOs make such choices, they are practicing medicine and should, therefore, be held accountable. The HMOs counter that these are administrative decisions and deny that they are practicing medicine.

The legal climate, however, began to change for HMOs during the mid-1990s. Both the Third Circuit Federal Court of Appeals in *Dukes v. U.S. Healthcare* (57 F.3d 350 [1995]) and the 10th Circuit Federal Court of Appeals in *PacifiCare of Oklahoma, Inc. v. Burrage* (59 F.3rd 151 [1995]) agreed that HMOs were liable for malpractice and negligence claims against the HMO and HMO physicians. In *Frappier Estate v. Wishnov* (678 So.2d 884 [1996]), the Florida District Court of Appeals, Fourth District, agreed with the earlier findings. It appeared that these court decisions would be backed by a new federal law when both houses of Congress passed legislation (the Patients' Bill of Rights) that would give patients more recourse to contest the decisions of HMOs, even though the U.S. House of Representatives and the U.S. Senate disagreed about the specific rights and actions patients could take to enforce their rights. By August 2002, however, the prospects for a patients' rights law passing by the end of that year dimmed as the House and Senate failed to resolve their differences about the legislation. The central issue that stalled the negotiations about the bill was the question of how much recourse patients should have in court when they believe their HMO has not provided adequate care.

In June 2004 the U.S. Supreme Court struck down a law in California and in several other states that allowed patients to sue their health plans for denying them health care services. Even though patients can still sue in federal court for reimbursement of denied benefits, they are no longer able to sue for damages in federal or state courts.

California Is the First State to Limit HMO Wait Times

In response to complaints from California HMO members about delays in obtaining appointments with HMO physicians, state regulators established guidelines in January 2010 to reduce wait times. Duke Helfand reports in "California Limits HMO Wait Times" (*Los Angeles Times*, January 19, 2010) that HMOs were given until January 2011 to implement the new guidelines, which require that people seeking care from a primary care physician be seen within 10 business days of requesting an appointment and within 15 days of requesting an appointment with a physician specialist.

PPOs

In response to HMOs and other efforts by insurance groups to cut costs, physicians began forming or joining PPOs during the 1990s. PPOs are managed care organizations that offer integrated delivery systems (networks of providers) available through a wide array of health plans and are readily accountable to purchasers for access, cost, quality, and services of their networks. They use provider selection standards, utilization management, and quality assessment programs to complement negotiated fee reductions (discounted rates from participating physicians, hospitals, and other health care providers) as effective strategies for long-term cost control. Under a PPO benefit plan, covered people retain the freedom of choice of providers but are offered financial incentives such as lower out-of-pocket costs to use the preferred provider network. PPO members may use other physicians and hospitals, but they usually have to pay a higher proportion of the costs. PPOs are marketed directly to employers and to third-party administrators who then market PPOs to their employer clients.

Exclusive provider organizations (EPOs) are a more restrictive variation of PPOs in which members must seek care from providers on the EPO panel. If a member visits an outside provider who is not on the EPO panel, then the EPO will offer either limited or no coverage for the office or hospital visit.

According to the Kaiser Family Foundation, in "Employer Health Benefits 2009 Annual Survey" (September 15, 2009, http://ehbs.kff.org/?page=charts &id=2&sn=20&p=1), 60% of U.S. workers were enrolled in PPO plans in 2009. By contrast, only 20% of U.S. workers were enrolled in HMO plans and 10% in POS plans.

Health Care Reform Will Affect Managed Care Plans

Brian Boyle, David Deaton, and Michael Maddigan of O'Melveny & Myers LLP note in "United States: The

Health Care Reform Legislation and Its Impact on the Health Care and Life Sciences Industries" (March 30, 2010, http://www.mondaq.com/unitedstates/article.asp?articleid=97086) that the Patient Protection and Affordable Care Act will have a significant impact on the benefits provided by managed care plans and other insurers. In the short term, the legislation requires insurers to change certain underwriting practices and benefit structures. The act requires the plans to cover children with preexisting conditions, forbids them from canceling coverage when enrollees require costly treatment, prohibits caps on lifetime benefits, and permits children to remain on their parents' insurance until they turn 27 years old.

Boyle, Deaton, and Maddigan explain that other changes will occur in 2014. When the requirement that most Americans will have to obtain health coverage or face penalties takes effect, managed care plans and other insurers will doubtless experience increased enrollment. Because the act limits the extent to which premiums can vary in response to enrollee characteristics, such as age, tobacco use, and whether coverage is for an individual or family, the plans may experience reduced revenue from premiums. Presumably, this reduced revenue would be offset by larger numbers of enrollees.

According to Boyle, Deaton, and Maddigan, plans that offer coverage to Medicaid and Medicare beneficiaries will also experience changes in enrollment. Because the act extends Medicaid eligibility to more low-income people, Medicaid managed care plans will experience increased enrollment. By contrast, the act reduces reimbursement to Medicare managed care plans, and these will lose enrollees should they reduce benefits in response to the reduced reimbursement.

In the article "Experts Talk Health-Care Reform Bill Impact" (*BusinessWeek*, March 22, 2010), Phillip Seligman of Standard & Poor's Equity Research opines that the health care reform legislation will ultimately have a favorable effect on managed care organizations. Seligman believes that while managed care plans "will face fees, which are delayed until 2014, and will have restrictions such as the ban on rescissions, no lifetime caps, and inability to bar coverage based on health status, which can pressure margins," these potential losses will "be offset by enrollment gains, providing economies of scale, leverage over general and administrative costs, and greater negotiating clout with providers. We also see potential opportunities for consolidation."

CHAPTER 4
RESEARCHING, MEASURING, AND MONITORING
THE QUALITY OF HEALTH CARE

There are hundreds of agencies, institutions, and organizations dedicated to researching, quantifying (measuring), monitoring, and improving health in the United States. Some are federally funded public entities such as the many institutes and agencies governed by the U.S. Department of Health and Human Services (HHS). Others are professional societies and organizations that develop standards of care, represent the views and interests of health care providers, and ensure the quality of health care facilities such as the American Medical Association and the Joint Commission on Accreditation of Healthcare Organizations. Still other voluntary health organizations, such as the American Heart Association, the American Cancer Society, and the March of Dimes, promote research and education about prevention and treatment of specific diseases.

U.S. DEPARTMENT OF HEALTH
AND HUMAN SERVICES

The HHS is the nation's lead agency for ensuring the health of Americans by planning, operating, and funding delivery of essential human services, especially for society's most vulnerable populations. According to the HHS, in "HHS: What We Do" (2010, http://www.hhs.gov/about/whatwedo.html/), it consists of more than 300 programs that are operated by 11 divisions, including eight agencies in the U.S. Public Health Service and three human services agencies. It is the largest grant-making agency in the federal government, funding several thousand grants each year as well as the HHS Medicare program, the nation's largest health insurer, which processes over 1 billion claims per year. For fiscal year (FY) 2011, the HHS had a budget of $910.7 billion, which was an increase of $50.9 billion from FY 2010. (See Table 4.1.)

HHS Milestones

The HHS notes in "Historical Highlights" (2010, http://www.hhs.gov/about/hhshist.html) that it began with the 1798 opening of the first Marine Hospital in Boston, Massachusetts, to care for sick and injured merchant seamen. Under President Abraham Lincoln (1809–1865) the agency that would become the U.S. Food and Drug Administration was established in 1862. The National Institutes of Health (NIH) dates back to 1887 and later became part of the Public Health Service. The 1935 enactment of the Social Security Act spurred the development of the Federal Security Agency in 1939 to direct programs in health, human services, insurance, and education. In 1946 the Communicable Disease Center, which would become the Centers for Disease Control and Prevention (CDC), was established, and 19 years later, in 1965, Medicare (a federal health insurance program for older adults and people with disabilities) and Medicaid (state and federal health insurance for low-income people) were enacted to improve access to health care for older, disabled, and low-income Americans. That same year the Head Start program was developed to provide education, health, and social services to preschool-aged children.

In 1970 the National Health Service Corps was established to help meet the health care needs of underserved areas and populations. The following year the National Cancer Act became law, which established cancer research as a national research priority. In 1984 the human immunodeficiency virus (HIV), the virus that causes the acquired immunodeficiency syndrome (AIDS), was identified by the Public Health Service and French research scientists. The National Organ Transplant Act became law in 1984, and in 1990 the Human Genome Project was initiated.

In 1994 NIH-funded research isolated the genes responsible for inherited breast cancer, colon cancer, and the most frequently occurring type of kidney cancer. In 1998 efforts were launched to eliminate racial and ethnic disparities (differences) in health, and in 2000 the human genome sequencing was published. In 2001

TABLE 4.1

U.S. Department of Health and Human Services budget, fiscal years 2009–11

[Dollars in millions]

	2009	2010	2011	2011 +/− 2010
Budget authority (excluding Recovery Act)	779,419	800,271	880,861	+80,591
Recovery Act budget authority	55,087	45,162	21,066	−24,096
Total budget authority	**834,506**	**845,432**	**901,927**	**+56,495**
Total outlays	**794,234**	**859,763**	**910,679**	**+50,916**
Full-time equivalents	67,875	70,028	72,923	+2,895

SOURCE: "FY 2011 President's Budget for HHS," in *U.S. Department of Health and Human Services Budget in Brief, Fiscal Year 2011*, U.S. Department of Health and Human Services, 2010, http://dhhs.gov/asfr/ob/docbudget/2011budgetinbrief.pdf (accessed May 18, 2010)

FIGURE 4.1

Cycle of health care research

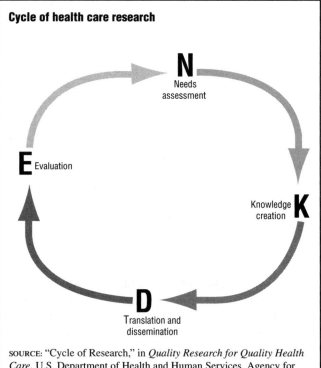

SOURCE: "Cycle of Research," in *Quality Research for Quality Health Care*, U.S. Department of Health and Human Services, Agency for Healthcare Research and Quality, March 2001, http://www.ahcpr.gov/about/qualres.pdf (accessed May 18, 2010)

the Health Care Financing Administration was replaced by the Centers for Medicaid and Medicare Services, and the HHS responded to the first reported cases of bioterrorism (the 2001 anthrax attacks) and developed new strategies to detect and prevent threats of bioterrorism.

According to the HHS, in *U.S. Department of Health and Human Services Budget in Brief, Fiscal Year 2011* (2010, http://dhhs.gov/asfr/ob/docbudget/2011budgetinbrief.pdf), significant initiatives funded in the FY 2011 budget include addressing the shortage of health care providers in underserved areas; enhancing health information technology, including the adoption of electronic medical records; improving public health through science to protect food supplies; and continuing to address the health and human service needs of low-income families, children, and other vulnerable populations.

HHS Agencies and Institutes Provide Comprehensive Health and Social Services

Besides the CDC and the NIH, the HHS explains in *U.S. Department of Health and Human Services Budget in Brief, Fiscal Year 2011* that the following agencies research, plan, direct, oversee, administer, and provide health care services:

- The Administration on Aging (AoA) provides services aimed at helping older Americans retain their independence. The AoA develops policies that support older adults and directs programs that provide transportation, in-home services, and other health and social services. For FY 2011 the AoA planned for a budget of $1.6 billion and 112 employees.

- The Administration for Children and Families (ACF) provides services for families and children in need, administers Head Start, and works with state foster care and adoption programs. The ACF was allotted a budget of $58.8 billion and 1,471 employees for FY 2011.

- The Agency for Healthcare Research and Quality (AHRQ) researches access to health care, quality of care, and efforts to control health care costs. It also looks at the safety of health care services and the ways to prevent medical errors. Figure 4.1 shows how the AHRQ researches health system problems by performing a continuous process of needs assessment, gaining knowledge, interpreting and communicating information, and evaluating the effects of this process on the health problem. Figure 4.2 shows the process that transforms new information about health care issues into actions to improve access, costs, outcomes (how patients fare as a result of the care they receive), and quality. For FY 2011 the AHRQ planned for a budget of $611 million and 315 employees. The AHRQ budgeted $65 million for patient safety research and activities and $34 million to reduce and prevent health care–associated infections.

- The Agency for Toxic Substances and Disease Registry (ATSDR) seeks to prevent exposure to hazardous waste. The agency's FY 2011 budget of $76 million represented a decrease of $500,000 from FY 2010.

- The Centers for Medicare and Medicaid Services (CMS) administers programs that provide health insurance for about 92 million Americans who are either aged 65 years and older or in financial need. It also operates the Children's Health Insurance Program, which covers about 10 million uninsured children, and regulates all

FIGURE 4.2

Health care research pipeline

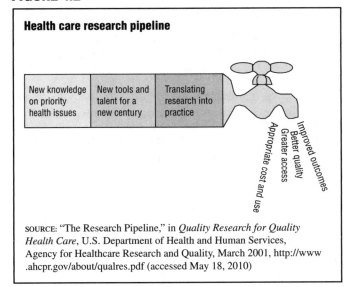

SOURCE: "The Research Pipeline," in *Quality Research for Quality Health Care*, U.S. Department of Health and Human Services, Agency for Healthcare Research and Quality, March 2001, http://www.ahcpr.gov/about/qualres.pdf (accessed May 18, 2010)

FIGURE 4.3

Budgeted net outlays, Centers for Medicare and Medicaid Services (CMS), fiscal year 2011

$784.3 billion

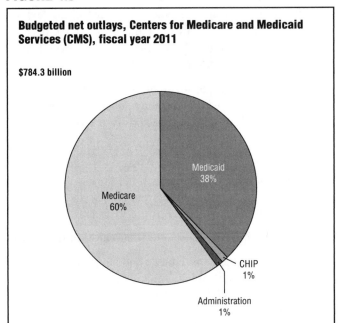

Note: State grants and demos accounts for 0.14 percent of net outlays.
CHIP = Children's Health Insurance Program

SOURCE: "CMS FY 2011 Net Outlays, Proposed Law $784.3 Billion," in *U.S. Department of Health and Human Services Budget in Brief, Fiscal Year 2011*, U.S. Department of Health and Human Services, 2010, http://dhhs.gov/asfr/ob/docbudget/2011budgetinbrief.pdf (accessed May 18, 2010)

laboratory testing, except testing performed for research purposes, in the United States. For FY 2011 the CMS planned for a $784.3 billion budget. Figure 4.3 shows the allocation of the CMS budget—more than half (60%) was devoted to Medicare, just over one-third (38%) to Medicaid, and 1% each to the Children's Health Insurance Plan and administration.

- The U.S. Food and Drug Administration (FDA) acts to ensure the safety and efficacy (the ability of an intervention to produce the intended diagnostic or therapeutic effect in optimal circumstances) of dietary supplements, pharmaceutical drugs, and medical devices and monitors food safety and purity. The FDA planned for a budget of $4 billion in FY 2011 and 13,677 employees. The FDA budget included an increase of $748 million over the 2010 budget of $3.3 billion to ensure the safety and security of the food supply and to provide other biodefense activities.

- The Health Resources and Services Administration (HRSA) provides services for medically underserved populations such as migrant workers, the homeless, and public housing residents. The HRSA oversees the nation's organ transplant program, directs efforts to improve maternal and child health, and delivers services to people with AIDS through the Ryan White CARE Act. In FY 2011 it planned to have 1,518 employees and a budget of $7.6 billion.

- The Indian Health Service (IHS) serves nearly 560 tribes through a network of 45 hospitals, 313 health stations, and 288 health centers. In FY 2011 the IHS planned to employ 15,649 workers and have a budget of $5.4 billion.

- The General Departmental Management provides the HHS's leadership and oversees the 11 operating divisions of the HHS. It also advises the president about

health, welfare, human service, and income security issues. In FY 2011 it was allotted 1,417 employees and a budget of $668 million.

- The Program Support Center (PSC) administers operations, financial management, and human resources for the HHS as well as for 31 other federal agencies. The PSC staff of 1,312 processes grant payments, provides personnel and payroll services for HHS employees, and performs accounting, management, information technology, and telecommunication services.

- The Substance Abuse and Mental Health Services Administration (SAMHSA) seeks to improve access to, and availability of, substance abuse prevention and treatment programs as well as other mental health services. The SAMHSA was budgeted $3.7 billion in FY 2011 and had 553 employees.

The HHS agencies work with state, local, and tribal governments as well as with public and private organizations to coordinate and deliver a wide range of services including:

- Conducting preventive health services such as surveillance to detect outbreaks of disease and immunization programs through efforts directed by the CDC and the NIH

- Ensuring food, drug, and cosmetic safety through efforts of the FDA

- Improving maternal and child health and preschool education in programs such as Head Start, which served more than 1 million children in 2010, according to the National Head Start Association (2010, http://www.nhsa.org/about_nhsa)

- Preventing child abuse, domestic violence, and substance abuse, as well as funding substance abuse treatment through programs directed by the ACF

- Ensuring the delivery of health care services to more than 1.9 million Native Americans and Alaskan Natives through the IHS, a network of hospitals, health centers, and other programs and facilities (2010, http://info.ihs.gov/Profile2010.asp)

- Administering Medicare and Medicaid via the CMS

- Providing financial assistance and support services for low-income and older Americans, such as home-delivered meals (Meals on Wheels) coordinated by the AoA

SUBSTANTIAL BUDGET HELPS THE HHS TO ACHIEVE ITS OBJECTIVES. Table 4.2 displays how the FY 2011 HHS budget was allocated and provides comparisons between 2009, 2010, and 2011 outlays. The FY 2011 budget is a net increase of $50.9 billion over the FY 2010 budget and aims to provide funds to help improve access to and quality of health care, prevent disease, and support scientific research. It provides funds to advance the adoption of information technologies and electronic health records. The budget is also intended to strengthen emergency preparedness and improve public health by intensifying prevention programs to reduce the occurrence of diabetes, asthma, and obesity.

The FY 2011 budget also addresses health reform. The HHS states in *U.S. Department of Health and Human Services Budget in Brief, Fiscal Year 2011* that "the Administration is committed to reforming the health care system to assure affordable, quality, health coverage for all Americans." It recounts the progress that has been made toward health insurance reform, such as:

- Reducing the cost of COBRA by 65% between February 2009 and May 2010 so laid-off workers and their families could continue their health benefits. (The U.S. Department of Labor explains in "Continuation of Health Coverage—COBRA" [2010, http://www.dol.gov/dol/topic/health-plans/cobra.htm] that "the Consolidated Omnibus Budget Reconciliation Act (COBRA) gives workers and their families who lose their health benefits the right to choose to continue group health benefits provided by their group health plan for limited periods of time under certain circumstances such as voluntary or involuntary job loss, reduction in the hours worked, transition between jobs, death, divorce, and other life events.")

- Allocating $2 billion to upgrade health centers and expand their service capabilities.

- Ameliorating the shortage of health care workers by investing $500 million to the National Health Service Corp.

- Improving health care quality and efficiency by investing in the adoption of electronic health records.

U.S. PUBLIC HEALTH SERVICE COMMISSIONED CORPS. The U.S. Public Health Service Commissioned Corps (October 28, 2008, http://www.usphs.gov/aboutus/history.aspx) was originally the uniformed service component of the early Marine Hospital Service, which adopted a military model for a group of career health professionals who traveled from one marine hospital to another as their services were needed. It also assisted the Marine Hospital Service to prevent infectious diseases from entering the country by examining newly arrived immigrants and directing state quarantine (the period and place where people suspected of having contagious diseases are detained and isolated) functions. A law enacted in 1889 established this group as the Commissioned Corps, and in 1912 the Marine Hospital Service was renamed the Public Health Service (PHS) to reflect its broader scope of activities.

Throughout the 20th century the corps grew to include a wide range of health professionals. Besides physicians, the corps employed nurses, dentists, research scientists, planners, pharmacists, sanitarians, engineers, and other public health professionals. These PHS-commissioned officers played important roles in disease prevention and detection, acted to ensure food and drug safety, conducted research, provided medical care to underserved groups such as Native Americans and Alaskan Natives, and assisted in disaster relief programs. As one of the seven uniformed services in the United States (the other six are the U.S. Navy, U.S. Army, U.S. Marine Corps, U.S. Air Force, U.S. Coast Guard, and the National Oceanic and Atmospheric Administration Commissioned Corps), the PHS Commissioned Corps continues to perform all these functions and identifies environmental threats to health and safety, promotes healthy lifestyles for Americans, and is involved with international agencies to help address global health problems.

The Office of the Surgeon General notes in "About the Office of the Surgeon General" (http://www.surgeongeneral.gov/about/index.html) that as of 2010 the PHS Commissioned Corps numbered approximately 6,500 health professionals. These people report to the U.S. surgeon general, who holds the rank of vice admiral in the PHS. Corps officers work in PHS agencies and at other agencies including the U.S. Bureau of Prisons, the U.S. Coast Guard, the U.S. Environmental Protection Agency, and

TABLE 4.2

Health and Human Services budget, by operating division, 2009–11

[Mandatory and discretionary dollars in millions]

	2009	2010	2011	2011+/− 2010
Food and Drug Administration:				
Program level	2,751	3,287	4,033	746
Budget authority	2,062	2,365	2,510	145
Outlays	1,843	2,349	2,429	80
Health Resources and Services Administration:				
Budget authority (excl. Recovery Act)[c]	7,328	7,587	7,635	48
Recovery Act budget authority[a]	2,500	—	—	—
Outlays	7,267	8,488	8,532	44
Indian Health Service:				
Budget authority (excl. Recovery Act)	3,731	4,202	4,556	354
Recovery Act budget authority[a]	500	—	—	—
Outlays	3,644	4,505	4,612	107
Centers for Disease Control and Prevention:				
Budget authority (excl. Recovery Act)[e]	6,370	6,477	6,342	−135
Recovery Act budget authority[a]	300	—	—	—
Outlays	6,247	6,581	6,491	−90
National Institutes of Health:				
Budget authority (excl. Recovery Act)	30,096	31,255	32,255	1,000
Recovery Act budget authority[a]	10,400	—	—	—
Outlays	29,847	31,807	37,189	5,382
Substance Abuse and Mental Health Services:				
Budget authority	3,335	3,432	3,541	110
Outlays	3,369	3,349	3,457	108
Agency for Healthcare Research and Quality:				
Program level[f]	372	397	611	214
Budget authority (excl. Recovery Act)	3	—	—	—
Recovery Act budget authority[b]	700	—	—	—
Outlays	−80	141	317	176
Centers for Medicare and Medicaid Services:				
Budget authority (excl. Recovery Act)[e]	657,147	696,077	763,290	67,213
Recovery Act budget authority[a, g]	31,887	39,865	20,138	−19,727
Outlays	686,791	733,457	781,713	48,256
Administration for Children and Families:				
Budget authority (excl. Recovery Act)	56,564	46,337	57,897	11,560
Recovery Act budget authority	5,933	5,284	913	−4,371
Outlays	52,211	61,281	58,472	−2,809
Administration on Aging:				
Budget authority (excl. Recovery Act)	1,488	1,513	1,625	112
Recovery Act budget authority[a]	100	—	—	—
Outlays	1,453	1,596	1,583	−13
Office of the National Coordinator:				
Budget authority (excl. Recovery Act)	44	42	78	36
Recovery Act budget authority[d]	2,000	—	—	—
Outlays	21	639	851	212
Medicare Hearings and Appeals:				
Budget authority	65	71	78	7
Outlays	67	71	78	7
Office for Civil Rights				
Budget authority	40	43	45	2
Outlays	32	38	42	4
Departmental Management:				
Budget authority (excl. Recovery Act)[e]	384	490	594	104
Recovery Act budget authority[a]	—	—	—	—
Outlays	355	443	543	100
Prevention and Wellness				
Recovery Act budget authority[a]	700			
Outlays		158	314	156
Public Health Social Service Emergency Fund:				
Budget authority (excl. Recovery Act)	10,611	738	735	−3
Recovery Act budget authority[a]	50	—	—	—
Outlays	1,868	5,179	4,325	−854
Office of Inspector General:				
Budget authority (excl. Recovery Act)	126	62	37	−26
Recovery Act budget authority[a]	17	13	16	3
Outlays	56	99	90	−9

the Commission on Mental Health of the District of Columbia. The surgeon general is a physician who is appointed by the U.S. president to serve in a medical leadership position for a four-year term of office. The surgeon general reports to the assistant secretary of health, and the Office of the Surgeon General (2010, http://www.surgeongeneral.gov/aboutoffice.html) is part of the Office of Public Health and Science. Eighteen

TABLE 4.2

Health and Human Services budget, by operating division, 2009–11 [CONTINUED]

[Mandatory and discretionary dollars in millions]

	2009	2010	2011	2011+/−2010
Program Support Center (Retirement pay, medical benefits, misc. trust funds):				
Budget authority	553	594	637	43
Outlays	466	590	633	43
Offsetting collections:				
Budget authority	−1,223	−1,008	−992	16
Outlays	−1,223	−1,008	−992	16
Budget authority (excl. Recovery Act)	**779,419**	**800,271**	**880,861**	**+80,591**
Total Recovery Act budget authority	**55,087**	**45,162**	**21,066**	**−24,096**
Total budget authority	**834,506**	**845,432**	**901,927**	**+56,495**
Outlays	**794,234**	**859,763**	**910,679**	**+50,916**
Full-time equivalents	67,875	70,028	72,923	+2,895

[a]Fiscal year 2009 Recovery Act appropriations were provided to fund programmatic costs in multiple fiscal years.
[b]The Recovery Act appropriated $1.1 billion for research that compares the effectiveness of medical options and transferred $400 million of this amount to the National Institute of Health (NIH). Of the remaining $700 million, $400 million is for allocation at the discretion of the Secretary.
[c]Does not include Congressional justification standards (C/J/S) vaccines.
[d]Total includes $20 million transfer to the National Institute of Standards and Technology (NIST).
[e]Levels are comparably adjusted to show transfer of Office of Global Health Affairs (OGHA) activities to Center of Disease Control and Prevention (CDC).
[f]The Agency for Healthcare Research and Quality (AHRQ) program level includes $3 million in mandatory budget authority from the Medicare Improvements for Patients and Providers Act of 2008 (MPIPPA).
[g]Budget authority for Centers of Medicaid and Medicare (CMS) defined as program outlays.

SOURCE: "HHS Budget by Operating Division," in *U.S. Department of Health and Human Services Budget in Brief, Fiscal Year 2011*, U.S. Department of Health and Human Services, 2010, http://dhhs.gov/asfr/ob/docbudget/2011budgetinbrief.pdf (accessed May 18, 2010)

surgeons general have served since the 1870s. In January 2010 Vice Admiral Regina M. Benjamin (1956–; http://www.usphs.gov/aboutus/VADMBenjamin_bio.aspx) began her term as the surgeon general.

CENTERS FOR DISEASE CONTROL AND PREVENTION

The CDC is the primary HHS agency responsible for ensuring the health and safety of the nation's citizens in the United States and abroad. The CDC's responsibilities include researching and monitoring health, detecting and investigating health problems, researching and instituting prevention programs, developing health policies, ensuring environmental health and safety, and offering education and training.

The CDC (February 25, 2010, http://www.cdc.gov/about/resources/facts.htm) states that it employs over 15,000 people in 168 disciplines and in 50 countries. Besides research scientists, physicians, nurses, and other health practitioners, the CDC employs epidemiologists, who study disease in populations as opposed to individuals. Epidemiologists measure disease occurrences, such as incidence and prevalence of disease, and work with clinical researchers to answer questions about causation (how particular diseases arise and the factors that contribute to their development), whether new treatments are effective, and how to prevent specific diseases.

The CDC states in "CDC Organization" (June 14, 2010, http://www.cdc.gov/about/organization/cio.htm) that

it is home to 17 national centers and various institutes and offices. Among the best known are the National Center for Health Statistics, which collects vital statistics, and the National Institute for Occupational Safety and Health, which seeks to prevent workplace injuries and accidents through research and prevention. Thomas R. Frieden (1960–) was named the director of the CDC in June 2009. Figure 4.4 shows the organization and leadership of the CDC in 2010.

CDC Actions to Protect the Health of the Nation

The CDC is part of the first response to natural disasters, outbreaks of disease, and other public health emergencies. For example, in May 2005 the agency joined the newly formed National Influenza Pandemic Preparedness Task Force, an interagency task force that was organized by the U.S. secretary of health and human services. The CDC's role in the task force is to monitor outbreaks and plan responses to the emerging threat of seasonal influenza and other influenza viruses. In 2009 the CDC tracked and reported the H1N1 flu outbreak. Table 4.3 shows the estimates of cases, hospitalizations, and deaths attributable to the H1N1 influenza from April 2009 to March 2010. Other examples of CDC initiatives are identification and education about effective strategies for preventing school and domestic violence as well as programs to promote a healthy diet and increase physical activity to prevent overweight and obesity.

FIGURE 4.4

Centers for Disease Control and Prevention organization and leadership, 2010

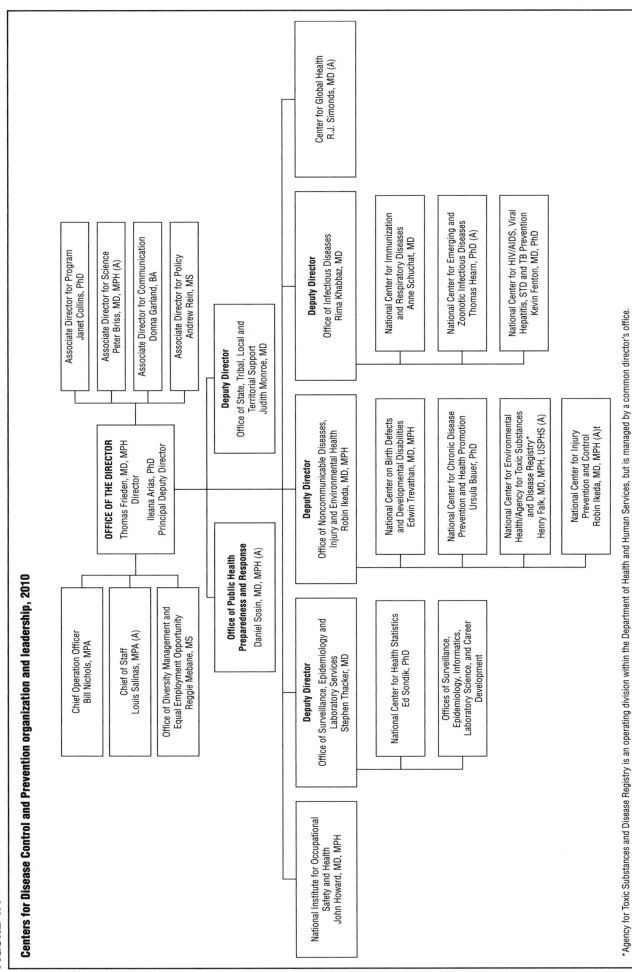

*Agency for Toxic Substances and Disease Registry is an operating division within the Department of Health and Human Services, but is managed by a common director's office.

SOURCE: "Department of Health and Human Services Centers for Disease Control and Prevention (CDC)," in *CDC Organization*, Centers for Disease Control and Prevention, 2010, http://www.cdc.gov/maso/pdf/CDC_Chart_wNames.pdf (accessed May 19, 2010)

TABLE 4.3

Centers for Disease Control and Prevention (CDC) estimates of H1N1 cases, hospitalizations and deaths by age group, April 2009 through March 2010

2009 H1N1	Mid-level range*	Estimated range*
Cases		
0–17 years	~19 million	~14 million to ~28 million
18–64 years	~35 million	~25 million to ~51 million
65 years and older	~6 million	~4 million to ~9 million
Cases total	~60 million	~43 million to ~88 million
Hospitalizations		
0–17 years	~86,000	~61,000 to ~127,000
18–64 years	~158,000	~112,000 to ~232,000
65 years and older	~26,000	~19,000 to ~39,000
Hospitalization total	~270,000	~192,000 to ~398,000
Deaths		
0–17 years	~1,270	~900 to ~1,870
18–64 years	~9,420	~6,700 to ~13,860
65 years and older	~1,580	~1,120 to ~2,320
Deaths total	~12,270	~8,720 to ~18,050

Note: Deaths have been rounded to the nearest ten. Hospitalizations have been rounded to the nearest thousand and cases have been rounded to the nearest million.

SOURCE: "CDC Estimates of 2009 H1N1 Cases and Related Hospitalizations and Deaths from April 2009 through March 13, 2010, by Age Group," in *2009 H1N1 Flu*, Centers for Disease Control and Prevention, 2010, http://www.cdc.gov/h1n1flu/pdf/graph_March%202010.pdf (accessed May 19, 2010)

Among the many recent CDC initiatives to combat the obesity epidemic is the surgeon general report *The Surgeon General's Vision for a Healthy and Fit Nation, 2010* (January 2010, http://www.surgeongeneral.gov/library/obesityvision/obesityvision2010.pdf), which includes strategies to help individuals make healthy choices and to create healthy home environments, child care settings, schools, and work sites. The surgeon general also exhorts physicians and other health care providers to teach patients about the relationship between obesity and disease risk and to refer overweight and obese patients to "resources ... that will help them meet their psychological, nutritional, and physical activity needs."

The CDC LEAN Works identifies and promotes worksite interventions to combat obesity as well as interventions that target school-age children and women. The CDC also educates and communicates vital health information via its publications *Morbidity and Mortality Weekly Report* and *Emerging Infectious Disease Journal*, which alert the medical community to the presence of health risks, outbreaks, and preventive measures. Besides providing vital statistics (births, deaths, and related health data), the CDC monitors Americans' health using surveys to measure the frequency of behaviors that increase health risk (such as smoking, substance abuse, and physical inactivity) and compiles data about the use of health care resources (such as inpatient hospitalization rates and visits to hospital emergency departments).

The CDC partners with national, state, local, public, and private agencies and organizations to deliver services. Examples of these collaborative efforts include the global battle against HIV/AIDS by way of the Leadership and Investment in Fighting an Epidemic initiative and the CDC Coordinating Center for Health Information and Service, which was created to improve public health through increased efficiencies and to foster stronger collaboration between the CDC and international health foundations, health care practitioners, community and philanthropic organizations, schools and universities, nonprofit and voluntary organizations, and state and local public health departments.

NATIONAL INSTITUTES OF HEALTH

The NIH (May 18, 2010, http://www.nih.gov/about/history.htm) began as a one-room laboratory in 1887 and eventually became the world's premier medical research center. The NIH conducts research in its own facilities and supports research in universities, medical schools, and hospitals throughout and outside the United States. The NIH trains research scientists and other investigators and serves to communicate medical and health information to professional and consumer audiences.

The NIH (May 18, 2010, http://www.nih.gov/about/organization.htm) consists of 27 centers and institutes and is housed in more than 75 buildings on a 300-acre (121-ha) campus in Bethesda, Maryland. Among the better-known centers and institutes are the National Cancer Institute, the National Human Genome Research Institute, the National Institute of Mental Health, and the National Center for Complementary and Alternative Medicine.

In "Facts at a Glance" (March 24, 2010, http://clinicalcenter.nih.gov/about/welcome/fact.shtml), the NIH explains that patients arrive at the NIH Warren Grant Magnuson Clinical Center in Bethesda to participate in clinical research trials. About 6,000 patients per year are treated as inpatients, and an additional 95,000 receive outpatient treatment. The National Library of Medicine—which produces the *Index Medicus*, a monthly listing of articles from the world's top medical journals, and maintains *MEDLINE*, a comprehensive medical bibliographic database—is in the NIH Lister Hill Center.

According to the NIH, in "The NIH Almanac—Historical Data" (September 1, 2009, http://www.nih.gov/about/almanac/historical/chronology_of_events.htm), the American Recovery and Reinvestment Act (ARRA), which was signed by President Barack Obama (1961–) in February 2009, gave the NIH a one-time 34% budget increase of $10.4 billion. This increase was intended to stimulate scientific research and create jobs. Also, funds totaling close to $430 million from ARRA provided funding for four major renovation projects at the NIH.

FIGURE 4.5

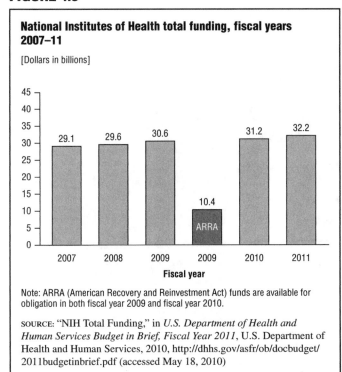

National Institutes of Health total funding, fiscal years 2007–11

[Dollars in billions]

Note: ARRA (American Recovery and Reinvestment Act) funds are available for obligation in both fiscal year 2009 and fiscal year 2010.

SOURCE: "NIH Total Funding," in *U.S. Department of Health and Human Services Budget in Brief, Fiscal Year 2011*, U.S. Department of Health and Human Services, 2010, http://dhhs.gov/asfr/ob/docbudget/2011budgetinbrief.pdf (accessed May 18, 2010)

FIGURE 4.6

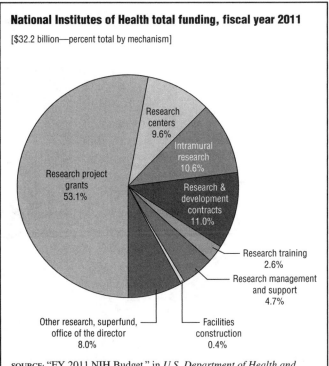

National Institutes of Health total funding, fiscal year 2011

[$32.2 billion—percent total by mechanism]

SOURCE: "FY 2011 NIH Budget," in *U.S. Department of Health and Human Services Budget in Brief, Fiscal Year 2011*, U.S. Department of Health and Human Services, 2010, http://dhhs.gov/asfr/ob/docbudget/2011budgetinbrief.pdf (accessed May 18, 2010)

The NIH budget for FY 2011 was $32.2 billion. Figure 4.5 shows how NIH funding increased by $3.1 billion between FYs 2007 and 2011. The NIH (2010, http://science.education.nih.gov/supplements/nih1/Genetic/about/about-nih.htm) works to achieve its ambitious research objectives "to acquire new knowledge to help prevent, detect, diagnose, and treat disease and disability, from the rarest genetic disorder to the common cold" by investing in promising biomedical research. The NIH makes grants and contracts to support research and training in every state in the country, at more than 2,000 institutions. The NIH allocated more than half (53.1%) of its FY 2011 budget to research project grants, 11% to research and development contracts, 10.6% to intramural research, and 9.6% to research centers. (See Figure 4.6.)

Establishing Research Priorities

By law, all 27 institutes of the NIH must be funded, and each institute must allocate its funding to specific areas and aspects of research within its domain. About half of each institute's budget is dedicated to supporting the best research proposals presented, in terms of their potential to contribute to advances that will combat the diseases the institute is charged with researching. Some of the other criteria used to determine research priorities include:

- Public health need—the NIH responds to health problems and diseases based on their incidence (the rate of

development of a disease in a group during a given period) and severity and on the costs associated with them. Examples of other measures used to weigh and assess need are the mortality rate (the number of deaths caused by disease), the morbidity rate (the degree of disability caused by disease), the economic and social consequences of the disease, and whether rapid action is required to control the spread of the disease.

- Rigorous peer review—proposals are scrutinized by accomplished researchers to determine their potential return on the investment of resources.

- Flexibility and expansiveness—the NIH experience demonstrates that important findings for commonly occurring diseases may come from research on rarer ones. The NIH attempts to fund the broadest possible array of research opportunities to stimulate creative solutions to pressing problems.

- Commitment to human resources and technology—the NIH invests in people and equipment in the pursuit of scientific advancement.

Because not even the most gifted scientists can accurately predict the next critical discovery or stride in biomedical research, the NIH must analyze each research opportunity in terms of competition for the same resources,

FIGURE 4.7

Views taken into consideration when setting research priorities at the National Institutes of Health, 2006

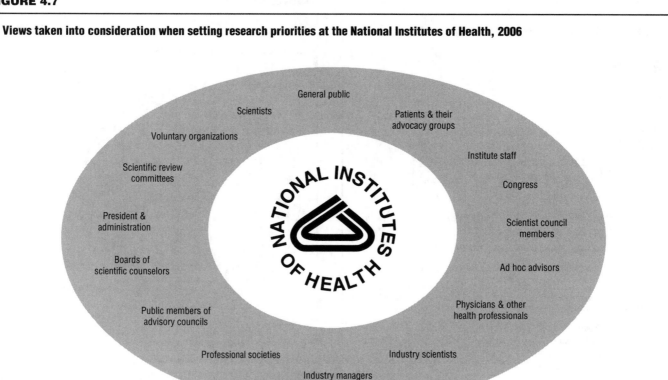

SOURCE: Norka Ruiz Bravo, "Setting Research Priorites: Every Voice Counts," in *How COPR Can Help Advance Biomedical Reasearch*, U.S. Department of Health and Human Services, National Institutes of Health, 2006, http://0-copr.nih.gov.library.law.suffolk.edu/meetings/presentations/bravo.pdf (accessed May 19, 2010)

public interest, scientific merit, and the potential to build on current knowledge. Figure 4.7 shows all the stakeholders whose interests and opinions are considered when NIH resource allocation and grant funding decisions are made.

NIH Achievements

The HHS notes in *U.S. Department of Health and Human Services Budget in Brief, Fiscal Year 2011* that in FY 2011 the NIH had 18,784 employees. The NIH recruits and attracts the most capable research scientists in the world. In fact, the NIH states in "The NIH Almanac—Nobel Laureates" (January 26, 2010, http://www.nih.gov/about/almanac/nobel/index.htm#scientists) that 129 scientists who conducted NIH research or were supported by NIH grants have received Nobel Prizes. Several Nobel Prize winners made their prize-winning discoveries in NIH laboratories.

Equally important, NIH research has contributed to great improvements in the health of the nation. The following are some of the NIH's (June 19, 2007, http://www.nih.gov/about/NIHoverview.html) achievements:

• Death rates from heart disease and stroke fell by 40% and 51%, respectively, between 1975 and 2000.

• The overall five-year survival rate for childhood cancers rose to nearly 80% during the 1990s from under 60% in the 1970s.

• The number of AIDS-related deaths fell by about 70% between 1995 and 2001.

• Sudden infant death syndrome rates fell by more than 50% between 1994 and 2000.

• Infectious diseases—such as rubella, whooping cough, and pneumococcal pneumonia—that once killed and disabled millions of people are now prevented by vaccines.

• Quality of life for 19 million Americans suffering with depression has improved as a result of more effective medication and psychotherapy.

• The sequencing of the human genome set a new course for developing ways to diagnose and treat diseases like cancer, Parkinson's disease, and Alzheimer's disease, as well as rare diseases.

• In response to the anthrax attacks of 2001, the NIH launched and expanded research to prevent, detect, diagnose, and treat diseases caused by potential bioterrorism agents.

• New and improved imaging techniques let scientists painlessly look inside the body and detect disease in its earliest stages when it is often most effectively treated.

- Researchers aggressively pursue ways to make effective vaccines for deadly diseases like HIV/AIDS, tuberculosis, malaria, and potential agents of bioterrorism.

- Progress in understanding the immune system may lead to new ways to treat and cure diabetes, arthritis, asthma, and allergies.

- New, more precise ways to treat cancer are emerging, such as drugs that zero in on abnormal proteins in cancer cells.

- Novel research methods are being developed that can identify the causes of outbreaks, such as Severe Acute Respiratory Syndrome (SARS), in weeks rather than months or years.

Francis S. Collins (1950–), the director of the NIH, explains in "The Future of Personalized Medicine" (*NIH MedlinePlus*, Winter 2010) that personalized medicine—understanding how family history influences an individual's risk of developing specific diseases—can help people take specific actions to reduce their risk of developing certain diseases. Collins describes several NIH websites where people can assess their risk and learn about actions to reduce risk:

- Smoking—http://www.cancer.gov/cancertopics/smoking offers smokers information about the risks associated with tobacco use and how to quit

- Breast cancer—http://www.cancer.gov/cancertopics/factsheet/estimating-breast-cancer-risk helps women assess their risk of developing breast cancer and http://www.cancer.gov/cancertopics/factsheet/Risk/BRCA provides information about cancer risk and genetic testing

- Colorectal cancer—http://www.cancer.gov/colorectalcancerrisk helps individuals assess their risks of developing colorectal cancer

- Cancer risk—http://www.cancer.gov/cancertopics/prevention-genetics-causes offers people at increased risk of developing cancer updated information about prevention and early detection

ACCREDITATION

Accreditation of health care providers (facilities and organizations) offers consumers, payers, and other stakeholders the assurance that accredited facilities and organizations have been certified as meeting or exceeding predetermined standards. Accreditation refers to both the process during which the quality of care delivered is measured and the resulting official endorsement that quality standards have been met. Besides promoting accreditation to health care consumers and other purchasers of care such as employer groups, accreditation assists health care facilities and organizations to recruit and retain qualified staff, increase organizational efficiencies

to reduce costs, identify ways to improve service delivery, and reduce liability insurance premiums.

Joint Commission on Accreditation of Healthcare Organizations

The Joint Commission on Accreditation of Healthcare Organizations (JCAHO; October 13, 2009, http://www.jointcommission.org/NewsRoom/faqs.htm) surveys and accredits more than 17,000 health care organizations and programs throughout the United States. The JCAHO is a not-for-profit organization and is headquartered in Oakbrook Terrace, Illinois, with a satellite office in Washington, D.C. The JCAHO (2010, http://www.jointcommission.org/AboutUs/CareerOpportunities/default.htm) has more than 1,000 surveyors—physicians, nurses, pharmacists, hospital and health care organization administrators, and other health professionals—who are qualified and trained to evaluate specific aspects of health care quality.

Working closely with medical and other professional societies, purchasers of health care services, and management experts as well as other accrediting organizations, the JCAHO develops the standards that health care organizations are expected to meet. Besides developing benchmarks and standards of organizational quality, the JCAHO is credited with promoting improvement in infection control, safety, and patients' rights.

THE JCAHO GROWS TO BECOME THE PREEMINENT ACCREDITING BODY. In "A Journey through the History of the Joint Commission" (August 25, 2009, http://www.jointcommission.org/AboutUs/joint_commission_history.htm), the JCAHO explains that early efforts to standardize and evaluate care delivered in hospitals began in 1913 by the American College of Surgeons. Thirty-eight years later, in 1951, the Joint Commission on Accreditation of Hospitals (JCAH) was established. In 1966 the JCAH began to offer accreditation to long-term care facilities, and in 1972 the Social Security Act was amended to require the U.S. secretary of health and human services to validate JCAH findings and include them in the HHS annual report to Congress. In subsequent years the JCAH's mandate was expanded to include a variety of other health care facilities, and in 1987 it was renamed the Joint Commission on Accreditation of Healthcare Organizations.

In 1992 the JCAHO instituted a requirement that accredited hospitals prohibit smoking in the hospital, and in 1993 it began performing random, surprise surveys (unannounced site visits) on 5% of accredited organizations. The JCAHO also moved to emphasize performance improvement standards by revising its policies on medical errors.

In 1999 the JCAHO required hospitals to begin collecting and reporting data about the care they provide for five specific diagnoses: acute myocardial infarction (heart attack), congestive heart failure, pneumonia, pregnancy and related medical conditions, and surgical procedures and complications. The JCAHO calls these diagnoses "core measure data" and uses these data to compare facilities and assess the quality of service delivered. In 2002 the JCAHO moved to make its recommendations more easily understood by consumers so they can make informed choices about health care providers.

In 2006 the JCAHO shifted to an unannounced survey program—meaning that organizations receive no advanced notice of their survey date. Before this policy change, the leaders of the nation's more than 4,500 Medicare-participating hospitals had ample notice and time to prepare for JCAHO visits and inspections. The policy change was intended to shift hospitals' orientation from preparing for the next JCAHO survey to preparing for the next patient. The policy also required hospitals to conduct an annual periodic performance review using their own internal evaluators to assess their own level of standards compliance and to communicate the results of their audit to the JCAHO.

This policy change, presumably implemented to improve hospital vigilance about safety, care, and quality, coincided with another, seemingly contradictory JCAHO policy change, which allowed hospitals to accumulate a higher number of deficiencies (patient care lapses and other violations) before sanctions are imposed on them. The JCAHO defends this practice by explaining that it would rather identify more problems and have hospitals resolve them than deny hospitals accreditation.

In 2008 Amy Wilson-Stronks et al. of the JCAHO published *One Size Does Not Fit All: Meeting the Health Care Needs of Diverse Populations* (http://www.joint commission.org/NR/rdonlyres/88C2C901-6E4E-4570 -95D8-B49BD7F756CF/0/HLCOneSizeFinal.pdf), which exhorts health care organizations to assess and enhance their capacity to meet patients' unique cultural and language needs to better accommodate specific populations. The researchers encourage organizational commitment to the provision of culturally competent care, which entails valuing diversity, engaging in self-assessment activities, acquiring cultural knowledge, and adapting to diversity in the communities they serve. Examples of specific ways to accommodate diverse patient populations include recruiting a diversified staff, using professional health care interpreters, and helping patients to better navigate the health care system.

In "Statement from the Joint Commission Regarding Enactment of Health Care Reform Bill" (March 26, 2010, http://www.jointcommission.org/NewsRoom/state ment_tjc_health_care_reform.htm), a statement about the Patient Protection and Affordable Care Act of 2010, the

JCAHO asserts that "the United States has the most technologically sophisticated care in the world, and a cadre of dedicated and skilled health professionals beyond rival. At the same time, there are persistent issues in health care delivery that keep the health care system from attaining the highest achievable levels of quality and safety for every patient in every setting." The JCAHO explains that it is working with health care facilities, providers, the CMS, safety advocates, Congress, and other stakeholders to effectively address urgent health and safety issues.

National Committee for Quality Assurance

The National Committee for Quality Assurance (NCQA) is another well-respected accrediting organization that focuses its attention on the managed care industry. The NCQA began surveying and accrediting managed care organizations (MCOs) in 1991. The NCQA notes in "Accreditation" (http://www.ncqa.org/tabid/66/ Default.aspx) that by 2010 most health maintenance organizations (HMOs) in the United States had been reviewed by the NCQA and that 70.5% of Americans enrolled in health plans were covered by NCQA-accredited plans. In addition, the NCQA indicates in *The State of Health Care Quality 2009* (2009, http://www.ncqa.org/ Portals/0/Newsroom/SOHC/SOHC_2009.pdf) that a growing number of health plans voluntarily submitted Health Plan Employer Data and Information Set (HEDIS) data to the NCQA in 2009: 702 HMOs and 277 preferred provider organizations (PPOs). This represented a 127% increase from 2000.

When an MCO undergoes an NCQA survey, it is assessed by more than 60 different standards, each focusing on a specific aspect of health plan operations. The standards address access and service, the qualifications of providers, the organization's commitment to prevention programs and health maintenance, the quality of care delivered to members when they are ill or injured, and the organization's approach to helping members manage chronic diseases such as diabetes, heart disease, and asthma. To ensure fair comparisons between managed health care plans and to track their progress and improvement over time, the NCQA considers many standards, including:

- Management of asthma and effective use of medication

- Controlling hypertension (high blood pressure)

- Effective and appropriate use of antidepressant medications

- The frequency and consistency with which smokers are counseled to quit

- Rates of breast cancer screening

- The frequency and consistency with which beta blocker (drug treatment) is used following heart attack

- Rates of immunization among children and teens

The NCQA combines HEDIS data with national and regional benchmarks of quality in a national database called the Quality Compass. This national database enables employers and health care consumers to compare health plans to one another and make choices about coverage based on quality and value rather than simply on price and participating providers (physicians, hospitals, and other providers that offer services to the managed care plan members).

The NCQA issues health plan report cards that rate HMOs and MCOs, and health care consumers and other stakeholders can access them at the NCQA website. After the NCQA review, the MCOs may be granted the NCQA's full accreditation for three years, indicating a level of excellence that exceeds NCQA standards. Those that need some improvement are granted one-year accreditation with recommendations about areas that need improvement, and those MCOs that meet some but not all NCQA standards may be denied accreditation or granted provisional accreditation.

In *State of Health Care Quality 2009*, the NCQA reports that "after more than a decade of steady, sometimes remarkable progress, the quality of care in America appears to have reached a plateau. With a few key exceptions, quality measures in the three major sectors of our system—commercial insurance, Medicare and Medicaid—were flat." The NCQA explains that "while some HEDIS measures have plateaued at a relatively high level, far too many are lodged at an unacceptable level of mediocrity." An example of a successful measure is that Americans with asthma receive appropriate medications 90% of the time, independent of the type of health care coverage they have. Less successful measures include chlamydia (a sexually transmitted bacterial disease) screening at 40.1% and follow-up care for children prescribed attention deficit hyperactivity disorder (a disorder that is characterized by troublesome inattentiveness, impulsivity, and overactivity) medication at 40.2%.

Accreditation Association for Ambulatory Health Care

Another accrediting organization, the Accreditation Association for Ambulatory Health Care (AAAHC), was formed in 1979 and focuses exclusively on ambulatory (outpatient) facilities and programs. Outpatient clinics, group practices, college health services, occupational medicine clinics, and ambulatory surgery centers are among the organizations that are evaluated by the AAAHC. The AAAHC accreditation process involves a self-assessment by the organization seeking accreditation and a survey conducted by AAAHC surveyors who are all practicing professionals. The AAAHC grants accreditation for periods ranging from six months to three years.

In 2002 the AAAHC and the JCAHO signed a collaborative accreditation agreement that permits ambulatory health care organizations to use their AAAHC accreditation to satisfy JCAHO requirements. That same year the CMS granted the AAAHC authority to review health plans that provide coverage for Medicare beneficiaries. HMOs, PPOs, and ambulatory surgery centers are now considered Medicare-certified on their receipt of accreditation from the AAAHC.

In 2009 the AAAHC established standards for reviewing so-called medical homes—primary care practices that aim to serve as centralized overseers all the health care needs of individuals. The term *medical home* is a relatively new descriptor of the long-standing practice of having a primary care practitioner (for adults usually an internist or family practitioner and for children a pediatrician) provide and coordinate needed care. By 2010 the AAAHC (http://www.aaahc.org/eweb/dynamic page.aspx?site=aaahc_site&webcode=about_aaahc) was accrediting over 4,600 organizations.

National Quality Forum

In 2006 two other national quality organizations, the National Quality Forum and the National Committee on Quality Health Care, merged to become a new organization, also named the National Quality Forum (NQF; http://www.qualityforum.org/). The NQF is a private, not-for-profit membership organization created to develop and implement a national strategy for health care quality measurement and reporting. Its mission is to improve U.S. health care through the endorsement of consensus-based national standards for measurement and public reporting of health care performance data that provide meaningful information about whether care is safe, timely, beneficial, patient centered, equitable, and efficient.

In the press release "Practice Makes Perfect—Tips for Safer Healthcare" (March 11, 2010, http://www.quality forum.org/News_And_Resources/Press_Releases/2010/ Practice_Makes_Perfect_-_Tips_for_Safer_Healthcare.aspx), the NQF states that beginning in March 2010 it endorsed the use of 34 best practices to address areas including medication use, radiation safety, and health care–associated infections to improve delivery of safe, effective health care. The NQF also produces the patient guide "Safe Practices for Better Healthcare" to help consumers obtain safer health care services.

PROFESSIONAL SOCIETIES

There are professional and membership organizations and societies for all health professionals, such as physicians, nurses, psychologists, and hospital administrators, as well as for institutional health care providers, such as hospitals, managed care plans, and medical groups. These professional organizations represent the interests and concerns of their members, advocate on their behalf, and frequently compile data and publish information about working conditions, licensing, accreditation, compensation, and scientific advancements of interest to members.

American Medical Association

The American Medical Association (AMA) is a powerful voice for U.S. physicians' interests. The AMA concerns itself with a wide range of health-related issues including medical ethics, medical education, physician and patient advocacy, and development of national health policy. The AMA publishes the highly regarded *Journal of the American Medical Association* and the *AMNews*, as well as journals in 10 specialty areas called *Archives Journals*.

Founded in 1847, the AMA has worked to upgrade medical education by expanding medical school curricula and establishing standards for licensing and accreditation of practitioners and postgraduate training programs. Recent activities of the AMA include campaigning to avert a Medicare pay cut for physicians, combating childhood obesity, and supporting the 2010 health care reform legislation. In the March 2010 statement "President Obama Signs Historic Health System Reform Bill for Health of Our Nation" (http://www.ama-assn.org/ama/pub/health-system-reform/news/march-2010/obama-signs-health-reform-bill.shtml), J. James Rohack, the president of the AMA, averred that "physicians see firsthand the pain and heartbreak that being uninsured causes in the lives of America's patients. Today, we move forward to start to ease that pain." Rohack praised the legislation's move to increase Medicaid reimbursement for primary care physicians and offer bonuses to physicians practicing in underserved areas. He also observed that insurance reforms—the elimination of lifetime caps and of insurance companies' ability to cancel insurance except in instances of fraud or abuse—will benefit patients.

American Nurses Association

The American Nurses Association (ANA; 2010, http://www.nursingworld.org/FunctionalMenuCategories/AboutANA.aspx) is a professional organization that represents more than 3.1 million registered nurses and promotes high standards of nursing practice and education as well as the roles and responsibilities of nurses in the workplace and the community. On behalf of its members, the ANA works to protect patients' rights, lobbies to advocate for nurses' interests, champions workplace safety, and provides career and continuing education opportunities. The ANA publishes the *American Journal of Nursing* and actively seeks to improve the public

image of nurses among health professionals and the community at large.

American Hospital Association

The American Hospital Association (AHA; 2010, http://www.aha.org/aha/about/index.html) represents nearly 5,000 hospitals, health care systems, networks, and other health care providers and 37,000 individual members. Originally established as a membership organization for hospital superintendents in 1898, the AHA eventually expanded its mission to address all facets of hospital care and quality. Besides national advocacy activities and participation in the development of health policy, the AHA oversees research and pilot programs to improve health service delivery. It also gathers and disseminates hospital and other related health care data, publishes information of interest for its members, and sponsors educational opportunities for health care managers and administrators.

VOLUNTARY HEALTH ORGANIZATIONS
American Heart Association

The American Heart Association's mission is to decrease disability and death from cardiovascular disease and stroke. The association's national headquarters is in Dallas, Texas, and eight regional affiliate offices serve the balance of the United States. The American Heart Association explains in "History of the American Heart Association" (2010, http://www.americanheart.org/presenter.jhtml?identifier=10860) that it was started by a group of physicians and social workers in New York City in 1915. The early efforts of this group, called the Association for the Prevention and Relief of Heart Disease, were to educate physicians and the general public about heart disease. The first fund-raising efforts were launched in 1948 during a radio broadcast, and since then the association has raised millions of dollars to fund research, education, and treatment programs.

Besides research, fund-raising, and generating public awareness about reducing the risk of developing heart disease, the American Heart Association has published many best-selling cookbooks featuring heart-healthy recipes and meal planning ideas. The association is also considered one of the world's most trusted authorities about heart health among physicians and scientists. It publishes five print journals and one online professional journal, including *Circulation, Stroke, Hypertension*, and *Atherosclerosis, Thrombosis, and Vascular Biology*.

The American Heart Association supports many initiatives to prevent heart disease and educate the community-at-large about the importance of timely treatment for heart attacks and stroke. For example, in April 2010, in "Statement by American Heart Association President Clyde Yancy, M.D. on Menu Labeling Measures in

New Health Reform Bill" (http://www.newsroom.heart.org/index.php?s=43&item=1015), the American Heart Association commended legislation requiring public restaurants to provide nutrition information about their offerings.

The American Heart Association also educates consumers about the warning signs of heart attacks and the importance of seeking medical care immediately when symptoms arise. For example, in the press release "Some Women More Likely to Miss or Ignore Heart Attack Warning Signs" (May 2010, http://www.newsroom.heart.org/index.php?s=43&item=409), the association notes that women may be less able or likely to identify their heart attack symptoms because they may experience atypical symptoms. American Heart Association research focuses on multiple factors that delay women from seeking needed care. These range from uncertainty about signs and symptoms to underestimating their risk of having heart disease.

American Cancer Society

The American Cancer Society (ACS; 2010, http://www.cancer.org/AboutUs/WhoWeAre/index) is headquartered in Atlanta, Georgia, and has more than 3,400 offices across the country. The ACS's (November 11, 2008, http://www.cancer.org/docroot/AA/content/AA_1_1_ACS_Mission_Statements.asp) mission is "eliminating cancer as a major health problem by preventing cancer, saving lives, and diminishing suffering from cancer, through research, education, advocacy, and service."

The ACS is the biggest source of private, not-for-profit funding for cancer research—second only to the federal government. In "ACS Fact Sheet" (2010, http://www.cancer.org/docroot/AA/content/AA_1_2_ACS_Fact_Sheet.asp), the ACS states that by the close of FY 2008 it had invested over $3 billion in cancer research at leading centers throughout the United States and had funded 44 Nobel Prize winners early in their careers. It also supports epidemiological research to provide cancer surveillance information about occurrence rates, risk factors, mortality, and availability of treatment services. The ACS publishes an array of patient information brochures and four clinical journals for health professionals: *Cancer, Cancer Cytopathology, CA: A Cancer Journal for Clinicians*, and

Cancer Practice. The ACS also maintains a 24-hour consumer telephone line that is staffed by trained cancer information specialists and a website with information for professionals, patients and families, and the media.

Besides education, prevention, and patient services, the ACS advocates for cancer survivors, their families, and every potential cancer patient. The ACS seeks to obtain support and passage of laws, policies, and regulations that benefit people affected by cancer. The ACS is especially concerned with developing strategies to better serve the poor and people with little formal education, who historically have been disproportionately affected by cancer.

March of Dimes

The March of Dimes was founded in 1938 by President Franklin D. Roosevelt (1882–1945) to help protect American children from polio. Besides supporting the research that produced the polio vaccine, it has advocated birth defects research and the fortification of food supplies with folic acid to prevent neural tube defects. It has also supported increasing access to quality prenatal care and the growth of neonatal intensive care units to help improve the chances of survival for babies born prematurely or those with serious medical conditions.

The March of Dimes continues to partner with volunteers, scientific researchers, educators, and community outreach workers to help prevent birth defects. It funds genetic research, investigates the causes and treatment of premature birth, educates pregnant women, and provides health care services for women and children, such as immunization, checkups, and treatment for childhood illnesses.

In *2008 Annual Report* (2010, http://www.marchofdimes.com/files/2008AnnualReport.pdf), the March of Dimes notes that in 2008 it provided support to more than 50,000 families with infants in newborn intensive care units, succeeded in expanding newborn screening so that every state requires testing for 21 treatable conditions, took action to prevent premature births, and invested $26.8 million in research to prevent birth defects, premature birth, and infant deaths.

CHAPTER 5
THE INCREASING COST OF HEALTH CARE

HOW MUCH DOES HEALTH CARE COST?

American society places a high value on human life and generally wants—and expects—quality medical care. However, quality care comes with an increasingly high cost. In 1970 the United States spent 7.2% of its gross domestic product (GDP; the total market value of final goods and services produced within an economy in a given year) on health care. By 2007 health care expenditures reached 16.2% of the GDP. Table 5.1 shows the growth in health care expenditures, the growth in the GDP, and the annual percent change from the previous year from 1960 to 2007.

For many years the consumer price index (CPI; a measure of the average change in prices paid by consumers) increased at a greater rate for medical care than for any other commodity. In 1990 the average annual increase in the overall CPI was 4.7%, whereas the average annual increase in the medical care index stood at 8.1%. (See Table 5.2.) In 2000 the average annual growth in the medical care index fell to 3.5%, but in 2008 it rose again to 4.2%, outpacing overall inflation, which was 3.8%. The medical care index has consistently outpaced the CPI in each decade. Of all the components of health care delivery, the sharpest price increase in 2008 was in hospital services at 7.4%.

The Centers for Medicare and Medicaid Services (CMS) projects that by 2019 the national health expenditure will grow to nearly $4.5 trillion—19.3% of the GDP, from 17.3% in 2010. (See Table 5.3.) (Because the numbers in Table 5.3 are projections, they may differ from the actual numbers presented in some other tables and figures that appear in this chapter.) In *National Health Expenditures Projections 2009–2019* (2009, http://www.cms.gov/NationalHealthExpendData/downloads/proj2009.pdf), the CMS indicates that Medicare accounted for a staggering 20.1% of national care expenditures in 2008.

Generally, projections are most accurate for the near future and less accurate for the distant future. For example, predictions for 2030 should be viewed more warily than predictions for 2012, because it is unlikely that the conditions on which the projections are based will remain the same. As a result, the CMS cautions that its projections should not be viewed as predictions for the future. Rather, they are intended to help policy makers evaluate the costs or savings of proposed legislative or regulatory changes.

Total Health Care Spending

The CMS, along with the Centers for Disease Control and Prevention and the U.S. Government Accountability Office, maintain most of the nation's statistics on health care costs. The CMS reports that the United States spent $2.3 trillion for health care in 2008, up 4.4% from $2.2 trillion in 2007. (See Table 5.3.) This rate has decreased since the 6.9% increase in 2005 and is projected to rise slightly and then remain relatively constant, although it will likely be as high as three times the rate of inflation through 2019.

Over $1.2 trillion of the 2008 health care expenditures came from private funds (out-of-pocket payments, private health insurance, and other private funds), and the balance was paid with public money. (See Table 5.4.) The 2008 per capita cost for health care (the average per individual if spending was divided equally among all people in the country) was $7,681.

Of the $2.3 trillion that was spent on health care in 2008, more than $1.9 trillion was spent on personal health services (expenses incurred by individuals as opposed to institutions). (See Table 5.5.) Some of the services included hospital care, physician and dental services, nursing and home health care, prescription drugs, and durable medical equipment.

Table 5.5 shows the trends and annual percent changes in personal health care expenditures by category. In 2008 the nation spent $731.2 billion on professional

TABLE 5.1

Gross domestic product (GDP), federal, state, and local government health expenditures and average annual percent change, selected years 1960–2007

[Data are compiled from various sources by the Centers for Medicare & Medicaid Services]

Gross domestic product, government expenditures, and national health expenditures	1960	1970	1980	1990	2000	2005	2006	2007
					Amount in billions			
Gross domestic product (GDP)	$ 526	$1,039	$2,790	$ 5,803	$ 9,817	$ 12,422	$ 13,178	$ 13,808
Implicit price deflator for GDP*	21.0	27.5	54.0	81.6	100.0	113.0	116.7	119.8
All federal government expenditures	$ 86.7	$201.1	$585.7	$1,253.5	$1,864.4	$2,558.6	$2,711.6	$2,880.5
All state and local government expenditures	40.2	113.0	329.4	730.5	1,269.5	1,684.9	1,765.3	1,892.4
National health expenditures	$ 27.5	$ 74.9	$253.4	$ 714.1	$1,353.2	$1,980.6	$2,112.7	$2,241.2
Private	20.7	46.8	147.0	427.4	756.4	1,081.6	1,139.7	1,205.5
Public	6.8	28.1	106.3	286.8	596.8	899.0	973.0	1,035.7
Federal government	2.9	17.7	71.6	193.9	417.7	640.3	707.6	754.4
State and local government	3.9	10.4	34.8	92.8	179.0	258.7	265.4	281.3
					Amount per capita			
National health expenditures	$ 148	$ 356	$1,100	$ 2,814	$ 4,789	$ 6,687	$ 7,062	$ 7,421
Private	111	222	638	1,684	2,677	3,652	3,810	3,991
Public	36	134	462	1,130	2,112	3,035	3,252	3,429
Federal government	15	84	311	764	1,479	2,162	2,365	2,498
State and local government	21	49	151	366	634	873	887	931
					Percent			
National health expenditures as percent of GDP	5.2	7.2	9.1	12.3	13.8	15.9	16.0	16.2
Health expenditures as a percent of total government expenditures								
All federal government	3.3	8.8	12.2	15.5	22.4	25.0	26.1	26.2
All state and local government	9.7	9.2	10.6	12.7	14.1	15.4	15.0	14.9
					Percent distribution			
National health expenditures	100.0	100.0	100.0	100.0	100.0	100.0	100.0	100.0
Private	75.3	62.4	58.0	59.8	55.9	54.6	53.9	53.8
Public	24.7	37.6	42.0	40.2	44.1	45.4	46.1	46.2
Federal government	10.4	23.7	28.2	27.2	30.9	32.3	33.5	33.7
State and local government	14.3	13.9	13.7	13.0	13.2	13.1	12.6	12.6
					Average annual percent change from previous year shown			
GDP	—	7.0	10.4	7.6	5.4	4.8	6.1	4.8
Federal government expenditures	—	8.8	11.3	7.9	4.0	6.5	6.0	6.2
State and local government expenditures	—	10.9	11.3	8.3	5.7	5.8	4.8	7.2
National health expenditures	—	10.5	13.0	10.9	6.6	7.9	6.7	6.1
Private	—	8.5	12.1	11.3	5.9	7.4	5.4	5.8
Public	—	15.3	14.2	10.4	7.6	8.5	8.2	6.4
Federal government	—	20.0	15.0	10.5	8.0	8.9	10.5	6.6
State and local government	—	10.2	12.8	10.3	6.8	7.6	2.6	6.0
National health expenditures, per capita	—	9.2	11.9	9.8	5.5	6.9	5.6	5.1
Private	—	7.2	11.1	10.2	4.7	6.4	4.3	4.8
Public	—	14.0	13.2	9.4	6.5	7.5	7.1	5.4
Federal government	—	18.8	14.0	9.4	6.8	7.9	9.4	5.6
State and local government	—	8.8	11.9	9.3	5.6	6.6	1.6	5.0

—Category not applicable.
Year 2000 = 100. Last revised December 23, 2008 by the Bureau of Economic Analysis.
Notes: Dollar amounts shown are in current dollars. Percents are calculated using unrounded data. Estimates may not add to totals because of rounding.

SOURCE: "Table 123. Gross Domestic Product, Federal, and State and Local Government Expenditures, National Health Expenditures, and Average Annual Percent Change: United States, Selected Years 1960–2007," in *Health, United States, 2009: With Special Feature on Medical Technology*, U.S. Department of Health and Human Services, Centers for Disease Control and Prevention, National Center for Health Statistics, 2010, http://www.cdc.gov/nchs/data/hus/hus09 .pdf (accessed May 21, 2010)

services, by far the largest amount of personal health care spending, followed by $718.4 billion on hospital care. This expense was followed by $496.2 billion on physician and clinical services, $299.6 billion on retail outlet sales of medical products, $234.1 billion on prescription drugs, and $203.1 billion on nursing home and home health care.

WHO PAYS THE BILL?

In general, the government is the fastest-growing payer of health care expenses. From 2004 to 2008 the public share of the nation's total health care bill rose from 45.3% to 47.3%, and it is projected to rise to 51.9% by 2019. (See Table 5.4.) In 2008 private health insurance, the major nongovernmental payer of health care costs, paid

TABLE 5.2

Consumer price index and average annual percent change for all items, selected items, and medical care costs, selected years 1960–2008

[Data are based on reporting by samples of providers and other retail outlets]

Items and medical care components	1960	1970	1980	1990	1995	2000	2005	2007	2008
	Consumer Price Index (CPI)								
All items	29.6	38.8	82.4	130.7	152.4	172.2	195.3	207.3	215.3
All items less medical care	30.2	39.2	82.8	128.8	148.6	167.3	188.7	200.1	207.8
Services	24.1	35.0	77.9	139.2	168.7	195.3	230.1	246.8	255.5
Food	30.0	39.2	86.8	132.4	148.4	167.8	190.7	202.9	214.1
Apparel	45.7	59.2	90.9	124.1	132.0	129.6	119.5	119.0	118.9
Housing	—	36.4	81.1	128.5	148.5	169.6	195.7	209.6	216.3
Energy	22.4	25.5	86.0	102.1	105.2	124.6	177.1	207.7	236.7
Medical care	22.3	34.0	74.9	162.8	220.5	260.8	323.2	351.1	364.1
Components of medical care									
Medical care services	19.5	32.3	74.8	162.7	224.2	266.0	336.7	369.3	384.9
Professional services	—	37.0	77.9	156.1	201.0	237.7	281.7	300.8	311.0
Physicians' services	21.9	34.5	76.5	160.8	208.8	244.7	287.5	303.2	311.3
Dental services	27.0	39.2	78.9	155.8	206.8	258.5	324.0	358.4	376.9
Eyeglasses and eye care[a]	—	—	—	117.3	137.0	149.7	163.2	171.6	174.1
Services by other medical professionals[a]	—	—	—	120.2	143.9	161.9	186.8	197.4	205.5
Hospital and related services	—	—	69.2	178.0	257.8	317.3	439.9	498.9	534.0
Hospital services[2]	—	—	—	—	—	115.9	161.6	183.6	197.2
Inpatient hospital services[b, c]	—	—	—	—	—	113.8	156.6	178.1	190.8
Outpatient hospital services[a, c]	—	—	—	138.7	204.6	263.8	373.0	424.2	456.8
Hospital rooms	9.3	23.6	68.0	175.4	251.2	—	—	—	—
Other inpatient services[a]	—	—	—	142.7	206.8	—	—	—	—
Nursing homes and adult day care[b]	—	—	—	—	—	117.0	145.0	159.6	165.3
Health insurance[d]	—	—	—	—	—	—	—	113.5	114.2
Medical care commodities	46.9	46.5	75.4	163.4	204.5	238.1	276.0	290.0	296.0
Prescription drugs[e]	54.0	47.4	72.5	181.7	235.0	285.4	349.0	369.2	378.3
Nonprescription drugs and medical supplies[a]	—	—	—	120.6	140.5	149.5	151.7	156.8	158.3
Internal and respiratory over-the-counter drugs	—	42.3	74.9	145.9	167.0	176.9	179.7	186.4	188.7
Nonprescription medical equipment and supplies	—	—	79.2	138.0	166.3	178.1	180.6	185.1	185.6
	Average annual percent change from previous year shown								
All items	...	2.7	7.8	4.7	3.1	2.5	2.5	3.0	3.8
All items excluding medical care	...	2.6	7.8	4.5	2.9	2.4	2.4	3.0	3.8
All services	...	3.8	8.3	6.0	3.9	3.0	3.3	3.6	3.5
Food	...	2.7	8.3	4.3	2.3	2.5	2.6	3.1	5.5
Apparel	...	2.6	4.4	3.2	1.2	−0.4	−1.6	−0.2	−0.1
Housing	...	—	8.3	4.7	2.9	2.7	2.9	3.5	3.2
Energy	...	1.3	12.9	1.7	0.6	3.4	7.3	8.3	13.9
Medical care	...	4.3	8.2	8.1	6.3	3.4	4.4	4.2	3.7
Components of medical care									
Medical care services	...	5.2	8.8	8.1	6.6	3.5	4.8	4.7	4.2
Professional services	...	—	7.7	7.2	5.2	3.4	3.5	3.3	3.4
Physicians' services	...	4.6	8.3	7.7	5.4	3.2	3.3	2.7	2.7
Dental services	...	3.8	7.2	7.0	5.8	4.6	4.6	5.2	5.1
Eyeglasses and eye care[a]	...	—	—	—	3.2	1.8	1.7	2.5	1.4
Services by other medical professionals[a]	...	—	—	—	3.7	2.4	2.9	2.8	4.1
Hospital and related services	...	—	—	9.9	7.7	4.2	6.8	6.5	7.0
Hospital services[b]	...	—	—	—	—	—	6.9	6.6	7.4
Inpatient hospital services[b, c]	...	—	—	—	—	—	6.6	6.6	7.1
Outpatient hospital services[a, c]	...	—	—	—	8.1	5.2	7.2	6.6	7.7
Hospital rooms	...	9.8	11.2	9.9	7.4	—	—	—	—
Other inpatient services[a]	...	—	—	—	7.7	—	—	—	—
Nursing homes and adult day care[b]	...	—	—	—	—	—	4.4	4.9	3.6
Health insurance[d]	...	—	—	—	—	—	—	—	0.6

33.5% of all health expenditures. The share of health care spending from private, out-of-pocket (paid by the patient) funds declined from 12.7% in 2004 to 11.9% in 2008.

Personal Health Care Bill

Much of the increase in government spending has occurred in the area of personal health care. In 2004 government sources paid 44.5% of personal health care expenditures; by 2008 they covered 46.5% of the $1.9 trillion spent on personal health care services. (See Table 5.6.) Of the total expenditures, 36.8% came from the federal government and 9.7% came from state and local governments. Some of the federal increase was attributed to Medicare spending, which grew from

TABLE 5.2

Consumer price index and average annual percent change for all items, selected items, and medical care costs, selected years 1960–2008 [CONTINUED]

[Data are based on reporting by samples of providers and other retail outlets]

Items and medical care components	1960	1970	1980	1990	1995	2000	2005	2007	2008
Medical care commodities	...	−0.1	5.0	8.0	4.6	3.1	3.0	2.5	2.1
Prescription drugs[e]	...	−1.3	4.3	9.6	5.3	4.0	4.1	2.9	2.5
Nonprescription drugs and medical supplies[a]	...	—	—	—	3.1	1.2	0.3	1.7	0.9
Internal and respiratory over-the-counter drugs	...	—	5.9	6.9	2.7	1.2	0.3	1.8	1.2
Nonprescription medical equipment and supplies	...	—	—	5.7	3.8	1.4	0.3	1.2	0.3

—Data not available
. . .Category not applicable.
[a]December 1986 = 100.
[b]December 1996 = 100.
[c]Special index based on a substantially smaller sample.
[d]December 2005 = 100.
[e]Prior to 2006 this category included medical supplies.
Notes: CPI for all urban consumers (CPI-U) U.S. city average, detailed expenditure categories. 1982–1984 = 100, except where noted. Data are not seasonally adjusted.

SOURCE: "Table 124. Consumer Price Index and Average Annual Percent Change for All Items, Selected Items, and Medical Care Components: United States, Selected Years 1960–2008," in *Health, United States, 2009: With Special Feature on Medical Technology*, U.S. Department of Health and Human Services, Centers for Disease Control and Prevention, National Center for Health Statistics, 2010, http://www.cdc.gov/nchs/data/hus/hus09.pdf (accessed May 21, 2010)

19.4% of all personal health care expenditures in 2004 to 22.8% in 2008.

WHY HAVE HEALTH CARE COSTS AND SPENDING INCREASED?

The increase in the cost of medical care is challenging to analyze, because the methods and quality of health care change constantly and as a result are often not comparable. A hospital stay in 1970 did not include the same services offered in 2010. Furthermore, the care received in a physician's office in 2010 is not comparable to that received a generation ago. One contributing factor to the rising cost of health care is the increase in biomedical technology, much of which is now available for use outside of a hospital.

Many other factors also contribute to the increase in health care costs. These include population growth, high salaries for physicians and some other health care workers, and the expense of malpractice insurance. Escalating malpractice insurance costs and professional liability premiums have prompted some physicians and other health care practitioners to refrain from performing high-risk procedures that increase their vulnerability or have caused them to relocate to states where malpractice premiums are lower. Furthermore, to protect themselves from malpractice suits, many health care practitioners routinely order diagnostic tests and prescribe treatments that are not medically necessary and do not serve to improve their patients' health. This practice is known as defensive medicine, and even though its precise contribution to rising health care costs is difficult to gauge, industry observers agree that it is a significant factor.

Marc R. Nuwer et al. assert in "The US Health Care System: Part 1: Our Current System" (*Neurology*, vol. 71, no. 23, December 2008) that defensive medicine accounts for about 10% of U.S. health care system costs, which means that in 2001 defensive medicine cost between $70 billion and $126 billion. In "National and Surgical Health Care Expenditures, 2005–2025" (*Annals of Surgery*, vol. 251, no. 2, February 2010), Eric Muñoz et al. attribute unabated health care spending in part to defensive medicine. However, other industry observers, such as Tom Baker in "Liability = Responsibility" (*New York Times*, July 11, 2009) and Daphne Eviatar in "Tort Reform Unlikely to Cut Health Care Costs" (*Washington Independent*, August 19, 2009), assert that defensive medicine makes a very small contribution to health care expenditures. They also suggest that malpractice liability costs are just a scant 1.5% of U.S. health care system costs and that the medical errors that malpractice liability tries to prevent pose greater costs—to injured patients and to the health care system.

Other factors for the increase in health care costs include advanced biomedical procedures that require high-technology expertise and equipment, redundant (excessive and unnecessary) technology in hospitals, cumbersome medical insurance programs and consumer demand for less restrictive insurance plans (ones that offer more choices, benefits, and coverage, but usually mean higher premiums), and consumer demand for the latest and most comprehensive testing and treatment. Legislation that increased Medicare spending and the growing number of older adults who use a disproportionate amount of health care services have also accelerated health care spending.

TABLE 5.3

National health expenditures and annual percent change, 2004–19

Item	2004	2005	2006	2007	2008	2009	2010	2011	2012	2013	2014	2015	2016	2017	2018	2019
						Projected										
National health expenditures (billions)	$1,855.4	$1,982.5	$2,112.5	$2,239.7	$2,338.7	$2,472.2	$2,569.6	$2,702.9	$2,850.2	$3,024.7	$3,225.3	$3,441.9	$3,683.8	$3,936.0	$4,203.6	$4,482.7
National health expenditures as a percent of gross domestic product	15.6%	15.7%	15.8%	15.9%	16.2%	17.3%	17.3%	17.3%	17.2%	17.3%	17.4%	17.7%	18.1%	18.5%	18.9%	19.3%
National health expenditures per capita	$6,327.5	$6,701.3	$7,071.1	$7,423.1	$7,680.7	$8,046.7	$8,289.9	$8,643.4	$9,035.2	$9,505.1	$10,048.0	$10,630.8	$11,281.4	$11,952.0	$12,658.1	$13,387.2
Gross domestic product (billions)	$11,867.8	$12,638.4	$13,398.9	$14,077.6	$14,441.4	$14,282.5	$14,853.8	$15,611.4	$16,563.7	$17,524.4	$18,488.2	$19,431.1	$20,344.4	$21,280.2	$22,259.1	$23,283.0
Gross domestic product (billions of 2005 $)	$12,263.8	$12,638.4	$12,976.2	$13,254.1	$13,312.2	$12,992.7	$13,343.5	$13,823.9	$14,404.5	$14,923.0	$15,370.7	$15,785.7	$16,148.8	$16,504.1	$16,867.2	$17,238.3
Gross domestic product implicit price deflator (chain weighted 2005 base year)	0.968	1.000	1.033	1.062	1.085	1.099	1.113	1.130	1.151	1.177	1.206	1.235	1.265	1.295	1.326	1.358
Consumer price index (CPI-W)—1982–1984 base	1.889	1.953	2.016	2.073	2.153	2.131	2.168	2.218	2.277	2.348	2.421	2.489	2.558	2.630	2.704	2.779
CMS implicit medical price deflator*	0.966	1.000	1.034	1.069	1.102	1.137	1.169	1.200	1.237	1.277	1.321	1.369	1.418	1.469	1.523	1.579
U.S. population	293.2	295.8	298.8	301.7	304.5	307.2	310.0	312.7	315.5	318.2	321.0	323.8	326.5	329.3	332.1	334.8
Population age less than 65 years	257.3	259.5	261.8	264.0	265.8	267.9	270.0	271.9	273.5	274.9	276.4	277.8	279.2	280.6	281.8	283.0
Population age 65 years and older	36.0	36.3	37.0	37.7	38.7	39.3	40.0	40.8	42.0	43.3	44.6	45.9	47.3	48.8	50.3	51.9
Private health insurance—NHE (billions)	$646.1	$691.0	$727.6	$759.7	$783.2	$808.7	$829.3	$862.3	$894.3	$942.2	$1,004.8	$1,075.9	$1,149.4	$1,220.4	$1,290.8	$1,360.6
Private health insurance—PHC (billions)	560.3	599.8	634.6	665.1	691.2	718.5	732.9	753.9	782.7	824.4	878.4	939.5	1,001.2	1,059.7	1,118.7	1,177.9
National health expenditures as a percent of gross domestic product (change)	—	6.9	6.6	6.0	4.4	5.7	3.9	5.2	5.5	6.1	6.6	6.7	7.0	6.8	6.8	6.6
National health expenditures as a percent of gross domestic product (change)	—	0.1%	0.1%	0.1%	0.3%	1.1%	0.0%	0.0%	-0.1%	0.1%	0.2%	0.3%	0.4%	0.4%	0.4%	0.4%
National health expenditures per capita	—	5.9	5.5	5.0	3.5	4.8	3.0	4.3	4.5	5.2	5.7	5.8	6.1	5.9	5.9	5.8
Gross domestic product (billions)	—	6.5	6.0	5.1	2.6	-1.1	4.0	5.1	6.1	5.8	5.5	5.1	4.7	4.6	4.6	4.6
Gross domestic product (billions of 2005 $)	—	3.1	2.7	2.1	0.4	-2.4	2.7	3.6	4.2	3.6	3.0	2.7	2.3	2.2	2.2	2.2
Gross domestic product implicit price deflator (chain weighted 2005 base year)	—	3.3	3.3	2.9	2.1	1.3	1.3	1.5	1.9	2.2	2.5	2.4	2.4	2.4	2.4	2.4
Consumer price index (CPI-W)—1982–1984 base	—	3.4	3.2	2.8	3.8	-1.0	1.7	2.3	2.7	3.1	3.1	2.8	2.8	2.8	2.8	2.8
CMS implicit medical price deflator*	—	3.6	3.4	3.4	3.0	3.2	2.8	2.7	3.0	3.3	3.5	3.6	3.6	3.6	3.7	3.7
U.S. population	—	0.9	1.0	1.0	0.9	0.9	0.9	0.9	0.9	0.9	0.9	0.9	0.9	0.9	0.8	0.8
Population age less than 65 years	—	0.9	0.9	0.8	0.7	0.8	0.8	0.7	0.6	0.5	0.5	0.5	0.5	0.5	0.4	0.4
Population age 65 years and older	—	1.1	1.8	2.0	2.5	1.8	1.6	2.1	3.0	3.2	3.0	2.9	3.0	3.1	3.1	3.2
Private health insurance—NHE	—	6.9	5.3	4.4	3.1	3.3	2.5	4.0	3.7	5.4	6.7	7.1	6.8	6.2	5.8	5.4
Private health insurance—PHC	—	7.0	5.8	4.8	3.9	4.0	2.0	2.9	3.8	5.3	6.6	7.0	6.6	5.8	5.6	5.3

CPI = Consumer Price Index for Urban Wage Earners and Clerical Workers.
CMS = Centers for Medicare and Medicaid Services.
NHE = National Health Expenditure.
PHC = Primary Health Care.

*2005 base year. Calculated as the difference between nominal personal health care spending and real personal health care spending. Real personal health care spending is produced by deflating spending on each service type by the appropriate deflator (Producer Price Index, Consumer Price Index, etc.) and adding real spending by service type.

Note: Numbers and percents may not add to totals because of rounding.

SOURCE: "Table 1. National Health Expenditures and Selected Economic Indicators, Levels and Annual Percent Change: Calendar Years 2004–2019," in *National Health Expenditures Projections 2009–2019*, U.S. Department of Health and Human Services, Centers for Medicare and Medicaid Services, 2009, http://www.cms.gov/NationalHealthExpendData/downloads/proj2009.pdf (accessed May 21, 2010)

TABLE 5.4

National health expenditures, by source of funds, 2004–19

Year	Total	Out-of-pocket payments	Third-party payments Total	Private health insurance	Other private funds	Public Total	Federal[a]	State and local[a]	Medicare[b]	Medicaid[c]
Historical estimates					Amount in billions					
2004	$1,855.4	$234.8	$1,620.6	$646.1	$134.5	$839.9	$599.8	$240.2	$311.3	$290.5
2005	1,982.5	247.5	1,735.0	691.0	144.3	899.8	641.4	258.4	339.8	311.5
2006	2,112.5	254.9	1,857.6	727.6	154.3	975.7	709.6	266.1	403.4	310.0
2007	2,239.7	270.3	1,969.4	759.7	171.0	1,038.7	755.3	283.4	432.2	328.9
2008	2,338.7	277.8	2,061.0	783.2	171.1	1,106.7	816.9	289.8	469.2	344.3
Projected										
2009	2,472.2	283.5	2,188.7	808.7	176.5	1,203.4	918.6	284.8	507.1	378.3
2010	2,569.6	292.1	2,277.5	829.3	182.5	1,265.7	965.7	300.0	514.7	412.0
2011	2,702.9	299.9	2,402.9	862.3	190.8	1,349.8	984.8	365.0	544.4	447.0
2012	2,850.2	311.1	2,539.2	894.3	201.2	1,443.6	1,057.3	386.3	585.7	478.3
2013	3,024.7	327.3	2,697.5	942.2	214.6	1,540.7	1,130.6	410.0	626.8	513.2
2014	3,225.3	348.1	2,877.2	1,004.8	230.7	1,641.6	1,206.9	434.8	672.8	551.7
2015	3,441.9	371.6	3,070.2	1,075.9	249.9	1,744.5	1,282.2	462.3	714.0	593.3
2016	3,683.8	395.0	3,288.8	1,149.4	269.6	1,869.8	1,376.4	493.4	767.4	638.3
2017	3,936.0	417.3	3,518.6	1,220.4	288.5	2,009.8	1,483.1	526.7	830.0	686.8
2018	4,203.6	440.8	3,762.8	1,290.8	308.3	2,163.7	1,601.1	562.5	900.8	739.0
2019	4,482.7	465.6	4,017.1	1,360.6	328.2	2,328.3	1,728.5	599.8	977.8	794.3
Historical estimates					Per capita amount					
2004	$6,327	$801	$5,527	$2,204	$459	$2,864	$2,045	$819	d	d
2005	6,701	837	5,865	2,336	488	3,041	2,168	873	d	d
2006	7,071	853	6,218	2,435	517	3,266	2,375	891	d	d
2007	7,423	896	6,527	2,518	567	3,443	2,503	939	d	d
2008	7,681	912	6,768	2,572	562	3,635	2,683	952	d	d
Projected									d	d
2009	8,047	923	7,124	2,632	574	3,917	2,990	927	d	d
2010	8,290	942	7,348	2,676	589	4,083	3,115	968	d	d
2011	8,643	959	7,684	2,757	610	4,317	3,149	1,167	d	d
2012	9,035	986	8,049	2,835	638	4,576	3,352	1,225	d	d
2013	9,505	1,028	8,477	2,961	674	4,841	3,553	1,289	d	d
2014	10,048	1,085	8,964	3,130	719	5,114	3,760	1,354	d	d
2015	10,631	1,148	9,483	3,323	772	5,388	3,960	1,428	d	d
2016	11,281	1,210	10,072	3,520	826	5,726	4,215	1,511	d	d
2017	11,952	1,267	10,685	3,706	876	6,103	4,503	1,600	d	d
2018	12,658	1,327	11,331	3,887	928	6,515	4,821	1,694	d	d
2019	13,387	1,390	11,997	4,063	980	6,953	5,162	1,791	d	d
Historical estimates					Percent distribution					
2004	100.0	12.7	87.3	34.8	7.2	45.3	32.3	12.9	16.8	15.7
2005	100.0	12.5	87.5	34.9	7.3	45.4	32.4	13.0	17.1	15.7
2006	100.0	12.1	87.9	34.4	7.3	46.2	33.6	12.6	19.1	14.7
2007	100.0	12.1	87.9	33.9	7.6	46.4	33.7	12.7	19.3	14.7
2008	100.0	11.9	88.1	33.5	7.3	47.3	34.9	12.4	20.1	14.7
Projected										
2009	100.0	11.5	88.5	32.7	7.1	48.7	37.2	11.5	20.5	15.3
2010	100.0	11.4	88.6	32.3	7.1	49.3	37.6	11.7	20.0	16.0
2011	100.0	11.1	88.9	31.9	7.1	49.9	36.4	13.5	20.1	16.5
2012	100.0	10.9	89.1	31.4	7.1	50.7	37.1	13.6	20.5	16.8
2013	100.0	10.8	89.2	31.1	7.1	50.9	37.4	13.6	20.7	17.0
2014	100.0	10.8	89.2	31.2	7.2	50.9	37.4	13.5	20.9	17.1
2015	100.0	10.8	89.2	31.3	7.3	50.7	37.3	13.4	20.7	17.2
2016	100.0	10.7	89.3	31.2	7.3	50.8	37.4	13.4	20.8	17.3
2017	100.0	10.6	89.4	31.0	7.3	51.1	37.7	13.4	21.1	17.4
2018	100.0	10.5	89.5	30.7	7.3	51.5	38.1	13.4	21.4	17.6
2019	100.0	10.4	89.6	30.4	7.3	51.9	38.6	13.4	21.8	17.7

According to Christopher J. Truffer et al., in "Health Spending Projections through 2019: The Recession's Impact Continues" (*Health Affairs*, vol. 29, no. 3, March–April 2010), national health spending grew by 5.7%, from $2.3 trillion in 2008 to $2.5 trillion in 2009, rising to 17.3% of the GDP. This steep rate increase was the largest one-year increase in the health share of the GDP since the National Health Expenditure Accounts started tracking health spending in 1960. Truffer et al. explain that the economic recession, high rates of unemployment that reduced private health insurance enrollment, and the aging U.S. population contributed to this

| | | | Third-party payments | | | | | | | |
| | | | | | | Public | | | | |
Year	Total	Out-of-pocket payments	Total	Private health insurance	Other private funds	Total	Federal[a]	State and local[a]	Medicare[b]	Medicaid[c]
Historical estimates					Annual percent change from previous year shown					
2004	—	—	—	—	—	—	—	—	—	—
2005	6.9	5.4	7.1	6.9	7.3	7.1	6.9	7.6	9.2	7.2
2006	6.6	3.0	7.1	5.3	7.0	8.4	10.6	3.0	18.7	−0.5
2007	6.0	6.0	6.0	4.4	10.8	6.5	6.4	6.5	7.1	6.1
2008	4.4	2.8	4.7	3.1	0.1	6.5	8.2	2.2	8.6	4.7
Projected										
2009	5.7	2.1	6.2	3.3	3.2	8.7	12.4	−1.7	8.1	9.9
2010	3.9	3.0	4.1	2.5	3.4	5.2	5.1	5.3	1.5	8.9
2011	5.2	2.7	5.5	4.0	4.6	6.6	2.0	21.7	5.8	8.5
2012	5.5	3.7	5.7	3.7	5.5	7.0	7.4	5.8	7.6	7.0
2013	6.1	5.2	6.2	5.4	6.7	6.7	6.9	6.1	7.0	7.3
2014	6.6	6.4	6.7	6.7	7.5	6.6	6.7	6.0	7.3	7.5
2015	6.7	6.7	6.7	7.1	8.3	6.3	6.2	6.3	6.1	7.5
2016	7.0	6.3	7.1	6.8	7.9	7.2	7.4	6.7	7.5	7.6
2017	6.8	5.6	7.0	6.2	7.0	7.5	7.7	6.8	8.2	7.6
2018	6.8	5.6	6.9	5.8	6.9	7.7	8.0	6.8	8.5	7.6
2019	6.6	5.6	6.8	5.4	6.5	7.6	8.0	6.6	8.6	7.5

[a]Includes Medicaid SCHIP (State Children's Health Insurance Program) Expansion and SCHIP.
[b]Subset of federal funds.
[c]Subset of federal and state and local funds.
[d]Calculation of per capita estimates is inappropriate.
Note: Numbers and percents may not add to totals because of rounding.

SOURCE: "Table 3. National Health Expenditures; Aggregate and per Capita Amounts, Percent Distribution and Annual Percent Change by Source of Funds: Calendar Years 2004–2019," in *National Health Expenditures Projections 2009–2019*, U.S. Department of Health and Human Services, Centers for Medicare and Medicaid Services, 2009, http://www.cms.gov/NationalHealthExpendData/downloads/proj2009.pdf (accessed May 21, 2010)

increase and will continue to influence health care expenditures from 2009 to 2019. The researchers observe that public health care spending rates will exceed private spending for hospital, physician, and clinical services from 2009 to 2012 and that by 2012 "public spending will account for more than half (52%) of all U.S. health care spending."

Truffer et al. indicate that from 2009 to 2019 health care spending is projected to grow at an average rate of 6.1% per year, which is a full 1.7% faster than the GDP. By 2019 spending for hospital care will be 6.6%, spending for physician and clinical services will be 6.4%, and spending on prescription drugs will be 7.3%. A significant proportion of this increase is attributable to the enormous baby-boom generation (people born between 1946 and 1964), much of which is now eligible for government-sponsored health care. The first wave of baby boomers is eligible for Medicare in 2011.

CONTROLLING HEALTH CARE SPENDING

In an effort to control health expenditures, the nation's health care system underwent some dramatic changes. Beginning in the late 1980s employers began looking for new ways to contain health benefit costs for their employees. Many enrolled their employees in managed care programs as alternatives to traditional, fee-for-service insurance.

Managed care programs offered lower premiums by keeping a tighter control on costs and utilization and by emphasizing the importance of preventive care. Insurers negotiated discounts with providers (physicians, hospitals, clinical laboratories, and others) in exchange for guaranteed access to employer-insured groups. In 2008 private insurance (33.5%) and other private funds (7.3%) paid for 40.8% of the nation's health costs. (See Table 5.4.) Public sources covered 47.3% of the nation's costs, and 11.9% of the costs came directly from consumers' pockets.

How Will the 2010 Health Care Reform Legislation Influence Health Care Spending?

Phil Galewitz explains in "Consumers Guide to Health Reform" (April 13, 2010, http://www.kaiserhealthnews.org/stories/2010/march/22/consumers-guide-health-reform.aspx) that the Patient Protection and Affordable Care Act (PPACA) of 2010 is projected to cost $938 billion over 10 years. Furthermore, the Congressional Budget Office (CBO; March 20, 2010, http://www.cbo.gov/ftpdocs/113xx/doc11379/AmendReconProp.pdf) anticipates that the legislation will produce a net reduction in federal deficits of $143 billion from 2010 to 2019 in response to changes in spending and revenues.

Revenues will be generated through higher taxes and fees and cost savings will be realized as a result of reduced Medicare payments to health care providers. For example,

TABLE 5.5

National health expenditures, by type of expenditures, 2004–19

										Projected					
Type of expenditure	2004	2005	2006	2007	2008	2009	2010	2011	2012	2013	2014	2015	2016	2017	2018	2019
	Amount in billions															
National health expenditures	$1,855.4	$1,982.5	$2,112.5	$2,239.7	$2,338.7	$2,472.2	$2,569.6	$2,702.9	$2,850.2	$3,024.7	$3,225.3	$3,441.9	$3,683.8	$3,936.0	$4,203.6	$4,482.7
Health services and supplies	1733.6	1851.9	1975.4	2089.7	2181.3	2306.2	2395.0	2518.7	2655.5	2817.3	3003.2	3202.4	3426.1	3660.2	3908.8	4169.7
Personal health care	1549.9	1655.2	1762.9	1866.4	1952.3	2068.3	2141.7	2244.6	2368.0	2512.1	2677.1	2853.8	3050.8	3256.7	3477.0	3709.0
Hospital care	566.5	607.5	649.4	687.6	718.4	760.6	788.9	827.3	875.8	932.4	996.3	1063.2	1137.7	1213.2	1292.4	1374.5
Professional services	581.2	621.5	658.4	697.5	731.2	777.3	797.2	832.8	877.9	930.4	989.7	1053.4	1125.5	1202.1	1284.4	1370.7
Physician and clinical services	393.6	422.4	446.5	472.6	496.2	527.6	535.8	556.1	582.3	612.3	646.8	684.0	728.3	776.6	828.1	882.0
Other professional services	52.9	55.9	58.4	62.2	65.7	69.6	71.4	74.6	79.3	84.3	90.0	96.0	102.3	109.0	116.1	123.7
Dental services	81.5	86.3	90.7	96.4	101.2	104.4	107.9	111.8	118.1	126.5	135.7	145.2	154.3	162.6	171.4	180.4
Other personal health care	53.3	56.9	62.7	66.3	68.1	75.7	82.2	90.3	98.2	107.2	117.2	128.2	140.5	154.0	168.9	184.6
Nursing home and home health	157.9	168.8	178.1	191.7	203.1	216.3	226.4	239.0	252.8	268.8	286.9	306.3	327.3	349.5	373.7	399.7
Home health care	42.7	48.1	53.0	59.3	64.7	72.2	77.1	82.8	89.1	96.2	104.2	112.6	121.8	131.7	142.3	153.8
Nursing home care	115.2	120.7	125.1	132.4	138.4	144.1	149.3	156.2	163.7	172.6	182.7	193.7	205.4	217.8	231.4	245.9
Retail outlet sales of medical products	244.3	257.4	277.0	289.7	299.6	314.1	329.1	345.4	361.4	380.5	404.3	430.9	460.4	491.9	526.5	564.1
Prescription drugs	188.8	199.7	217.0	226.8	234.1	246.3	260.1	274.5	287.5	302.9	322.1	343.8	368.4	395.4	425.2	457.8
Other medical products	55.5	57.7	60.0	62.9	65.5	67.8	69.1	70.9	73.9	77.6	82.2	87.1	92.1	96.5	101.3	106.4
Durable medical equipment	22.8	23.8	24.7	25.5	26.6	27.0	27.4	28.1	29.2	30.7	32.6	34.7	36.9	38.8	40.9	43.0
Other non-durable medical products	32.7	34.0	35.3	37.4	39.0	40.8	41.6	42.8	44.7	46.9	49.5	52.4	55.2	57.7	60.4	63.3
Program administration and net cost of private health insurance	129.8	140.3	152.0	158.4	159.6	162.8	172.6	189.5	198.2	210.3	225.1	240.6	260.0	280.5	300.6	320.3
Government public health activities	53.8	56.4	60.6	64.8	69.4	75.2	80.8	84.6	89.4	94.9	101.0	107.9	115.2	123.0	131.3	140.3
Investment	121.8	130.6	137.1	150.0	157.5	166.0	174.6	184.2	194.7	207.4	222.1	239.5	257.8	275.8	294.8	313.0
Research*	38.9	40.7	41.8	42.5	43.6	48.0	51.3	54.2	57.7	61.6	65.9	70.4	75.2	80.3	85.6	91.2
Structures & equipment	83.0	90.0	95.3	107.5	113.9	117.9	123.3	130.0	137.1	145.8	156.2	169.1	182.5	195.5	209.2	221.8
	Percent distribution															
National health expenditures	—	6.9	6.6	6.0	4.4	5.7	3.9	5.2	5.5	6.1	6.6	6.6	7.0	6.8	6.8	6.6
Health services and supplies	—	6.8	6.7	5.8	4.4	5.7	3.8	5.2	5.4	6.1	6.6	6.6	7.0	6.8	6.8	6.7
Personal health care	—	6.8	6.5	5.9	4.6	5.9	3.5	4.8	5.5	6.1	6.6	6.6	6.9	6.7	6.8	6.7
Hospital care	—	7.2	6.9	5.9	4.5	5.9	3.7	4.9	5.9	6.5	6.9	6.7	7.0	6.6	6.5	6.3
Professional services	—	6.9	5.9	5.9	4.8	6.3	2.6	4.5	5.4	6.0	6.4	6.4	6.8	6.8	6.8	6.7
Physician and clinical services	—	7.3	5.7	5.8	5.0	6.3	1.5	3.8	4.7	6.0	5.6	5.7	6.5	6.6	6.5	6.5
Other professional services	—	5.8	4.4	6.5	5.6	5.9	2.7	4.4	6.3	6.4	6.7	6.6	6.5	6.5	6.5	6.5
Dental services	—	6.0	5.1	6.2	5.1	3.2	3.3	3.6	5.7	7.1	7.2	7.1	6.2	5.4	5.4	5.2
Other personal health care	—	6.8	10.3	5.8	2.6	11.2	8.5	9.9	8.8	9.2	9.3	9.4	9.6	9.6	9.6	9.3
Nursing home and home health	—	6.9	5.6	7.6	6.0	6.5	4.7	5.6	5.8	6.3	6.7	6.8	6.8	6.8	6.9	7.0
Home health care	—	12.6	10.3	11.8	9.0	11.7	6.8	7.4	7.6	8.0	8.3	8.1	8.2	8.1	8.1	8.0
Nursing home care	—	4.8	3.7	5.8	4.6	4.1	3.6	4.6	4.8	5.4	5.9	6.0	6.1	6.0	6.2	6.3
Retail outlet sales of medical products	—	5.4	7.6	4.6	3.4	4.8	4.8	5.0	4.6	5.3	6.2	6.6	6.8	6.8	7.0	7.2
Prescription drugs	—	5.8	8.7	4.5	3.2	5.2	5.6	5.6	4.7	5.4	6.3	6.7	7.1	7.3	7.5	7.7
Other medical products	—	4.0	4.0	4.8	4.1	3.5	1.8	2.7	4.2	5.1	5.9	6.0	5.7	4.9	4.9	5.0
Durable medical equipment	—	4.1	4.0	3.3	4.1	1.7	1.5	2.4	3.9	5.2	6.4	6.5	6.1	5.2	5.3	5.3
Other non-durable medical products	—	3.9	4.0	5.9	4.2	4.7	2.0	2.9	4.3	5.0	5.6	5.7	5.4	4.6	4.7	4.8
Program administration and net cost of private health insurance	—	8.1	8.3	4.3	0.7	2.0	6.0	9.8	4.6	6.1	7.0	6.9	8.1	7.9	7.2	6.6
Government public health activities	—	4.7	7.4	7.1	7.1	8.2	7.5	4.8	5.6	6.2	6.5	6.8	6.7	6.8	6.8	6.9
Investment	—	7.2	5.0	9.4	5.0	5.4	5.2	5.5	5.7	6.5	7.1	7.8	7.6	7.0	6.9	6.2
Research*	—	4.6	2.9	1.6	2.6	10.2	6.7	5.8	6.4	6.8	7.0	6.8	6.8	6.7	6.7	6.5
Structures & equipment	—	8.5	5.9	12.9	5.9	3.6	4.6	5.4	5.5	6.4	7.1	8.3	8.0	7.1	7.0	6.1

*Research and development expenditures of drug companies and other manufacturers and providers of medical equipment and supplies are excluded from research expenditures. These research expenditures are implicitly included in the expenditure class in which the product falls, in that they are covered by the payment received for that product.

Note: Numbers may not add to totals because of rounding.

SOURCE: "Table 2. National Health Expenditure Amounts, and Annual Percent Change by Type of Expenditure: Calendar Years 2004–2019," in National Health Expenditures Projections 2009–2019, U.S. Department of Health and Human Services, Centers for Medicare and Medicaid Services, 2009, http://www.cms.gov/NationalHealthExpendData/downloads/proj2009.pdf (accessed May 21, 2010)

TABLE 5.6

Personal health expenditures, by source of funds, 2004–19

Year	Total	Out-of-pocket payments	Third-party payments Total	Private health insurance	Other private funds	Public Total	Federal[a]	State and local[a]	Medicare[b]	Medicaid[c]
Historical estimates					Amount in billions					
2004	$1,549.9	$234.8	$1,315.1	$560.3	$65.3	$689.4	$527.3	$162.1	$300.3	$269.9
2005	1,655.2	247.5	1,407.7	599.8	68.7	739.3	562.3	176.9	326.3	288.8
2006	1,762.9	254.9	1,508.0	634.6	74.6	798.8	620.1	178.7	382.1	285.9
2007	1,866.4	270.3	1,596.1	665.1	81.0	850.1	661.3	188.7	408.2	303.4
2008	1,952.3	277.8	1,674.5	691.2	75.5	907.8	718.0	189.8	444.3	316.7
Projected										
2009	2,068.3	283.5	1,784.8	718.5	77.1	989.2	808.3	180.9	481.2	348.1
2010	2,141.7	292.1	1,849.6	732.9	78.6	1,038.1	847.9	190.2	488.8	379.1
2011	2,244.6	299.9	1,944.6	753.9	81.1	1,109.6	863.1	246.4	517.2	411.0
2012	2,368.0	311.1	2,056.9	782.7	85.1	1,189.1	927.2	262.0	556.5	439.8
2013	2,512.1	327.3	2,184.9	824.4	90.3	1,270.2	991.2	279.0	595.3	472.0
2014	2,677.1	348.1	2,329.0	878.4	96.8	1,353.7	1,057.4	296.3	638.7	507.4
2015	2,853.8	371.6	2,482.2	939.5	104.2	1,438.4	1,123.0	315.4	678.0	545.7
2016	3,050.8	395.0	2,655.8	1,001.2	111.7	1,543.0	1,205.6	337.3	728.5	587.0
2017	3,256.7	417.3	2,839.4	1,059.7	118.8	1,660.9	1,299.9	361.0	788.0	631.6
2018	3,477.0	440.8	3,036.2	1,118.7	126.1	1,791.3	1,404.8	386.5	855.4	679.6
2019	3,709.0	465.6	3,243.4	1,177.9	133.8	1,931.8	1,518.3	413.5	928.7	730.5
Historical estimates					Per capita amount					
2004	$5,286	$801	$4,485	$1,911	$223	$2,351	$1,798	$553	d	d
2005	5,595	837	4,758	2,027	232	2,499	1,901	598	d	d
2006	5,901	853	5,047	2,124	250	2,674	2,076	598	d	d
2007	6,186	896	5,290	2,204	268	2,817	2,192	626	d	d
2008	6,411	912	5,499	2,270	248	2,981	2,358	623	d	d
Projected									d	d
2009	6,732	923	5,809	2,339	251	3,220	2,631	589	d	d
2010	6,909	942	5,967	2,364	254	3,349	2,736	613	d	d
2011	7,178	959	6,219	2,411	260	3,548	2,760	788	d	d
2012	7,506	986	6,520	2,481	270	3,770	2,939	831	d	d
2013	7,894	1,028	6,866	2,591	284	3,991	3,115	877	d	d
2014	8,340	1,085	7,256	2,737	302	4,217	3,294	923	d	d
2015	8,814	1,148	7,667	2,902	322	4,443	3,469	974	d	d
2016	9,343	1,210	8,133	3,066	342	4,725	3,692	1,033	d	d
2017	9,889	1,267	8,622	3,218	361	5,044	3,947	1,096	d	d
2018	10,470	1,327	9,143	3,369	380	5,394	4,230	1,164	d	d
2019	11,077	1,390	9,686	3,518	399	5,769	4,534	1,235	d	d
Historical estimates					Percent distribution					
2004	100.0	15.2	84.8	36.2	4.2	44.5	34.0	10.5	19.4	17.4
2005	100.0	15.0	85.0	36.2	4.1	44.7	34.0	10.7	19.7	17.4
2006	100.0	14.5	85.5	36.0	4.2	45.3	35.2	10.1	21.7	16.2
2007	100.0	14.5	85.5	35.6	4.3	45.5	35.4	10.1	21.9	16.3
2008	100.0	14.2	85.8	35.4	3.9	46.5	36.8	9.7	22.8	16.2
Projected										
2009	100.0	13.7	86.3	34.7	3.7	47.8	39.1	8.7	23.3	16.8
2010	100.0	13.6	86.4	34.2	3.7	48.5	39.6	8.9	22.8	17.7
2011	100.0	13.4	86.6	33.6	3.6	49.4	38.5	11.0	23.0	18.3
2012	100.0	13.1	86.9	33.1	3.6	50.2	39.2	11.1	23.5	18.6
2013	100.0	13.0	87.0	32.8	3.6	50.6	39.5	11.1	23.7	18.8
2014	100.0	13.0	87.0	32.8	3.6	50.6	39.5	11.1	23.9	19.0
2015	100.0	13.0	87.0	32.9	3.7	50.4	39.4	11.1	23.8	19.1
2016	100.0	12.9	87.1	32.8	3.7	50.6	39.5	11.1	23.9	19.2
2017	100.0	12.8	87.2	32.5	3.6	51.0	39.9	11.1	24.2	19.4
2018	100.0	12.7	87.3	32.2	3.6	51.5	40.4	11.1	24.6	19.5
2019	100.0	12.6	87.4	31.8	3.6	52.1	40.9	11.1	25.0	19.7

Galewitz notes that beginning in 2013 individuals and couples with an income in excess of between $200,000 and $250,000 will pay a Medicare payroll tax of 2.3%, which is an increase from the 2010 rate of 1.4%. High-income taxpayers also will be required to pay a 3.8% tax on unearned income over the earning limits. The act levies a 40% excise tax (often referred to as a Cadillac tax because it applies to higher cost plans) starting in 2018 on richer, more costly health coverage—the portion of employer sponsored plans that is more than $10,200 per year for individuals and $27,500 for families. The CBO estimates this excise tax will raise $32 billion over a decade.

According to Galewitz, the act also raises the threshold for deducting out-of-pocket unreimbursed medical

TABLE 5.6

Personal health expenditures, by source of funds, 2004–19 [CONTINUED]

Year	Total	Out-of-pocket payments	Third-party payments Total	Private health insurance	Other private funds	Public Total	Federal[a]	State and local[a]	Medicare[b]	Medicaid[c]
Historical estimates				Annual percent change from previous year shown						
2004	—	—	—	—	—	—	—	—	—	—
2005	6.8	5.4	7.0	7.0	5.1	7.2	6.6	9.2	8.7	7.0
2006	6.5	3.0	7.1	5.8	8.7	8.1	10.3	1.0	17.1	−1.0
2007	5.9	6.0	5.8	4.8	8.5	6.4	6.6	5.6	6.8	6.1
2008	4.6	2.8	4.9	3.9	−6.7	6.8	8.6	0.6	8.9	4.4
Projected										
2009	5.9	2.1	6.6	4.0	2.0	9.0	12.6	−4.7	8.3	9.9
2010	3.5	3.0	3.6	2.0	2.0	4.9	4.9	5.1	1.6	8.9
2011	4.8	2.7	5.1	2.9	3.3	6.9	1.8	29.6	5.8	8.4
2012	5.5	3.7	5.8	3.8	4.8	7.2	7.4	6.3	7.6	7.0
2013	6.1	5.2	6.2	5.3	6.2	6.8	6.9	6.5	7.0	7.3
2014	6.6	6.4	6.6	6.6	7.2	6.6	6.7	6.2	7.3	7.5
2015	6.6	6.7	6.6	7.0	7.6	6.3	6.2	6.5	6.2	7.5
2016	6.9	6.3	7.0	6.6	7.2	7.3	7.4	6.9	7.5	7.6
2017	6.7	5.6	6.9	5.8	6.3	7.6	7.8	7.0	8.2	7.6
2018	6.8	5.6	6.9	5.6	6.2	7.9	8.1	7.1	8.5	7.6
2019	6.7	5.6	6.8	5.3	6.0	7.8	8.1	7.0	8.6	7.5

[a]Includes Medicaid State Children's Health Insurance Program (SCHIP) Expansion and SCHIP.
[b]Subset of federal funds.
[c]Subset of federal and state and local funds.
[d]Calculation of per capita estimates is inappropriate.
Note: Numbers and percents may not add to totals because of rounding.

SOURCE: "Table 5. Personal Health Care Expenditures; Aggregate and per Capita Amounts, Percent Distribution and Annual Percent Change by Source of Funds: Calendar Years 2004–2019," in *National Health Expenditures Projections 2009–2019*, U.S. Department of Health and Human Services, Centers for Medicare and Medicaid Services, 2009, http://www.cms.gov/NationalHealthExpendData/downloads/proj2009.pdf (accessed May 21, 2010)

expenses from 7.5% of a taxpayer's adjusted gross income to 10%. Beginning in 2013 it also limits contributions to flexible spending accounts, which may be used to pay medical expenses to $2,500, and charges tanning salon users a 10% tax.

Prescription Drug Prices Continue to Rise

One of the fastest-growing components of health care is the market for prescription drugs. In 2008 Americans spent $234.1 billion on prescription medication—this was a 3.2% increase from $226.8 billion in 2007. (See Table 5.5.) A large part of the increase was financed by private insurers, who paid $98.5 billion of the drug costs in 2008, slightly more than the previous year's $97.8 billion. (See Table 5.7.) The aging population and the fact that prescription drugs are increasingly substituted for other types of health care have fueled growth in this sector of health services. For example, antidepressant drugs have demonstrated effectiveness in place of more expensive psychotherapy.

In *Rx Watchdog Report Trends in Manufacturer Prices of Prescription Drugs Used by Medicare Beneficiaries 2008 Year-End Update* (April 2009, http://assets.aarp .org/rgcenter/health/2009_07_rxq408.pdf), Leigh Purvis, Stephen W. Schondelmeyer, and David J. Gross note that the average annual increase in manufacturer prices for selected drugs widely used by Medicare beneficiaries

consistently surpasses the general inflation rate. For example, in 2008 the average rate of increase for these widely used drugs was 4.5%, which was higher than the general inflation rate of 3.8%. All but seven of the 219 brand-name drugs the researchers considered had price increases that exceeded the rate of general inflation in 2008.

The Medicare drug benefit, which was implemented in 2006, was intended to increase government spending for prescription drugs and provide prescription drug savings for older Americans and people with disabilities. The voluntary program allows Medicare beneficiaries to choose from dozens of plans that are offered by health insurers and health plans called pharmacy benefit managers.

Purvis, Schondelmeyer, and Gross observe that manufacturers' drug price increases produce higher pharmacy prices and higher out-of-pocket costs for Medicare beneficiaries who pay a percent of their drug costs as opposed to fixed co-payment per prescription. The higher prices also result in higher costs for drug plans, which in turn may serve to increase the plans' premiums or cause them to reduce benefits.

THE 2010 HEALTH CARE REFORM LEGISLATION STRENGTHENS MEDICARE DRUG BENEFIT. The PPACA reduced Medicare Part D enrollees' out-of-pocket drug costs when they reach the coverage gap, known as the

TABLE 5.7

Prescription drug expenditures, by source of funds, 2004–19

| | | | Third-party payments | | | | | | | |
| | | | | | | | Public | | | |
Year	Total	Out-of-pocket payments	Total	Private health insurance	Other private funds	Total	Federal[a]	State and local[a]	Medicare[b]	Medicaid[c]
Historical estimates					Amount in billions					
2004	$188.8	$46.2	$142.6	$90.0	$0.0	$52.5	$31.4	$21.1	$3.4	$36.3
2005	199.7	48.8	150.9	95.8	0.0	55.1	32.6	22.5	3.9	37.2
2006	217.0	46.9	170.1	96.2	0.0	73.9	58.7	15.2	39.6	19.1
2007	226.8	48.9	177.8	97.8	0.0	80.0	65.4	14.7	46.0	18.8
2008	234.1	48.5	185.5	98.5	0.0	87.0	72.5	14.5	52.1	19.4
Projected										
2009	246.3	49.0	197.3	100.8	0.0	96.5	82.8	13.7	57.8	21.2
2010	260.1	50.9	209.1	104.5	0.0	104.7	89.7	15.0	61.6	23.9
2011	274.5	52.3	222.2	108.3	0.0	113.9	95.0	18.9	67.2	25.8
2012	287.5	53.4	234.1	110.9	0.0	123.2	103.1	20.2	73.3	27.5
2013	302.9	55.4	247.5	114.9	0.0	132.6	111.1	21.5	79.5	29.3
2014	322.1	58.5	263.6	121.5	0.0	142.1	119.3	22.8	86.5	31.4
2015	343.8	62.0	281.8	129.1	0.0	152.6	128.4	24.2	93.8	33.6
2016	368.4	65.7	302.7	136.9	0.0	165.8	139.8	26.0	102.6	35.9
2017	395.4	69.6	325.8	145.5	0.0	180.3	152.4	27.9	112.4	38.3
2018	425.2	73.9	351.3	154.9	0.0	196.4	166.5	29.9	123.5	40.8
2019	457.8	78.6	379.2	165.0	0.0	214.2	182.1	32.1	135.8	43.5
Historical estimates					Per capita amount					
2004	$644	$158	$486	$307	$0	$179	$107	$72	d	d
2005	675	165	510	324	0	186	110	76	d	d
2006	726	157	569	322	0	247	196	51	d	d
2007	752	162	589	324	0	265	217	49	d	d
2008	769	159	609	324	0	286	238	48	d	d
Projected									d	d
2009	802	160	642	328	0	314	269	45	d	d
2010	839	164	675	337	0	338	289	48	d	d
2011	878	167	711	346	0	364	304	60	d	d
2012	911	169	742	351	0	391	327	64	d	d
2013	952	174	778	361	0	417	349	68	d	d
2014	1,003	182	821	378	0	443	372	71	d	d
2015	1,062	192	870	399	0	471	397	75	d	d
2016	1,128	201	927	419	0	508	428	80	d	d
2017	1,201	211	989	442	0	548	463	85	d	d
2018	1,280	223	1,058	466	0	591	501	90	d	d
2019	1,367	235	1,132	493	0	640	544	96	d	d
Historical estimates					Percent distribution					
2004	100.0	24.5	75.5	47.7	0.0	27.8	16.6	11.2	1.8	19.2
2005	100.0	24.4	75.6	48.0	0.0	27.6	16.3	11.3	2.0	18.6
2006	100.0	21.6	78.4	44.3	0.0	34.1	27.1	7.0	18.2	8.8
2007	100.0	21.6	78.4	43.1	0.0	35.3	28.8	6.5	20.3	8.3
2008	100.0	20.7	79.3	42.1	0.0	37.2	31.0	6.2	22.2	8.3
Projected										
2009	100.0	19.9	80.1	40.9	0.0	39.2	33.6	5.6	23.5	8.6
2010	100.0	19.6	80.4	40.2	0.0	40.2	34.5	5.8	23.7	9.2
2011	100.0	19.1	80.9	39.5	0.0	41.5	34.6	6.9	24.5	9.4
2012	100.0	18.6	81.4	38.6	0.0	42.9	35.9	7.0	25.5	9.6
2013	100.0	18.3	81.7	37.9	0.0	43.8	36.7	7.1	26.2	9.7
2014	100.0	18.2	81.8	37.7	0.0	44.1	37.0	7.1	26.8	9.8
2015	100.0	18.0	82.0	37.6	0.0	44.4	37.3	7.1	27.3	9.8
2016	100.0	17.8	82.2	37.2	0.0	45.0	37.9	7.1	27.8	9.7
2017	100.0	17.6	82.4	36.8	0.0	45.6	38.6	7.1	28.4	9.7
2018	100.0	17.4	82.6	36.4	0.0	46.2	39.2	7.0	29.0	9.6
2019	100.0	17.2	82.8	36.0	0.0	46.8	39.8	7.0	29.7	9.5

so-called donut hole. Most Medicare Part D basic drug benefit plans require enrollees to pay all their prescription drug costs after their drug spending exceeds the pre-designated dollar amount that is their initial coverage limit until they satisfy the dollar amount that qualifies them for catastrophic coverage. For example, for many Medicare beneficiaries the donut hole or gap during which Medicare beneficiaries must pay 100% of their prescription drug costs begins when total spending for drugs is $2,250 and closes when drug spending reaches $5,100. According to the Kaiser Family Foundation, in "Explaining Health Care Reform: Key Changes to the Medicare Part D Drug Benefit Coverage Gap" (March 2010, http://www.kff.org/healthreform/upload/8059.pdf), this gap was $3,610 in 2010 and is projected to exceed $6,000 by 2020.

TABLE 5.7

Prescription drug expenditures, by source of funds, 2004–19 [CONTINUED]

			Third-party payments			Public				
Year	Total	Out-of-pocket payments	Total	Private health insurance	Other private funds	Total	Federal[a]	State and local[a]	Medicare[b]	Medicaid[c]
Historical estimates				Annual percent change from previous year shown						
2004	—	—	—	—	—	—	—	—	—	—
2005	5.8	5.5	5.9	6.4	—	4.9	3.9	6.5	16.5	2.4
2006	8.7	−3.8	12.7	0.4	—	34.0	79.9	−32.5	905.2	−48.6
2007	4.5	4.3	4.5	1.7	—	8.3	11.3	−3.5	16.3	−1.7
2008	3.2	−0.8	4.3	0.7	—	8.7	10.9	−1.0	13.1	3.5
Projected										
2009	5.2	1.0	6.3	2.3	—	10.9	14.2	−5.6	10.9	9.1
2010	5.6	3.9	6.0	3.7	—	8.5	8.3	9.2	6.6	13.1
2011	5.6	2.8	6.2	3.7	—	8.8	5.9	25.9	9.1	7.7
2012	4.7	2.1	5.4	2.3	—	8.2	8.5	6.9	9.1	6.7
2013	5.4	3.8	5.7	3.6	—	7.6	7.8	6.7	8.5	6.7
2014	6.3	5.6	6.5	5.7	—	7.1	7.4	5.9	8.8	7.1
2015	6.7	6.0	6.9	6.3	—	7.4	7.6	6.4	8.5	6.9
2016	7.1	5.8	7.4	6.0	—	8.6	8.8	7.3	9.3	6.8
2017	7.3	6.0	7.6	6.2	—	8.8	9.1	7.2	9.6	6.7
2018	7.5	6.2	7.8	6.5	—	8.9	9.2	7.2	9.8	6.6
2019	7.7	6.3	7.9	6.6	—	9.0	9.4	7.2	10.0	6.5

[a]Includes Medicaid State Children's Health Insurance Program (SCHIP) Expansion and SCHIP.
[b]Subset of federal funds.
[c]Subset of federal and state and local funds.
[d]Calculation of per capita estimates is inappropriate.
Note: Numbers and percents may not add to totals because of rounding.

SOURCE: "Table 11. Prescription Drug Expenditures; Aggregate and per Capita Amounts, Percent Distribution and Annual Percent Change by Source of Funds: Calendar Years 2004–2019," in *National Health Expenditures Projections 2009–2019*, U.S. Department of Health and Human Services, Centers for Medicare and Medicaid Services, 2009, http://www.cms.gov/NationalHealthExpendData/downloads/proj2009.pdf (accessed May 21, 2010)

Effective in 2010, Part D enrollees who reach the coverage gap will receive a $250 rebate, and in 2011 Part D enrollees who reach the coverage gap will receive a 50% discount on the total cost of the brand-name drugs they purchase in the gap. Furthermore, Medicare will create subsidies for generic drugs in the coverage gap in 2011 and for brand-name drugs in 2013, thereby reducing the beneficiary coinsurance rate in the gap from 100% to 25% by 2020. The law also reduces the out-of-pocket spending required for enrollees' eligibility for catastrophic coverage, which further reduces out-of-pocket costs for people with high prescription drug expenses.

HEALTH CARE FOR OLDER ADULTS, PEOPLE WITH DISABILITIES, AND THE POOR

Despite passage of the groundbreaking PPACA, which promises to dramatically expand health care coverage, the United States remains one of the few industrialized nations that does not have a government-funded national health care program that provides coverage for all of its citizens. Government-funded health care exists, and it forms a major part of the health care system, but it is available only to specific segments of the U.S. population. In other developed countries government national medical care programs cover almost all their citizens' health-related costs, from maternity care to long-term care.

In the United States the major government health care entitlement programs are Medicare and Medicaid. They provide financial assistance for people aged 65 years and older, the poor, and people with disabilities. Before the existence of these programs, many older Americans could not afford adequate medical care. For older adults who are beneficiaries, the Medicare program provides reimbursement for hospital and physician care, whereas Medicaid pays for the cost of nursing home care.

Medicare

The Medicare program, which was enacted under Title XVIII (Health Insurance for the Aged) of the Social Security Act, was approved in 1965. The program consists of four parts:

- Part A provides hospital insurance. Coverage includes physicians' fees, nursing services, meals, semiprivate rooms, special-care units, operating room costs, laboratory tests, and some drugs and supplies. Part A also covers rehabilitation services, limited posthospital care in a skilled nursing facility, home health care, and hospice care for the terminally ill.

- Part B (Supplemental Medical Insurance [SMI]) is elective medical insurance; that is, enrollees must pay premiums to obtain coverage. SMI covers outpatient physicians' services, diagnostic tests, outpatient hospital services, outpatient physical therapy, speech pathology services, home health services, and medical equipment and supplies.

- Part C is the Medicare+Choice program, which was established by the Balanced Budget Act of 1997 to expand beneficiaries' options and allow them to participate in private-sector health plans.

- Part D is also elective and provides voluntary, subsidized access to prescription drug insurance coverage, for a premium, to individuals who are entitled to Part A or who are enrolled in Part B. Part D also has provisions (premium and cost-sharing subsidies) for low-income enrollees. Part D coverage began in 2006 and includes most of the prescription drugs that are approved by the U.S. Food and Drug Administration (FDA).

In general, Medicare reimburses physicians on a fee-for-service basis (paid for each visit, procedure, or treatment that is delivered), as opposed to per capita (per head) or per member per month. In response to the increasing administrative burden of paperwork, reduced compensation, and delays in reimbursements, some physicians opt out of Medicare participation—they do not provide services under the Medicare program and choose not to accept Medicare patients into their practice. Others still provide services to Medicare beneficiaries but do not "accept assignment," meaning that patients must pay out of pocket for services and then seek reimbursement from Medicare.

Because of these problems, the Tax Equity and Fiscal Responsibility Act of 1982 authorized a risk managed care option for Medicare, based on agreed-on prepayments. Beginning in 1985 the Health Care Financing Administration (now known as the CMS) could contract to pay health care providers, such as health maintenance organizations (HMOs) or health care prepayment plans, to serve Medicare and Medicaid patients. These groups are paid a predetermined cost per patient for their services.

Medicare-Risk HMOs Control Costs, but Some Senior Health Plans Do Not Survive

During the 1980s and 1990s the federal government, employers that provided health coverage for retiring employees, and many states sought to control costs by encouraging Medicare and Medicaid beneficiaries to enroll in HMOs. From the early 1980s through the late 1990s Medicare-risk HMOs did contain costs because, essentially, the federal government paid the health plans that operated them with fixed fees—a predetermined dollar amount per member per month (PMPM). For this fixed fee, Medicare recipients were to receive a fairly comprehensive, preset array of benefits. PMPM payment provided financial incentives for Medicare-risk HMO physicians to control costs, unlike physicians who were reimbursed on a fee-for-service basis.

Even though Medicare recipients were generally pleased with these HMOs (even when enrolling meant that they had to change physicians and thereby end long-standing relationships with their family doctors), many of the health plans did not fare well financially. The health plans suffered for a variety of reasons: some plans had underestimated the service utilization rates of older adults, and some were unable to provide the stipulated range of services as cost effectively as they had believed possible. Other plans found that the PMPM payment was simply not sufficient to enable them to cover all the clinical services and their administrative overhead.

Still, the health plans providing these senior HMOs competed fiercely to enroll older adults. Some health plans feared that closing their Medicare-risk programs would be viewed negatively by employer groups, which, when faced with the choice of plans that offered coverage for both younger workers and retirees or one that only covered the younger workers, would choose the plans that covered both. Despite losing money, most health plans maintained their Medicare-risk programs to avoid alienating the employers they depended on to enroll workers who were younger, healthier, and less expensive to serve than the older adults.

By the mid-1990s some of the Medicare-risk plans faced a challenge that proved daunting. Their enrollees had aged and required even more health care services than they had previously. For example, a senior HMO member who had joined as a healthy 65-year-old could now be a frail 75-year-old with multiple chronic health conditions requiring many costly health services. Even though the PMPM had increased over the years, for some plans it was simply insufficient to cover their costs. Some Medicare-risk plans, especially those operated by smaller health plans, were forced to end their programs abruptly, leaving thousands of older adults scrambling to join other health plans. Others endured by offering older adults comprehensive care and generating substantial cost savings for employers and the federal government.

The Balanced Budget Act of 1997 produced another plan for Medicare recipients called Medicare+Choice. This plan offers Medicare beneficiaries a wider range of managed care plan options than just HMOs—older adults may join preferred provider organizations (PPOs) and provider-sponsored organizations that generally offer greater freedom of choice of providers (physicians and hospitals) than what is available through HMO membership. These plans (as well as those formerly called Medicare-risk plans), are known as Medicare Advantage (MA) plans. MA plans include HMOs, PPOs, private fee-for-service plans, and medical savings account plans (which deposit money from Medicare into an account that can be used to pay medical expenses). According to the Kaiser Family Foundation, in "Total Medicare Advantage (MA)

Enrollment, 2010" (2010, http://www.statehealthfacts.org/comparetable.jsp?ind=327&cat=6), in 2010 these plans had nearly 11 million members.

Medicare Faces Challenges

With the dual challenges of providing increasingly expensive medical care to an aging population and keeping the program financially secure for the future, discussions about Medicare are likely to remain prominent on the nation's agenda in the years ahead.

—Kaiser Family Foundation, *Medicare: A Primer, 2010* (April 2010)

The Medicare program's continuing financial viability is in jeopardy. In 1995, for the first time since 1972, the Medicare trust fund lost money, a sign that the financial condition of Medicare was worse than previously assumed. The CMS did not expect a deficit until 1997; however, income to the trust fund, primarily from payroll taxes, was less than expected and spending was higher. The deficit is significant because losses are anticipated to grow from year to year. The Kaiser Family Foundation explains in *Medicare: A Primer, 2010* (April 2010, http://www.kff.org/medicare/upload/7615-03.pdf) that ensuring Medicare's long-term financial viability is a continuing and increasingly urgent challenge for policy makers. Medicare provides health coverage for 47 million beneficiaries, many of whom have multiple chronic conditions and significant health needs.

A NATIONAL BIPARTISAN COMMISSION CONSIDERS THE FUTURE OF MEDICARE. The National Bipartisan Commission on the Future of Medicare was created by Congress in the Balanced Budget Act of 1997. The commission was chaired by Senator John B. Breaux (1944–; D-LA) and Representative William M. Thomas (1941–; R-CA) and was charged with examining the Medicare program and drafting recommendations to avert a future financial crisis and reinforce the program in anticipation of the retirement of the baby boomers.

The commission observed that much like Social Security, Medicare would suffer because there would be fewer workers per retiree to fund it. Furthermore, it predicted that beneficiaries' out-of-pocket costs would rise and forecast soaring Medicare enrollment.

When the commission disbanded in March 1999, it was unable to forward an official recommendation to Congress because a plan endorsed by Senator Breaux fell one vote short of the required majority needed to authorize an official recommendation. The plan backed by Senator Breaux would have changed Medicare into a premium system, where instead of Medicare directly covering beneficiaries, the beneficiaries would be given a fixed amount of money to purchase private health insurance. The plan would have also raised the age of eligibility from 65 to 67 (as had already been done with Social Security in 1983) and provided prescription drug coverage for low-income beneficiaries, much like the Medicare Prescription Drug, Improvement, and Modernization Act of 2003.

In February 2010 President Barack Obama (1961–) established the National Commission on Fiscal Responsibility and Reform to suggest strategies to reduce the federal budget deficit. Among the commission's tasks is to recommend ways to slow the growth in entitlement program spending.

MEDICARE PRESCRIPTION DRUG, IMPROVEMENT, AND MODERNIZATION ACT AIMS TO REFORM MEDICARE. Supported by Senator Breaux, the Medicare Prescription Drug, Improvement, and Modernization Act of 2003 was a measure intended to introduce private-sector enterprise into a Medicare model in urgent need of reform.

The CMS explains in "2010 Part B Premium Amounts for Persons with Higher Income Levels" (October 19, 2009, http://questions.medicare.gov/app/answers/detail/a_id/2261) that older adults with substantial incomes face increasing Part B premium costs. In 2010 older adults with annual incomes below $85,000 (or $170,000 for couples) paid a monthly premium of $96.40; individuals earning $85,001 to $107,000 (or $170,001 to $214,000 for couples) paid $154.70; those earning $107,001 to $160,000 (or $214,001 to $320,000 for couples) paid $221.00; individuals making $160,001 to $214,000 (or $320,001 to $428,000 for couples) paid $287.30; and those earning more than $214,000 (or more than $428,000 for couples) paid $243.10.

The act also expands coverage of preventive medical services. According to the CMS, new beneficiaries will receive a free physical examination along with laboratory tests to screen for heart disease and diabetes. The act also provides employers with $89 billion in subsidies and tax breaks to help offset the costs associated with maintaining retiree health benefits.

Medicare reform continues to be hotly contested. The Kaiser Family Foundation indicates in "Democrats Push Three-Year Medicare 'Doc Fix' as Part of Larger Tax Bill" (May 21, 2010, http://www.kaiserhealthnews.org/Daily-Reports/2010/May/21/Doc-Fix-Medicare.aspx) that a major issue that attracted attention from policy makers, legislators, health care providers, and the public in 2010 was a proposed tax bill that would reduce Medicare payments to physicians and hospitals for three years. One of the controversial aspects of the proposal was the fact that in 2012 and 2013 primary care physicians would see higher rates of increase in payments than physician specialists.

IMPACT OF THE PPACA ON MEDICARE. In *Summary of New Health Reform Law* (June 18, 2010, http://www.kff.org/healthreform/upload/8061.pdf), the Kaiser Family Foundation indicates that besides changes in the prescription drug benefit (Part D) between 2014 and 2019, the health reform legislation reduces the out-of-pocket expenditures an individual must incur to become eligible for catastrophic coverage. It immediately extends Medicare coverage to individuals who have been exposed to environmental health hazards and have developed certain health conditions as a result of these exposures. For example, being exposed to asbestos (a group of minerals that are heat resistant and have been used in many industries) is considered an environmental health hazard because it is linked to the development of lung cancer, mesothelioma (a noncancerous tumor in the lining of the chest or abdomen), and other cancers. The act also gives a 10% bonus payment to primary care physicians practicing in underserved areas between 2011 and 2015 and in fiscal years (FYs) 2011 and 2012 it provides additional payments to hospitals with the lowest Medicare spending.

Medicaid

Medicaid was enacted by Congress in 1965 under Title XIX (Grants to States for Medical Assistance Programs) of the Social Security Act. It is a joint federal-state program that provides medical assistance to selected categories of low-income Americans: the aged, people who are blind or disabled, and financially struggling families with dependent children. Medicaid covers hospitalization, physicians' fees, laboratory and radiology fees, and long-term care in nursing homes. It is the largest source of funds for medical and health-related services for the poorest Americans and the second-largest public payer of health care costs, after Medicare.

The Deficit Reduction Act (DRA) was signed into law by President George W. Bush (1946–) in 2006. The DRA changed many aspects of the Medicaid program. Some of the changes are mandatory provisions that the states must enact, such as proof of citizenship and other criteria that will make it more difficult for people to qualify for or enroll in Medicaid. Other changes are optional; they allow the states to make drastic changes to the Medicaid program through state plan amendments. For example, states can choose to require anyone with a family income more than 150% of the poverty level to pay a premium of as much as 5% of their income. Before the DRA, the states had to provide a mandatory set of services to Medicaid recipients. As of March 31, 2006, the states could modify their Medicaid benefits such that they were comparable to those offered to federal and state employees, the benefits provided by the HMO with the largest non-Medicaid enrollment, or coverage approved by the U.S. secretary of health and human services.

Robert Pear reports in "New Medicaid Rules Allow States to Set Premiums and Higher Co-Payments" (*New York Times*, November 26, 2008) that a new federal rule was passed in November 2008 that permits states to charge premiums and higher co-payments to Medicaid recipients. The states can also deny coverage or services to people who do not pay their premiums or co-payments for specific health care services. This rule will enable states to increase revenues and contain losses that are associated with Medicaid. Between 2009 and 2014 the rule is anticipated to save the states about $1.1 billion and the federal government nearly $1.4 billion. Public health professionals as well as professional and consumer groups including the American Academy of Pediatrics, the National Association for Home Care, and the AARP (formerly the American Association of Retired Persons) fear that people unable to pay their premiums or co-payments may forgo or delay needed medical care.

According to Farhana Hossain and Kevin Quealy, in "How the Health Care Overhaul Could Affect You" (*New York Times*, March 21, 2010), the 2010 health care reform legislation prevents a state from dropping Medicaid coverage for beneficiaries until 2014, when insurance exchanges will be available, unless the state has a budget shortfall. States are prohibited from dropping children from Medicaid or the Children's Health Insurance Program until 2019. In 2014 people with incomes below 133% of the poverty level will be eligible for Medicaid coverage. Medicaid coverage will include preventive services at no cost, and payments to physicians will be increased to spur physicians to accept Medicaid patients into their practice.

LONG-TERM HEALTH CARE

One of the most urgent health care problems facing Americans in the 21st century is the growing need for long-term care. Long-term care refers to health and social services for people with chronic illnesses or mental or physical conditions so disabling that they cannot live independently without assistance—they require care daily. Longer life spans and improved life-sustaining technologies are increasing the likelihood that more people than ever before may eventually require costly, long-term care.

Limited and Expensive Options

Caring for chronically ill or elderly patients presents difficult and expensive choices for Americans: they must either provide long-term care at home or rely on a nursing home. Home health care was the fastest-growing segment of the health care industry during the first half of the 1990s. Even though the rate of growth slowed during the late 1990s, the CMS projects that the home health care sector will more than double, from $64.7 billion in 2008 to $153.8 billion in 2019. (See Table 5.5.)

High Cost of Long-Term Care

The options for quality, affordable long-term care in the United States are limited but improving. Nursing home costs average about $80,000 per year, depending on services and location. According to MetLife, in *The 2009 MetLife Market Survey of Nursing Home, Assisted Living, Adult Day Services, and Home Care Costs* (October 2009, http://www.metlife.com/assets/cao/mmi/publications/studies/mmi-market-survey-nursing-home-assisted-living.pdf), in 2009 nursing home care cost an average of $219 per day for a private room, or $79,935 per year. Many nursing home residents rely on Medicaid to pay these fees. In 2008 Medicaid covered 40.6% of nursing home costs for older Americans. (See Table 5.8.) The most common sources of payment at admission were Medicare (which pays only for short-term stays after hospitalization), private insurance, and other private funds. The primary source of payment changes as a stay lengthens. After their funds are exhausted, nursing home residents on Medicare shift to Medicaid.

To be eligible for Medicaid, a person must have no more than $2,500 in assets. (In the case of a married couple where only one spouse is in a nursing home, the remaining spouse can retain a house, a car, up to $75,000 in assets, and $2,000 in monthly income.) Many older adults must "spend down" to deplete their life savings to qualify for Medicaid assistance. This term refers to a provision in Medicaid coverage that provides care for seniors whose income exceeds eligibility requirements. For example, if their monthly income is $100 over the state Medicaid eligibility line, they can spend $100 per month on their medical care, and Medicaid will cover the remainder.

Nursing home care may seem cost-prohibitive, but even an unskilled caregiver who makes home visits earned an average of $18 per hour in 2009; skilled care costs much more, and most older adults cannot afford this expense. In *Genworth 2010 Cost of Care Survey: Home Care Providers, Adult Day Health Care Facilities, Assisted Living Facilities, and Nursing Homes* (April 2010, http://www.genworth.com/content/etc/medialib/genworth_v2/pdf/ltc_cost_of_care.Par.14625.File.dat/2010_Cost_of_Care_Survey_Full_Report.pdf), Genworth Financial indicates that in 2010 the average hourly rates were $18 for homemaker services and $19 for home health aide services, up about 3% from 2009.

It should be noted that lifetime savings may be exhausted long before the need for care ends. The National Health Policy Forum estimates in "National Spending for Long-Term Services and Supports" (April 30, 2010, http://www.nhpf.org/library/the-basics/Basics_LongTermServicesSupports_04-30-10.pdf) that the total expenditure for long-term care services for older adults in 2008 (excluding the value of donated care from relatives and friends) was $191.1 billion—nearly 10% of total U.S. personal health care spending. Approximately 6% of people who were aged 65 years in 2005 are likely to incur out-of-pocket long-term care expenses in excess of $100,000 over their remaining lifetime, and about 12% are likely to spend between $25,000 and $100,000.

The U.S. Census Bureau (March 18, 2004, http://www.census.gov/population/www/projections/usinterimproj/natprojtab02b.pdf) projects that the population over the age of 85 years (those most likely to require long-term care) will nearly triple by 2050. Even though disability rates among older adults have declined in recent years, reducing somewhat the need for long-term care, the CBO anticipates that the growing population of people likely to require long-term care will no doubt increase spending commensurate with this growth.

MENTAL HEALTH SPENDING

In *Projections of National Expenditures for Mental Health Services and Substance Abuse Treatment, 2004–2014* (2008, http://csat.samhsa.gov/IDBSE/spendEst/reports/MHSA_Est_Spending2003_2014.pdf), a study funded by the Substance Abuse and Mental Health Services Administration (SAMHSA), Katharine R. Levit et al. predict that spending for mental health and substance abuse (alcohol and chemical dependency) treatment in the United States will reach $239 billion in 2014, up from $121 billion in 2003, representing 6.9% of all health care spending. Even though mental health and substance abuse spending is projected to increase fourfold between 1986 and 2014, the rate of increase is less than the sixfold increase that is forecast for total health care spending. This is in part because mental health treatment does not involve the costly technology that drives overall health care costs. Figure 5.1 shows how mental health and substance abuse spending will account for a smaller share of total health care spending by 2014.

Levit et al. also report that:

- Mental health spending rose from an average of $136 per person in 1986 to $339 per person in 2003 and is forecast to reach $626 per person in 2014

- In 2014 Medicaid will pay 27% of mental health expenditures, private payers will pay 26%, and out-of-pocket costs will be 12%

- Prescription drug costs will increase from 23% in 2003 to 30% in 2014

- The largest contributors to the increase in mental health spending from 2003 to 2014 will be prescription drugs (37%), physician services (18%), and hospitals (17%) (see Figure 5.2)

Health care industry observers attribute the decrease in mental health inpatient services to the increased emphasis on

TABLE 5.8

Nursing home care expenditures, by source of funds, 2004–19

| | | | | | | Third-party payments | | | | |
| | | | | | | | Public | | | |
Year	Total	Out-of-pocket payments	Total	Private health insurance	Other private funds	Total	Federal[a]	State and local[a]	Medicare[b]	Medicaid[c]
Historical estimates						Amount in billions				
2004	$115.2	$30.9	$84.2	$8.7	$4.3	$71.3	$49.1	$22.2	$16.9	$51.5
2005	120.7	31.6	89.1	8.9	4.4	75.8	51.9	24.0	19.0	53.7
2006	125.1	32.6	92.5	9.2	4.5	78.8	54.3	24.5	21.0	54.5
2007	132.4	35.4	96.9	9.8	5.2	81.9	57.2	24.7	23.4	54.9
2008	138.4	36.9	101.5	10.3	5.1	86.2	62.1	24.1	25.7	56.3
Projected										
2009	144.1	37.0	107.1	10.4	5.2	91.5	70.6	20.9	27.6	59.5
2010	149.3	37.1	112.2	10.4	5.2	96.5	75.1	21.4	29.1	62.8
2011	156.2	37.8	118.4	10.5	5.4	102.5	72.6	29.9	30.7	66.9
2012	163.7	39.3	124.4	10.8	5.7	107.9	76.5	31.4	32.4	70.2
2013	172.6	41.3	131.2	11.3	6.1	113.8	80.8	33.0	34.5	73.8
2014	182.7	43.8	139.0	11.9	6.6	120.5	85.7	34.8	36.8	77.8
2015	193.7	46.5	147.2	12.5	7.1	127.6	90.8	36.9	39.0	82.3
2016	205.4	49.2	156.3	13.1	7.6	135.5	96.5	39.1	41.6	87.2
2017	217.8	51.7	166.1	13.6	8.2	144.3	102.8	41.5	44.5	92.6
2018	231.4	54.6	176.8	14.2	8.8	153.8	109.7	44.1	47.8	98.4
2019	245.9	57.7	188.2	14.8	9.5	163.9	117.0	46.9	51.3	104.6
Historical estimates						Per capita amount				
2004	$393	$106	$287	$30	$15	$243	$167	$76	(d)	(d)
2005	408	107	301	30	15	256	175	81	(d)	(d)
2006	419	109	310	31	15	264	182	82	(d)	(d)
2007	439	117	321	33	17	271	190	82	(d)	(d)
2008	455	121	333	34	17	283	204	79	(d)	(d)
Projected									(d)	(d)
2009	469	120	349	34	17	298	230	68	(d)	(d)
2010	482	120	362	34	17	311	242	69	(d)	(d)
2011	499	121	379	34	17	328	232	96	(d)	(d)
2012	519	125	394	34	18	342	242	99	(d)	(d)
2013	542	130	412	36	19	358	254	104	(d)	(d)
2014	569	136	433	37	20	375	267	108	(d)	(d)
2015	598	144	455	39	22	394	280	114	(d)	(d)
2016	629	151	479	40	23	415	295	120	(d)	(d)
2017	661	157	504	41	25	438	312	126	(d)	(d)
2018	697	164	532	43	27	463	330	133	(d)	(d)
2019	734	172	562	44	28	490	349	140	(d)	(d)
Historical estimates						Percent distribution				
2004	100.0	26.9	73.1	7.5	3.7	61.9	42.6	19.3	14.7	44.7
2005	100.0	26.2	73.8	7.3	3.6	62.9	43.0	19.9	15.8	44.5
2006	100.0	26.0	74.0	7.4	3.6	63.0	43.4	19.6	16.8	43.6
2007	100.0	26.8	73.2	7.4	3.9	61.9	43.2	18.6	17.6	41.4
2008	100.0	26.7	73.3	7.4	3.7	62.2	44.9	17.4	18.6	40.6
Projected										
2009	100.0	25.7	74.3	7.2	3.6	63.5	49.0	14.5	19.2	41.3
2010	100.0	24.9	75.1	7.0	3.5	64.6	50.3	14.3	19.5	42.1
2011	100.0	24.2	75.8	6.7	3.5	65.6	46.5	19.1	19.6	42.8
2012	100.0	24.0	76.0	6.6	3.5	65.9	46.7	19.2	19.8	42.9
2013	100.0	24.0	76.0	6.6	3.5	66.0	46.8	19.1	20.0	42.8
2014	100.0	24.0	76.0	6.5	3.6	66.0	46.9	19.1	20.1	42.6
2015	100.0	24.0	76.0	6.5	3.7	65.9	46.9	19.0	20.1	42.5
2016	100.0	23.9	76.1	6.4	3.7	66.0	47.0	19.0	20.3	42.5
2017	100.0	23.7	76.3	6.3	3.8	66.2	47.2	19.1	20.4	42.5
2018	100.0	23.6	76.4	6.1	3.8	66.5	47.4	19.1	20.6	42.5
2019	100.0	23.5	76.5	6.0	3.9	66.7	47.6	19.1	20.8	42.5

drug treatment of mental health disorders, the increasing frequency of outpatient treatment, the closure of psychiatric hospitals, and the cost containment efforts of managed care. Figure 5.2 shows an increasing share of mental health spending for prescription drugs. Levit et al. indicate that spending for prescription drugs increased from 7% in 1986 to 23% in 2003 and is projected to reach 30% in 2014. Despite the higher spending for these psychoactive prescription drugs, some industry observers believe the increased availability of effective drug therapy actually served to contain mental health spending by enabling providers to offer drug therapy instead of more costly inpatient treatment.

TABLE 5.8

Nursing home care expenditures, by source of funds, 2004–19 [CONTINUED]

Year	Total	Out-of-pocket payments	Total	Private health insurance	Other private funds	Total	Federal[a]	State and local[a]	Medicare[b]	Medicaid[c]
						Public				
Historical estimates			Annual percent change from previous year shown							
2004	—	—	—	—	—	—	—	—	—	—
2005	4.8	2.0	5.8	2.3	3.3	6.4	5.6	8.0	12.7	4.3
2006	3.7	3.1	3.8	4.0	3.4	3.8	4.6	2.2	10.6	1.5
2007	5.8	8.8	4.8	6.9	14.3	4.0	5.4	0.8	11.0	0.6
2008	4.6	4.2	4.7	4.6	−2.5	5.2	8.6	−2.5	10.2	2.6
Projected										
2009	4.1	0.1	5.5	1.2	1.9	6.2	13.6	−12.9	7.4	5.8
2010	3.6	0.4	4.7	0.1	1.3	5.4	6.5	2.0	5.2	5.6
2011	4.6	1.9	5.5	0.7	2.9	6.2	−3.4	39.8	5.4	6.5
2012	4.8	4.1	5.1	3.0	5.8	5.3	5.4	5.0	5.8	5.0
2013	5.4	5.0	5.5	4.5	6.9	5.5	5.7	5.2	6.4	5.1
2014	5.9	5.9	5.9	5.1	7.6	5.9	6.0	5.5	6.6	5.5
2015	6.0	6.2	5.9	5.3	8.0	5.9	5.9	5.8	6.0	5.8
2016	6.1	5.8	6.2	4.7	7.8	6.2	6.3	6.0	6.7	5.9
2017	6.0	5.2	6.3	4.0	7.4	6.5	6.5	6.2	7.0	6.2
2018	6.2	5.5	6.5	4.2	7.7	6.6	6.7	6.3	7.3	6.3
2019	6.3	5.8	6.5	4.0	7.8	6.6	6.7	6.3	7.3	6.3

[a]Includes Medicaid State Children's Health Insurance Program (SCHIP) Expansion and SCHIP.
[b]Subset of federal funds.
[c]Subset of federal and state and local funds.
[d]Calculation of per capita estimates is inappropriate.
Note: Numbers and percents may not add to totals because of rounding.

SOURCE: "Table 13. Nursing Home Care Expenditures; Aggregate and per Capita Amounts, Percent Distribution and Annual Percent Change by Source of Funds: Calendar Years 2004–2019," in *National Health Expenditures Projections 2009–2019*, U.S. Department of Health and Human Services, Centers for Medicare and Medicaid Services, 2009, http://www.cms.gov/NationalHealthExpendData/downloads/proj2009.pdf (accessed May 21, 2010)

SAMHSA Spending

In *Advancing the Health, Safety, and Well-Being of Our People* (2010, http://dhhs.gov/asfr/ob/docbudget/2011budgetinbrief.pdf), the U.S. Department of Health and Human Services (HHS) states that the FY 2011 budget request for SAMHSA was $3.7 billion, $110 million more than the FY 2010 budget. The funds were used to continue to prevent youth violence and reduce youth drug use, improve children's mental health, and help people with mental illness who face homelessness.

State Mental Health Agency Expenditures

A number of court rulings during the 1970s and an evolution in professional thinking prompted the release of many people with serious mental illness from institutions to community treatment programs. The census (the number of patients or occupants, which is frequently referred to as a rate) of public mental hospitals sharply declined, and there was increasing pressure on the states to deliver community-based treatment.

State mental health agencies (SMHAs) operate the public mental health system that acts as a safety net for poor, uninsured, and otherwise indigent people suffering from mental illness. In "A Primer on State Mental Health Agencies" (January 30, 2009, http://www.samhsa.gov/Financing/post/A-Primer-on-State-Mental-Health-Agencies.aspx), SAMHSA describes these public mental health

FIGURE 5.1

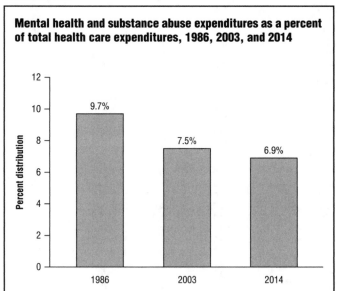

Mental health and substance abuse expenditures as a percent of total health care expenditures, 1986, 2003, and 2014

SOURCE: Katharine R. Levit et al., "Figure 2.1. MHSA Expenditures As a Percent of Total Health Care Expenditures: 1986, 2003, and 2014," in *Projections of National Expenditures for Mental Health and Substance Abuse Treatment 2004–2014*, Substance Abuse and Mental Health Services Administration, 2008, http://csat.samhsa.gov/IDBSE/spendEst/reports/MHSA_Est_Spending2003_2014.pdf (accessed May 24, 2010)

systems as "responsible for the delivery of mental health services to over 6 million persons each year and control

FIGURE 5.2

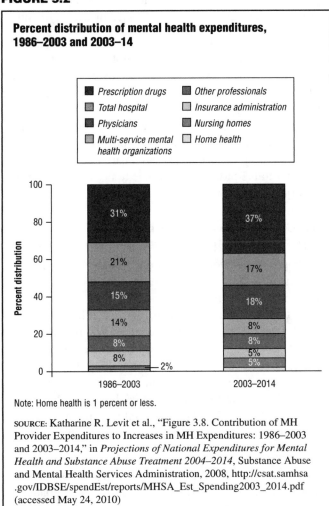

Percent distribution of mental health expenditures, 1986–2003 and 2003–14

Legend:
- Prescription drugs
- Total hospital
- Physicians
- Multi-service mental health organizations
- Other professionals
- Insurance administration
- Nursing homes
- Home health

Note: Home health is 1 percent or less.

SOURCE: Katharine R. Levit et al., "Figure 3.8. Contribution of MH Provider Expenditures to Increases in MH Expenditures: 1986–2003 and 2003–2014," in *Projections of National Expenditures for Mental Health and Substance Abuse Treatment 2004–2014*, Substance Abuse and Mental Health Services Administration, 2008, http://csat.samhsa.gov/IDBSE/spendEst/reports/MHSA_Est_Spending2003_2014.pdf (accessed May 24, 2010)

over $30 billion in expenditures for this care. The persons served by SMHAs are frequently minorities (31%), unemployed (22% were employed), lack private health insurance (54% receive Medicaid), and often have serious mental illnesses or emotional disturbances (66%)." The SMHAs vary from state to state—some purchase, regulate, administer, manage, and provide care and treatment; others simply purchase care using public funds that include general state revenues and federal funds. Generally, the federal funds are Medicare and Medicaid payments made to state-owned or state-operated facilities, although the SMHAs also administer additional Medicaid payments when the state Medicaid agency grants the SMHA control of all Medicaid mental health expenditures.

Similar to the movement of privately insured people into managed care, during the 1990s state Medicaid programs turned to managed care organizations (MCOs) and behavioral health services in an effort to contain costs. More than half the states have separated the administration and financing of physical health and mental health in their MCO contracts.

The SMHAs manage funds from the SAMHSA Mental Health Block Grant (MHBG) program. The MHBG was created in 1982 and its flexible funding enables states to innovate, develop, and expand successful community-based programs. Block grants (lump sums of money) are awarded based on a formula that considers each state's population, service costs, income, and taxable resources, and the funds enable the states to finance community mental health treatment programs. According to the HHS, in *Advancing the Health, Safety, and Well-Being of Our People*, the FY 2011 budget request included $421 million for MHBG funding.

HIGH COSTS OF RESEARCH

Medical and pharmaceutical research, disease prevention research, and the work to develop and conduct clinical trials of new drugs are expensive. The National Institutes of Health (NIH) reports in "Estimates of Funding for Various Research, Condition, and Disease Categories (RCDC)" (February 1, 2010, http://www.nih.gov/news/fundingresearchareas.htm) that its FY 2011 budget allocated an estimated $3.2 billion for human immunodeficiency virus (HIV) and acquired immunodeficiency syndrome (AIDS) research, compared with $784 million to investigate obesity prevention and treatment. Pharmaceutical manufacturers also spend billions of dollars every year researching and developing new medicines. For example, according to the Pharmaceutical Research and Manufacturers of America (PhRMA; 2010, http://www.phrma.org/about_phrma/), U.S. pharmaceutical companies spent $65.3 billion in 2009. By contrast, the entire NIH FY 2009 budget was $30.6 billion. (See Figure 4.5 in Chapter 4.)

Decisions about how much is spent to research a particular disease are not based solely on how many people develop the disease or die from it. Rightly or wrongly, economists base the societal value of an individual on his or her earning potential and productivity (the ability to contribute to society as a worker). The bulk of the people who die from heart disease, stroke, and cancer are older adults. Many have retired from the workforce, and their potential economic productivity is usually low or nonexistent. (This is not an observation about how society values older adults; instead, it is simply an economic measure of present and future financial productivity.)

In contrast, AIDS patients are often much younger and die in their 20s, 30s, and 40s. Until they developed AIDS, their potential productivity, measured in economic terms, was high. The number of work years lost when they die is considerable. Using this economic equation to determine how disease research should be funded, it may be considered economically wise to invest more money to research AIDS because the losses, which are measured in potential work years rather than in lives, is so much greater.

Once a new drug receives FDA approval, its manufacturer is ordinarily allowed to hold the patent on the drug to recoup its investment. During the life of the patent the drug is priced much higher than if other manufacturers were allowed to compete by producing generic versions of the same drug. After the patent expires, competition between pharmaceutical manufacturers generally lowers the price. For example, HIV/AIDS drugs are granted only seven years of exclusivity under legislation to encourage research and promote development of new treatments.

In *What Goes into the Cost of Prescription Drugs? ... and Other Questions about Your Medicines* (June 2005, http://www.phrma.org/files/attachments/Cost_of_Prescription_Drugs.pdf), PhRMA explains that the pharmaceutical manufacturer must cover the cost not only of research and development for the approximately three out of 10 drugs that succeed but also for many—seven out of 10—that fail. In contrast, the producer of generic drugs has the formula and must simply manufacture the drugs properly. On average, manufacturers spend over $800 million to bring brand-name drugs to market, including the expense of 12 to 15 years of product development. The generic manufacturer does not have to pay for successful and unsuccessful research and development of new drugs, nor does it have to pursue the complicated, time-consuming process of seeking and obtaining FDA approval. The generic manufacturer's FDA submission need only reference the original manufacturer's clinical data supporting the safety and efficacy (the ability of an intervention to produce the intended diagnostic or therapeutic effect in optimal circumstances) of the drug.

HARDSHIP OF HIGH HEALTH CARE COSTS ON FAMILIES

The Families USA Foundation is a national health care advocacy organization that is dedicated to achieving affordable, quality health care and long-term care for all American families. The organization contends that American families pay about two-thirds of the nation's health care bill, whereas American businesses pay the other one-third. This ratio is based on the premise that families and businesses pay for health care in several ways:

- Directly, through out-of-pocket payments and insurance expenses. These include premiums, deductibles (annual amounts that must be paid by the employee before the insurance plan begins paying), and co-payments.

- Indirectly, through Medicare payroll, income, and other federal, state, and local taxes that support public health programs. These include veterans' health benefits, military health benefits, the Medicaid program, and a variety of smaller public health programs.

As a result, the Families USA Foundation estimates of per capita health care spending differ from other reports, such as those from the CMS and the Census Bureau, which take into account only direct payments.

Families also purchase insurance themselves when they work for employers that do not offer group health insurance or when insurers refuse to insure certain groups they consider to be at high risk (such as people with chronic diseases). Workers who retire before reaching age 65 and are not yet eligible for Medicare coverage must also purchase insurance on their own. Furthermore, many Medicare beneficiaries pay insurance premiums for supplemental (Medigap) insurance to cover the difference in charges that Medicare does not pay.

High Cost of Prescription Drugs

Even though it has slowed somewhat in recent years, spending for prescription drugs remains the fastest-growing component of health care spending. In 2008 prescription drug expenditures reached $234.1 billion and were projected to more than double to $457.8 billion by 2019. (See Table 5.7.) Tauren Dyson observes in "Prices for Brand-Name Drugs Most Used by Medicare Patients Jump Almost 10 Percent" (*AARP Bulletin*, May 18, 2010) that the cost of brand-name prescription drugs most commonly used by those in Medicare rose 9.7% between March 2009 and March 2010. Expensive specialty drugs also rose by 9.2%; however, generic drug prices declined by 9.7%.

To control prescription drug expenditures, many hospitals, health plans, employers, and other group purchasers have attempted to obtain discounts and rebates for bulk purchases from pharmaceutical companies. Some have developed programs to encourage health care practitioners and consumers to use less costly generic drugs, and others have limited, reduced, or even eliminated prescription drug coverage.

The Kaiser Family Foundation explains in "Prescription Drug Costs" (February 2010, http://www.kaiseredu.org/topics_im.asp?id=352&parented=68&imID=1) that even though prescription drugs account for just 10% of total health care spending—with 90% of older adults and 58% of adults under the age of 65 years relying on prescription drugs—the costs will continue to mount for health insurers and government payers. There is also renewed attention to pharmaceutical company profits. For example, the article "Top Industries: Most Profitable" (CNNMoney.com, July 20, 2009) states that the pharmaceutical industry was the second-most profitable industry in the United States in 2008.

Generic Drugs Promise Cost Savings

When patents expire on popular brand-name drugs, the entry of generic versions of these drugs to the market promises cost savings for consumers and payers. Generic drugs usually cost 10% to 30% less when they first enter the market and even less once additional generic manufacturers join in the competition. According to Kathy Method, in "Going, Going, Gone" (August 10, 2009, http://drugtopics.modernmedicine.com/), among the drugs with patents that were set to expire in 2010 were Aricept (for early Alzheimer's disease), Lipitor (for lowering cholesterol), and Arimidex (for treatment of breast cancer). In 2011 patents will expire on many popular drugs including Advair (for asthma), the blood thinner Plavix (for people who have suffered a heart attack or stroke), and the antidepressant Effexor XR. Industry observers predict that consumers can expect to pay $5 to $20 less per prescription when they opt for generic drugs rather than for brand-name drugs. Several major chain stores, such as Walmart, Target, Walgreens, and Kroger, sell 30-day supplies of various generic drugs for a flat $4, and 90-day supplies for $10.

How Will Health Reform Legislation Affect Drug Costs?

The PPACA authorizes the FDA to approve generic versions of biologic drugs (drugs derived from living organisms that are used to prevent, diagnose, or treat diseases) and grant biologics manufacturers 12 years of exclusive use before generics can be developed. In "In Health Care Overhaul, Boons for Hospitals and Drug Makers" (*New York Times*, March 21, 2010), Reed Abelson asserts that because the legislation will provide insurance coverage for an additional 32 million Americans, there will be more customers for health services including prescription drugs. Abelson observes that even though pharmaceutical companies have been asked to "contribute $85 billion toward the cost of the bill in the form of industry fees and lower prices paid under government programs over 10 years," this will be more than offset by the revenues generated by millions of additional prescription drug purchases. Furthermore, because the legislation closes the Medicare coverage gap, older adults who may have delayed or deferred filling their prescriptions when they exhausted coverage will no longer have to do so, which will generate even more prescription sales.

Abelson reports that consumers are unlikely to realize prescription drug savings as a result of the legislation and quotes Jon Leibowitz, the chairman of the Federal Trade Commission, who said, "The big loser is the American consumer, who is going to have to pay an extra $3.5 billion a year in much-needed drugs." Nearly four out of 10 American consumers appear to understand that prescription drug prices will rise. According to Rasmussen Reports, in "43% Say Cost of Prescription Drugs Will Go up If Health Plan Becomes Law" (March 22, 2010, http://www.rasmussenreports.com/public_content/politics/current_events/healthcare/march_2010/), 43% of Americans anticipate a rise in drug costs and 23% believe prescription drug costs will decrease. Over one-third (36%) of respondents said they were paying more for prescription drugs than they had six months prior to the survey, whereas 52% said they were not paying more.

RATIONING HEALTH CARE

When health care rationing (allocating medical resources) is defined as "all care that is expected to be beneficial is not always available to all patients," most health care practitioners, policy makers, and consumers accept that rationing has been, and will continue to be, a feature of the U.S. health care system. Most American opinion leaders and industry observers accept that even a country as wealthy as the United States cannot afford all the care that is likely to benefit its citizens. The practical considerations of allocating health care resources involve establishing priorities and determining how these resources should be rationed.

Opponents of Rationing

There is widespread agreement among Americans that rationing according to patients' ability to pay for health care services or insurance is unfair. Ideally, health care should be equitably allocated on the basis of need and the potential benefit derived from the care. Those who argue against rationing fear that society's most vulnerable populations—older adults, the poor, and people with chronic illnesses—suffer most from the rationing of health care.

Many observers believe improving the efficiency of the U.S. health care system will save enough money to supply basic health care services to all Americans. They suggest that because expenditures for the same medical procedures vary greatly in different areas of the country, standardizing fees and costs could realize great savings. They also believe money could be saved if greater emphasis was placed on preventive care and on effective strategies to prevent or reduce behaviors that increase health risk such as smoking, alcohol and drug abuse, and unsafe sexual practices. Furthermore, they insist that the high cost of administering the U.S. health care system could be streamlined with a single payer for health care—as in the Canadian system.

Supporters of Rationing

Those who endorse rationing argue that the spiraling cost of the U.S. health care system stems from more than simple inefficiency. They attribute escalating costs to the aging population, rapid technological innovation, and the increasing costs for labor and supplies.

Not everyone who supports rationing thinks the U.S. health care system is working well. Some rationing supporters believe that the nation's health care system charges too much for the services it delivers and that it fails altogether to deliver to the millions of the uninsured. In fact, they point out that the United States already rations health care by not covering the uninsured. Other health care–rationing advocates argue that the problem is one of basic cultural assumptions, not the economics of the health care industry. Americans value human life, believe in the promise of health and quality health care for all, and insist that diseases can be cured. They contend the issue is not whether health care should be rationed but how care is rationed. They believe the United States spends too much on health compared with other societal needs, too much on the old rather than on the young, more on curing and not enough on caring, and too much on extending the length of life and not enough on enhancing the quality of life. Supporters of rationing argue instead for a system that guarantees a minimally acceptable level of health care for all, while reining in the expensive excesses of the current system, which often acts to prolong life at any cost.

The Oregon Health Plan: An Experiment in Rationing

In 1987 Oregon designed a new, universal health care plan that would simultaneously expand coverage and contain costs by limiting services. Unlike other states, which trimmed budgets by eliminating people from Medicaid eligibility, Oregon chose to eliminate low-priority services. Michael Janofsky reports in "Oregon Starts to Extend Health Care" (*New York Times*, February 19, 1994) that the Oregon Health Plan, which was approved in August 1993, aimed to provide Medicaid to 120,000 additional residents living below the federal poverty level. The plan also established a high-risk insurance pool for people who were refused health insurance coverage because of preexisting medical conditions, offered more insurance options for small businesses, and improved employees' abilities to retain their health insurance benefits when they changed jobs. A gradual increase in the state cigarette tax was expected to provide $45 million annually, which would help fund the additional estimated $200 million needed over the next several years.

Oregon developed a table of health care services and performed a cost-benefit analysis to rank them. It was decided that Oregon Medicaid would cover the top 565 services on a list of 696 medical procedures. Janofsky notes that services that fell below the cutoff point were "not deemed to be serious enough to require treatment, like common colds, flu, mild food poisoning, sprains, cosmetic procedures and experimental treatments for diseases in advanced stages."

As the Oregon Health Services Commission (HSC) prepared to establish the priorities, it decided that disease prevention and quality of well-being (QWB) were the factors that most influenced the ranking of the treatments. QWB drew fire from those who felt that such judgments could not be decided subjectively. Active medical or surgical treatment of terminally ill patients also ranked low on the QWB scale, whereas comfort and hospice care ranked

high. The HSC emphasized that its QWB judgments were not based on an individual's quality of life at a given time; such judgments were considered ethically questionable. Instead, it focused on the potential for change in an individual's life, posing questions such as: "After treatment, how much better or worse off would the patient be?"

Critics countered that the plan obtained its funding by reducing services that were currently offered to Medicaid recipients (often poor women and children) rather than by emphasizing cost control. Others objected to the ranking and the ethical questions raised by choosing to support some treatments over others.

According to Jonathan Oberlander of the University of North Carolina, Chapel Hill, in "Health Reform Interrupted: The Unraveling of the Oregon Health Plan" (*Health Affairs*, vol. 26, no. 1, 2007), the Oregon Health Plan initially did serve to reduce the percentage of uninsured Oregonians from 18% in 1992 to 11% in 1996, but its early success proved difficult to sustain. By 2003 the Oregon plan was not even close to achieving its goal of having no uninsured people in the state. In fact, the ranks of the uninsured were growing, so much so that by 2003 they reached 17%. An economic downturn in the state and the state's strategy of explicit rationing are cited by Oberlander as reasons for the ambitious plan's failure to achieve its goals.

The Oregon HSC continued to modify the plan's covered benefits. The HSC's most recent effort to refine the list of covered services began in January 2002. The HSC sought to reduce the overall costs of the plan by eliminating less effective treatments and determining if any covered medical conditions could be more effectively treated using standardized clinical practice guidelines (step-by-step instructions for diagnosis and treatment of specific illnesses or disorders) while preserving basic coverage. The benefit review process will be ongoing with the HSC submitting a new prioritized list of benefits on July 1 of each even-numbered year for review by the legislative assembly.

Oregon is credited with initiating health care reform earlier than other states. Regardless, the Office for Oregon Health Policy and Research observes in "Trends in Oregon's Health Care Market and the Oregon Health Plan" (February 2009, http://www.oregon.gov/OHPPR/RSCH/docs/Trends/Trends_in_Oregons_Health_Care3.pdf) that in 2006 one out of six (15.6%) Oregon residents remained uninsured and that uninsurance rates for children had been rising since 1996.

Rationing by HMOs

Until 2000, steadily increasing numbers of Americans received their health care from HMOs or other managed care systems. According to the Kaiser Family Foundation, in "Health Insurance & Managed Care" (http://statehealthfacts

.org/comparecat.jsp?cat=7&rgn=6&rgn=1), by July 2008 national enrollment in HMOs was 64.5 million, which was more than four times the enrollment rate two decades earlier (15.1 million). However, the number of enrollees has steadily declined since 2000. By contrast, the number of HMOs operating in the United States has risen slightly, from 560 in July 2000 to 577 in July 2008.

Managed care programs have sought to control costs by limiting coverage for experimental, duplicative, and unnecessary treatments. Before physicians can perform experimental procedures or prescribe new treatment plans, they must obtain prior authorization (approval from the patient's managed care plan) to ensure that the expenses will be covered.

Increasingly, patients and physicians are battling HMOs for approval to use and receive reimbursement for new technology and experimental treatments. Judges and juries, moved by the desperate situations of patients, have frequently decided cases against HMOs, regardless of whether the new treatment has been shown to be effective.

"SILENT RATIONING." Physicians and health care consumers are concerned that limiting coverage for new, high-cost technology will discourage research and development for new treatments before they have even been developed. This is called "silent rationing," because patients will never know what they have missed.

In an effort to control costs, some HMOs have discouraged physicians from informing patients about certain treatment options—those that are extremely expensive or not covered by the HMO. This has proved to be a highly controversial issue, both politically and ethically. In December 1996 the HHS ruled that HMOs and other health plans cannot prevent physicians from telling Medicare patients about all available treatment options.

Could Less Health Care Be Better Than More?

Even though health care providers and consumers fear that rationing sharply limits access to medical care and will ultimately result in poorer health among affected Americans, researchers are also concerned about the effects of too much care on the health of the nation. Several studies suggest that an oversupply of medical care may be as harmful as an undersupply.

John E. Wennberg, Elliott S. Fisher, and Jonathan S. Skinner of Dartmouth Medical School find in *Geography and the Debate over Medicare Reform* (February 13, 2002, http://content.healthaffairs.org/cgi/reprint/hlthaff.w2.96v1) tremendous regional variation in both the utilization and the cost of health care that they believe is explained, at least in part, by the distribution of health care providers. They also suggest that variations in physicians' practice styles—whether they favor outpatient treatment over hospitalization for specific procedures such as biopsies

(surgical procedures to examine tissue to detect cancer cells)—greatly affect demand for hospital care.

Variation in demand for health care services in turn produces variation in health care expenditures. Wennberg, Fisher, and Skinner report wide geographic variation in Medicare spending. Medicare paid more than twice as much to care for a 65-year-old in Miami, Florida, where the supply of health care providers is overabundant, than it spent on care for a 65-year-old in Minneapolis, Minnesota, a city with an average supply of health care providers. To be certain that the differences were not simply higher fees and charges in Miami, the researchers also compared rates of utilization. They find that older adults in Miami visited physicians and hospitals much more often than their counterparts in Minneapolis.

Wennberg, Fisher, and Skinner also wanted to be sure that the differences were not caused by the severity of illness, so they compared care during the last six months of life to control for any underlying regional differences in the health of the population. Remarkably, the widest variations were observed in care during the last six months of life, when older adults in Miami saw physician specialists six times as often as those in Minneapolis. The researchers assert that higher expenditures, particularly at the end of life, do not purchase better care. Instead, they finance generally unpleasant and futile interventions intended to prolong life rather than to improve the quality of patients' lives. Wennberg, Fisher, and Skinner conclude that areas with more medical care, higher utilization, and higher costs fared no better in terms of life expectancy, morbidity (illness), or mortality (death), and that the care that people received was no different in quality from care received by people in areas with average supplies of health care providers.

In *The Care of Patients with Severe Chronic Illness: An Online Report on the Medicare Program by the Dartmouth Atlas Project* (2006, http://www.dartmouthatlas .org/downloads/atlases/2006_Chronic_Care_Atlas.pdf), John E. Wennberg et al. of Dartmouth Medical School detail differences in the management of Medicare enrollees with severe chronic illnesses. The researchers find that average utilization and health care spending varied by state, region, and even by hospital in the same region. Expenditures were not linked with rates of illness in different parts of the country; instead, they reflected how intensively selected resources (e.g., acute care hospital beds, specialist physician visits, tests, and other services) were used to care for patients who were very ill but could not be cured. Because other research demonstrates that, for these chronically ill Americans, receiving more services does not result in improved health outcomes, and because most Americans say they prefer to avoid excessively high-tech end-of-life care, the researchers conclude that Medicare spending for the care of the chronically ill could be reduced by as much as 30%, while improving quality, patient satisfaction, and outcomes. Wennberg et al.'s research and similar studies pose two important and as yet unanswered questions: How much health care is needed to deliver the best health to a population? Are Americans getting the best value for the dollars spent on health care?

Elliot S. Fisher, Julie P. Bynum, and Jonathan S. Skinner of Dartmouth Medical School assert in "Slowing the Growth of Health Care Costs—Lessons from Regional Variation" (*New England Journal of Medicine*, vol. 360, no. 9, February 26, 2009) that "by learning from regions that have attained sustainable growth rates and building on successful models of delivery-system and payment-system reform, we might, with adequate physician leadership, manage to 'bend the cost curve.'" They also suggest that "such a change would not solve the country's long-term fiscal challenges. But it suggests that if we focus reform efforts on current areas of overspending—overuse of hospitals and unnecessary visits, consultations, tests, and minor procedures—we may be able to bend the cost curve while continuing to enjoy the benefits of technological advances."

Economic Impact of the 2010 Health Care Reform Legislation

According to the CBO (March 20, 2010, http://www.cbo.gov/ftpdocs/113xx/doc11379/AmendReconProp.pdf), the 2010 health care reform legislation has the capacity to reduce the budget deficit by half a percent of the GDP—more than a trillion dollars—between 2010 and 2019. The bill also serves to reduce the total cost of health care via changes in Medicare and Medicaid eligibility and in reimbursement, such as by reducing payments to insurance plans under the Medicare Advantage program. Furthermore, the bill funds comparative effectiveness research to identify the most cost-effective medical procedures.

The legislation generates revenues via new taxes and fees, including an excise tax on high-cost insurance plans, which the CBO estimates will raise $32 billion over 10 years. According to Galewitz, other tax changes slated to begin in 2013 and beyond include:

- Small companies with 25 or fewer employees will be eligible for tax credits up to 35% of the cost of premiums to help them purchase health insurance

- Companies with 50 employees or more that do not offer health care coverage will have to pay as much as $2,000 per full-time employee for each employee who obtains coverage from a government-subsidized insurance exchange

- People using indoor tanning salon services will pay a 10% tax

It also is anticipated that by enabling workers to seek new opportunities without the fear of losing their employer-sponsored health care coverage, the legislation may stimulate business growth.

CHAPTER 6
INSURANCE: THOSE WITH AND THOSE WITHOUT

In 1798 Congress established the U.S. Marine Hospital Services for seamen. It was the first time an employer offered health insurance in the United States. Payments for hospital services were deducted from the sailors' salary.

In the 21st century many factors affect the availability of health insurance, including an economic recession, employment, income, personal health status, and age. As a result, an individual's or family's health insurance status often changes as circumstances change. Carmen DeNavas-Walt, Bernadette D. Proctor, and Jessica C. Smith of the U.S. Census Bureau report in *Income, Poverty, and Health Insurance Coverage in the United States: 2008* (http://www.census.gov/hhes/www/hlthins/data/incpovhlth/2008/_g07.pdf) that in 2008, 66.7% of Americans were covered during all or part of the year by private health insurance and 58.5% were covered by employment-based health insurance. (See Figure 6.1.) The researchers note that the economic recession decreased the number of Americans who were covered by private and employment-based health insurance, from 67.5% in 2007 to 66.7% in 2008 and from 59.3% in 2007 to 58.5% in 2008, respectively. Medicare (a federal health insurance program for older adults and people with disabilities) covered 14.3% of Americans in 2008, and Medicaid (a federal health insurance program for the poor) covered 14.1%. Another 15.4% of Americans were without health coverage. DeNavas-Walt, Proctor, and Smith indicate that the percentage of the U.S. population without health coverage in 2008 was the highest it had been since 1997. The Centers for Disease Control and Prevention (CDC) reports that 46 million (15.3%) Americans were without health insurance in 2009. (See Figure 6.2.)

According to Michael E. Martinez and Robin A. Cohen of the National Center for Health Statistics (NCHS), in *Early Release of Estimates from the National Health Interview Survey, January–September 2009* (March 2010, http://www.cdc.gov/nchs/data/nhis/earlyrelease/insur201003.pdf), the percentage of adults aged 18 to 64 years without health care coverage at the time of the interview increased from 19.7% in 2008 to 21% in the first nine months of 2009. (See Figure 6.3.) The researchers indicate that from January to September 2009 there were 58.4 million (19.4%) people who were uninsured for at least part of the 12 months preceding the interview. Of this group, 57.8 million were under the age of 65, 48.2 million were aged 18 to 64 years, and 9.6 million were children under the age of 18. Figure 6.4 shows the percentages of children under the age of 18 and adults aged 18 to 64 years that were uninsured at the time of the interview, at least part of the year, and for more than a year, as well as the percentages of children and adults covered by public and private insurance.

WHO WAS UNINSURED IN 2009?

Not surprisingly, in 2009 poverty status was associated with a lack of health insurance coverage. Among people of all ages, those who were poor or near poor were more likely to be uninsured than the not poor. (The Census Bureau defines "poor" people as those below the poverty threshold; "near poor" people have incomes of 100% to less than 200% of the poverty threshold; and "not poor" people have incomes equal to or greater than 200% of the poverty threshold.) For example, among people under the age of 65, 43.2% of those who were poor and 39.7% of those who were near poor were uninsured at the time of the interview, compared with just 12.3% of those who were not poor in 2009. (See Table 6.1.)

The proportion of people who did not have health insurance in 2009 for at least part of the year preceding the interview varied by geography. It was greatest in the

FIGURE 6.1

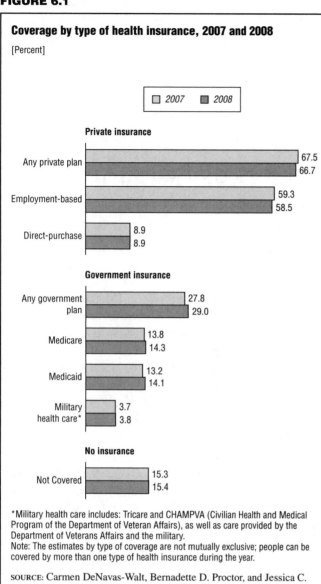

Coverage by type of health insurance, 2007 and 2008

[Percent]

☐ 2007 ■ 2008

Private insurance

Any private plan — 67.5 / 66.7

Employment-based — 59.3 / 58.5

Direct-purchase — 8.9 / 8.9

Government insurance

Any government plan — 27.8 / 29.0

Medicare — 13.8 / 14.3

Medicaid — 13.2 / 14.1

Military health care* — 3.7 / 3.8

No insurance

Not Covered — 15.3 / 15.4

*Military health care includes: Tricare and CHAMPVA (Civilian Health and Medical Program of the Department of Veteran Affairs), as well as care provided by the Department of Veterans Affairs and the military.
Note: The estimates by type of coverage are not mutually exclusive; people can be covered by more than one type of health insurance during the year.

SOURCE: Carmen DeNavas-Walt, Bernadette D. Proctor, and Jessica C. Smith, "Figure 7. Coverage by Type of Health Insurance: 2007 and 2008," in *Income, Poverty, and Health Insurance Coverage in the United States: 2008*, U.S. Census Bureau, September 2009, http://www.census.gov/hhes/www/hlthins/data/incpovhlth/2008/fig07.pdf (accessed May 29, 2010)

FIGURE 6.2

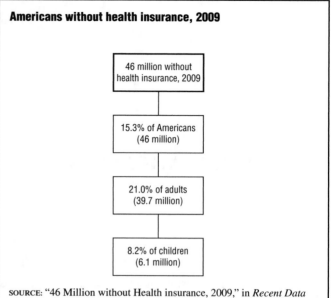

Americans without health insurance, 2009

46 million without health insurance, 2009

15.3% of Americans (46 million)

21.0% of adults (39.7 million)

8.2% of children (6.1 million)

SOURCE: "46 Million without Health insurance, 2009," in *Recent Data on Health Insurance*, National Center for Health Statistics, Division of Health Interview Statistics, May 26, 2010, http://www.cdc.gov/Features/dsInsuranceCoverage/ (accessed May 29, 2010)

FIGURE 6.3

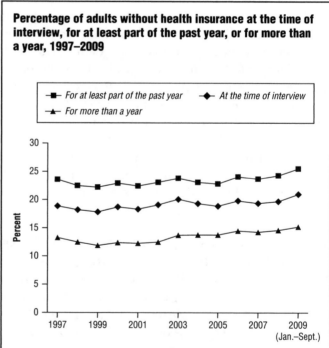

Percentage of adults without health insurance at the time of interview, for at least part of the past year, or for more than a year, 1997–2009

■ For at least part of the past year ◆ At the time of interview
▲ For more than a year

SOURCE: Michael E. Martinez and Robin A. Cohen, "Figure 7. Percentage of Adults Aged 18–64 Years Who Lacked Health Insurance Coverage at the Time of Interview, for at Least Part of the Past Year, or for More Than a Year: United States, 1997–September 2009," in *Health Insurance Coverage: Early Release of Estimates from the National Health Interview Survey, January–September 2009*, National Center for Health Statistics, March 2010, http://www.cdc.gov/nchs/data/nhis/earlyrelease/insur201003.pdf (accessed May 29, 2010)

South (22.8%) and West (21.4%), and less in the Midwest (16.6%) and Northeast (13.4%). (See Table 6.2.) Hispanics (35.3%) and non-Hispanic African-Americans (22.1%) were more likely to be uninsured in 2009 than Asian-Americans (17.2%) and non-Hispanic whites (15%).

The Uninsured by Gender and Age

Among people under 65 years old in 2009, the percentage of people without insurance at the time of the interview was highest among young adults aged 18 to 24 years (29.7%) and lowest among young people under the age of 18 (8.2%). (See Figure 6.5.) Among adults aged 18 to 64 years, men were more likely than women to be uninsured.

FIGURE 6.4

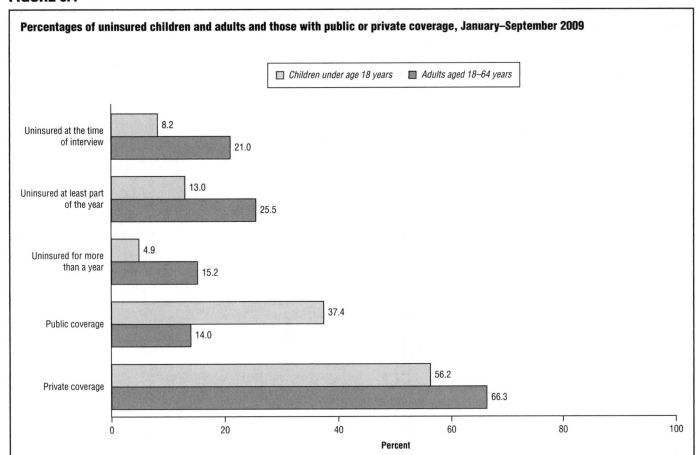

Percentages of uninsured children and adults and those with public or private coverage, January–September 2009

Legend: Children under age 18 years; Adults aged 18–64 years

- Uninsured at the time of interview: 8.2 / 21.0
- Uninsured at least part of the year: 13.0 / 25.5
- Uninsured for more than a year: 4.9 / 15.2
- Public coverage: 37.4 / 14.0
- Private coverage: 56.2 / 66.3

Percent

SOURCE: Michael E. Martinez and Robin A. Cohen, "Figure 1. Percentage of Persons without Health Insurance, by Three Measurements and Age Group, and Percentage of Persons with Health Insurance, by Coverage Type and Age Group: United States, January–September 2009," in *Health Insurance Coverage: Early Release of Estimates from the National Health Interview Survey, January–September 2009*, National Center for Health Statistics, March 2010, http://www.cdc.gov/nchs/data/nhis/earlyrelease/insur201003.pdf (accessed May 29, 2010)

LACK OF INSURANCE HAS SIGNIFICANT CONSEQUENCES

In *Sicker and Poorer: The Consequences of Being Uninsured* (May 2002, http://www.kff.org/uninsured/upload/Full-Report.pdf), a landmark report prepared for the Kaiser Commission on Medicaid and the Uninsured, Jack Hadley of the Urban Institute discusses an exhaustive review of the literature detailing the major findings of more than 25 years of health services research on the effects of health insurance. Hadley notes that the uninsured receive less preventive care, are diagnosed at more advanced stages of disease, and receive less treatment as measured in terms of pharmaceutical and surgical interventions.

Hadley concludes that if the uninsured were provided with health insurance, their mortality rates (the number of deaths caused by disease) would be reduced by between 10% and 15%. The reduction in mortality would largely result from improved access to timely and appropriate care. This finding is supported by the Institute of Medicine (IOM), which observes in *America's Uninsured Crisis:*

Consequences for Health and Health Care (February 2009, http://books.nap.edu/openbook.php?record_id=12511) that the economic downturn has exacerbated Americans' health problems because more Americans are uninsured. The IOM explains that "fewer people have access to coverage at work, more people find the costs of private coverage too expensive, and others lose public coverage because of changed personal circumstances, administrative barriers, and program cutbacks." The IOM also notes that rigorous research confirms that uninsurance has a profound negative affect on the health and mortality of adults and children.

In *Lives on the Line: The Deadly Consequences of Delaying Health Reform* (February 2010, http://www.familiesusa.org/assets/pdfs/delaying-reform.pdf), the Families USA Foundation, a national health care advocacy organization, provides state-level estimates of the number of deaths attributable to the lack of health insurance. For example, the foundation asserts that between 1995 and 2009 an estimated 38,400 Californians

TABLE 6.1

Percentage uninsured at the time of interview for persons under age 65 years, by age group and poverty status, 1997–2009

Age group and year	Total	Poverty status[a]			
		Poor	Near poor	Not poor	Unknown
		Percent uninsured[b]			
Under 65 years					
1997	17.4	32.7	30.4	8.9	21.6
1998	16.5	32.7	30.8	8.0	20.7
1999	16.0	32.1	30.7	7.8	20.1
2000	16.8	32.7	31.3	8.7	19.7
2001	16.2	31.0	28.6	8.4	20.3
2002	16.5	28.6	28.3	9.5	20.7
2003	17.2	29.4	30.2	9.1	21.3
2004 (Method 1)[c, d]	16.6	30.5	29.1	9.4	18.7
2004 (Method 2)[c, d]	16.4	30.1	28.9	9.4	18.6
2005[c]	16.0	28.4	28.6	9.1	18.5
2006[c, e]	16.8	29.2	30.8	9.7	17.5
2007[f]	16.4	28.0	30.2	9.8	20.8
2008[c]	16.7	27.9	30.6	10.2	21.0
2009[c] (Jan.–Sept.)	17.4	30.7	29.7	10.5	22.1
Under 18 years					
1997	13.9	22.4	22.8	6.1	18.3
1998	12.7	21.6	22.5	4.9	16.5
1999	11.8	21.4	21.6	4.4	14.9
2000	12.3	20.6	21.4	5.3	15.0
2001	11.0	18.8	17.0	4.4	15.5
2002	10.5	15.9	15.7	5.3	14.1
2003	10.1	15.4	14.7	4.8	13.5
2004 (Method 1)[c, d]	9.6	16.2	15.5	5.0	10.5
2004 (Method 2)[c, d]	9.4	15.3	15.1	5.0	10.3
2005[c]	8.9	13.0	14.7	4.6	11.0
2006[c, e]	9.3	12.7	16.5	4.8	10.0
2007[f]	8.9	11.4	15.5	4.9	11.8
2008[c]	8.9	12.4	15.6	4.8	11.0
2009[c] (Jan.–Sept.)	8.2	12.1	12.2	4.9	9.9
18–64 years					
1997	18.9	40.2	34.9	9.9	22.9
1998	18.2	40.8	36.0	9.2	22.2
1999	17.8	39.9	36.3	9.0	22.2
2000	18.7	41.1	37.4	10.0	21.5
2001	18.3	39.5	35.6	9.9	22.1
2002	19.1	37.0	36.2	11.0	23.2
2003	20.1	38.2	39.5	10.6	24.2
2004 (Method 1)[c, d]	19.4	40.1	36.9	11.0	21.7
2004 (Method 2)[c, d]	19.3	39.9	36.8	11.0	21.6
2005[c]	18.9	38.5	36.6	10.7	21.2
2006[c, e]	19.8	40.0	38.6	11.4	20.3
2007[f]	19.4	38.6	39.3	11.4	23.8
2008[c]	19.7	37.7	39.9	11.9	24.4
2009[c] (Jan.–Sept.)	21.0	43.2	39.7	12.3	26.3

[a]Poverty status is based on family income and family size, using the U.S. Census Bureau's poverty thresholds. "Poor" persons are defined as those below the poverty threshold; "near poor" persons have incomes of 100% to less than 200% of the poverty threshold; and "not poor" persons have incomes of 200% of the poverty threshold or greater. The percentage of respondents with unknown poverty status was 19.1% in 1997, 23.6% in 1998, 26.4% in 1999, 27.0% in 2000, 27.1% in 2001, 28.1% in 2002, 31.5% in 2003, 29.6% in 2004, 28.9% in 2005, 30.7% in 2006, 18.0% in 2007, 15.8% in 2008, and 12.5% in the first three quarters of 2009. Estimates may differ from estimates based on both reported and imputed income.
[b]A person was defined as uninsured if he or she did not have any private health insurance, Medicare, Medicaid, Children's Health Insurance Program (CHIP), state-sponsored or other government-sponsored health plan, or military plan at the time of the interview. A person was also defined as uninsured if he or she had only Indian Health Service coverage or had only a private plan that paid for one type of service, such as accidents or dental care.
[c]Beginning in the third quarter of 2004, two additional questions were added to the National Health Interview Survey (NHIS) insurance section to reduce potential errors in reporting Medicare and Medicaid status. Persons aged 65 years and over not reporting Medicare coverage were asked explicitly about Medicare coverage, and persons under age 65 with no reported coverage were asked explicitly about Medicaid coverage. Estimates of uninsurance for 2004 were calculated without using the additional information from these questions (noted as Method 1) and with the responses to these questions (noted as Method 2). Respondents who were reclassified as "covered" by the additional questions received the appropriate follow-up questions concerning periods of noncoverage for insured respondents. Beginning in 2005, all estimates were calculated using Method 2.
[d]In 2004, a much larger than expected proportion of respondents reported a family income of "$2." Based on extensive review, these "$2" responses were coded to "not ascertained" for the final 2004 NHIS data files. Effective with the March 2006 Early Release report, the 2004 estimates were recalculated to reflect this editing decision.
[e]In 2006, NHIS underwent a sample redesign. The impact of the new sample design on estimates presented in this report is minimal.
[f]In 2007, the income section of NHIS was redesigned, and estimates by poverty status may not be directly comparable with earlier years.

SOURCE: Michael E. Martinez and Robin A. Cohen, "Table 4. Percentage Uninsured at the Time of Interview for Persons under Age 65 Years, by Age Group, and Poverty Status: United States, 1997–September 2009," in *Health Insurance Coverage: Early Release of Estimates from the National Health Interview Survey, January–September 2009*, National Center for Health Statistics, March 2010, http://www.cdc.gov/nchs/data/nhis/earlyrelease/insur201003.pdf (accessed May 29, 2010)

TABLE 6.2

Percentage without health insurance by selected characteristics, January–September 2009

Selected characteristic	Uninsured[a] at the time of interview	Uninsured[a] for at least part of the past year[b]	Uninsured[a] for more than a year[b]
	Percent		
Age			
All ages	15.3	19.4	10.8
Under 65 years	17.4	22.0	12.3
Under 18 years	8.2	13.0	4.9
18–64 years	21.0	25.5	15.2
65 years and over	0.9	1.7	0.7
Sex			
Male	17.2	21.0	12.4
Female	13.5	17.9	9.2
Race/ethnicity			
Hispanic or Latino	31.1	35.3	24.7
Non-Hispanic			
White, single race	11.0	15.0	7.3
Black, single race	17.3	22.1	11.5
Asian, single race	14.1	17.2	10.7
Other races and multiple races	19.8	25.1	12.1
Region			
Northeast	9.9	13.4	7.0
Midwest	12.8	16.6	8.0
South	18.6	22.8	13.6
West	16.8	21.4	12.1
Education[c]			
Less than high school	33.3	36.7	27.8
High school diploma or GED[d]	21.0	24.8	15.4
More than high school	11.6	15.7	7.4
Employment status[e]			
Employed	17.9	22.1	13.6
Unemployed	52.3	59.5	32.2
Not in workforce	20.7	25.6	14.6
Marital status[c]			
Married	12.5	15.5	9.4
Widowed	5.3	6.4	4.3
Divorced or separated	20.9	26.1	15.4
Living with partner	31.6	38.4	21.9
Never married	28.2	33.5	19.5

[a]A person was defined as uninsured if he or she did not have any private health insurance, Medicare, Medicaid, Children's Health Insurance Program (CHIP), state-sponsored or other government-sponsored health plan, or military plan. A person was also defined as uninsured if he or she had only Indian Health Service coverage or had only a private plan that paid for one type of service, such as accidents or dental care.
[b]A year is defined as the 12 months prior to interview.
[c]Education and marital status are shown only for persons aged 18 years and over.
[d]GED is General Educational Development high school equivalency diploma.
[e]Employment status is shown only for persons aged 18–64 years.

SOURCE: Michael E. Martinez and Robin A. Cohen, "Table 7. Percentage of Persons Who Lacked Health Insurance Coverage at the Time of Interview, for at Least Part of the Past Year, or for More Than a Year, by Selected Demographic Characteristics: United States, January–September 2009," in *Health Insurance Coverage: Early Release of Estimates from the National Health Interview Survey, January–September 2009*, National Center for Health Statistics, March 2010, http://www.cdc.gov/nchs/data/nhis/earlyrelease/insur201003.pdf (accessed May 29, 2010).

died from the lack of health insurance. During this same period 32,300 people in Texas and 24,400 people in Florida died because they had no health care coverage. The Families USA Foundation observes that "every day in 2010, approximately 68 non-elderly adult Americans died prematurely due to lack of health coverage."

SOURCES OF HEALTH INSURANCE

People under the Age of 65

For people under the age of 65 there are two principal sources of health insurance coverage: private insurance (from employer or private policies) and Medicaid. From 1997 to 2009 the proportion of those covered by private insurance at the time of the interview declined from 70.8% to 63.4%. (See Table 6.3.) During this same period the percentage covered by public health plans grew from 13.6% in 1997 to 20.6% in 2009.

DeNavas-Walt, Proctor, and Smith report that the percentage of people covered by employment-based health insurance dropped from 59.3% in 2007 to 58.5% in 2008. (See Figure 6.1.) In contrast, during the 1980s close to 70% of workers obtained private health insurance through their employer. This decline is consistent with the continuing decline in all forms of private health coverage, which dropped from 67.5% in 2007 to 66.7% in 2008. For people under the age of 65, the overall decline in private health insurance coverage between 1997 and 2009 was just 7.4%, from 70.8% to 63.4%, but among people who were near poor the percentage covered by private insurance fell 17.5%, from 53.5% to 36%. (See Table 6.4.)

Two major factors contributed to the long-term decline in private health insurance. The first is the rising cost of health care, which frequently leads to greater cost sharing between employers and employees. Some workers simply cannot afford the higher premiums and co-payments (the share of the medical bill the employee pays for each health service). The second factor is the shift in U.S. commerce from the goods-producing sector, where health benefits have traditionally been provided, to the service sector, where many employers do not offer health insurance.

People Aged 65 Years and Older

There are three sources of health insurance for people aged 65 years and older: private insurance, Medicare, and Medicaid. Medicare is the federal government's primary health program for people who are aged 65 years and older, and all people in this age group are eligible for certain basic benefits under Medicare. Medicaid is the federal program for the poor and people with disabilities. In 2009 a scant 1.7% of adults aged 65 years and older went without some type of health insurance for at least part of the year preceding the interview. (See Table 6.2.)

Older adults may be covered by a combination of private health insurance and Medicare, or Medicare and Medicaid, depending on their income and level of disability. Nearly all adults over the age of 65 are covered by Medicare. In *Health, United States, 2009* (2010, http://www.cdc.gov/nchs/data/hus/hus09.pdf), the NCHS reports that in 2007, 19.5% of older adults were covered by a Medicare managed care plan, and 14.6% used Medicare to obtain care on a fee-for-service basis.

FIGURE 6.5

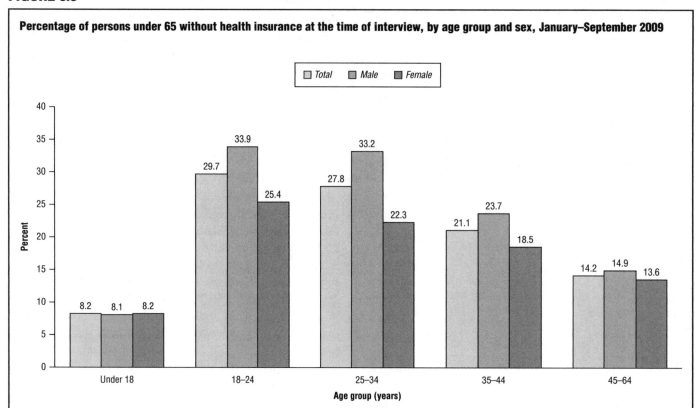

Percentage of persons under 65 without health insurance at the time of interview, by age group and sex, January–September 2009

Legend: ☐ Total ☐ Male ■ Female

SOURCE: Michael E. Martinez and Robin A. Cohen, "Figure 2. Percentage of Persons under 65 Years of Age without Health Insurance Coverage at the Time of Interview, by Age Group and Sex: United States, January–September 2009," in *Health Insurance Coverage: Early Release of Estimates from the National Health Interview Survey, January–September 2009*, National Center for Health Statistics, March 2010, http://www.cdc.gov/nchs/data/nhis/earlyrelease/insur201003.pdf (accessed May 29, 2010)

MEDICARE C

Medicare C, also known as Medicare+Choice, became available to Medicare recipients on January 1, 1999. Medicare C came about as a result of the Balanced Budget Act of 1997 and was designed to supplement Medicare Parts A and B. Medicare C offers beneficiaries a wider variety of health plan options than previously available. These options include traditional (fee-for-service) Medicare, Medicare provider-sponsored organizations, preferred provider organizations (PPOs), Medicare health maintenance organizations (HMOs), and medical savings accounts (MSAs).

Medicare provider-sponsored organizations are organized and operated the same way that HMOs are. However, they are administered by providers—physicians and hospitals. PPOs are similar to HMOs but permit patients to see providers outside the network and do not require their members to choose a network primary care physician to coordinate their care. Patients in PPOs may seek care from any physician who is associated with the plan. Medicare HMOs are more like traditional Medicare, except patients may pay more out-of-pocket expenses. MSAs have two parts: an insurance policy and a savings account. Medicare pays the insurance premium and deposits a fixed amount into an MSA each year to pay for an individual's health care.

CHANGING MEDICARE REIMBURSEMENT

Medicare reimbursement varies in different parts of the country, although everyone pays the same amount to Medicare through taxes. As a result, older adults in some geographic regions have access to a more comprehensive range of services (e.g., coverage for nursing home care and eyeglasses) than older adults in other regions.

Describing this practice as unfair and outdated, legislators have repeatedly called for more equitable reimbursement formulas. For example, since 2002 the Medi-Fair Act (previously called the Medicare Fairness in Reimbursement Act; the act aimed to improve the provision of items and services provided to Medicare beneficiaries residing in rural areas in part by improving reimbursement) has repeatedly failed to pass. Senator Patty Murray (1950–; D-WA) and Representative Adam Smith (1965–; D-WA) reintroduced the legislation in May 2008 in an effort to raise Washington State's Medicare reimbursement rates to the national average and to ensure that all states receive at least the national average of per-patient spending. The Medicare Improvements for Patients and Providers Act of 2008 aimed to stem declining reimbursement by postponing a provision to reduce some Medicare reimbursement rates. The bill became law in July 2008.

TABLE 6.3

Percentage of persons with public or private health insurance at time of interview, 1997–2009

Type of coverage and year	Under 65 years	Under 18 years	18–64 years
Public health plan coverage[a]		Percent	
1997	13.6	21.4	10.2
1998	12.7	20.0	9.5
1999	12.4	20.4	9.0
2000	12.9	22.0	9.1
2001	13.6	23.6	9.4
2002	15.2	27.1	10.3
2003	16.0	28.6	10.9
2004 (Method 1)[c]	16.1	28.5	11.1
2004 (Method 2)[c]	16.2	28.7	11.1
2005[c]	16.8	29.9	11.5
2006[c, d]	18.1	32.3	12.4
2007[c]	18.1	32.7	12.3
2008[c]	19.3	34.2	13.4
2009[c] (Jan.–Sept.)	20.6	37.4	14.0
Private health insurance coverage[b]			
1997	70.8	66.2	72.8
1998	72.0	68.5	73.5
1999	73.1	69.1	74.7
2000	71.8	67.1	73.8
2001	71.6	66.7	73.7
2002	69.8	63.9	72.3
2003	68.2	62.6	70.6
2004[c]	68.6	63.1	70.9
2005[c]	68.4	62.4	70.9
2006[c, d]	66.5	59.7	69.2
2007[c]	66.8	59.9	69.6
2008[c]	65.4	58.3	68.1
2009[c] (Jan.–Sept.)	63.4	56.2	66.3

[a]"Public health plan coverage" includes Medicaid, Children's Health Insurance Program (CHIP), state-sponsored or other government-sponsored health plan, Medicare (disability), and military plans.
[b]"Private health insurance coverage" excludes plans that paid for only one type of service, such as accidents or dental care. A small number of persons were covered by both public and private plans and were included in both categories.
[c]Beginning in the third quarter of 2004, two additional questions were added to the National Health Interview Survey (NHIS) insurance section to reduce potential errors in reporting Medicare and Medicaid status. Persons aged 65 years and over not reporting Medicare coverage were asked explicitly about Medicare coverage, and persons under age 65 with no reported coverage were asked explicitly about Medicaid coverage. Estimates of uninsurance for 2004 were calculated without using the additional information from these questions (noted as Method 1) and with the responses to these questions (noted as Method 2). Respondents who were reclassified as "covered" by the additional questions received the appropriate follow-up questions concerning periods of noncoverage for insured respondents. The two additional questions added beginning in the third quarter of 2004 did not affect the estimates of private coverage. Beginning in 2005, all estimates were calculated using Method 2.
[d]In 2006, NHIS underwent a sample redesign. The impact of the new sample design on estimates presented in this report is minimal.

SOURCE: Michael E. Martinez and Robin A. Cohen, "Table 3. Percentage of Persons under Age 65 Years with Public Health Plan or Private Health Insurance Coverage at the Time of Interview, by Age Group: United States, 1997–September 2009," in *Health Insurance Coverage: Early Release of Estimates from the National Health Interview Survey, January–September 2009*, National Center for Health Statistics, March 2010, http://www.cdc.gov/nchs/data/nhis/earlyrelease/insur201003.pdf (accessed May 29, 2010)

According to Patricia A. Davis et al. of the Congressional Research Service, in *Medicare Provisions in the Patient Protection and Affordable Care Act (PPACA)* (April 23, 2010, http://www.ncsl.org/documents/health/MCProv.pdf), the 2010 health care reform legislation, the Patient Protection and Affordable Care Act (PPACA), promises to further rectify persisting inequalities in Med-

icare reimbursement rates. The legislation creates an Independent Payment Advisory Board to institute changes in Medicare payment rates and permits some flexibility in the review and adjustment of Medicare payments for providers practicing in so-called frontier states—that is, sparsely populated rural areas that are isolated from population centers and services.

Medicare Prescription Drug, Improvement, and Modernization Act

In December 2003 President George W. Bush (1946–) signed the Medicare Prescription Drug, Improvement, and Modernization Act into law. Heralded as landmark legislation, the act provides older adults and people with disabilities with a prescription drug benefit, more choices, and improved benefits under Medicare. On June 1, 2004, seniors and people with disabilities began using their Medicare-approved drug discount cards to obtain savings on prescription medicines. Low-income beneficiaries qualified for a $600 credit to help pay for their prescriptions. Besides providing coverage for prescription drugs, this legislation offers seniors the opportunity to choose the coverage and care that best meets their needs. For example, some older adults may opt for traditional Medicare coverage along with the new prescription benefit. Others may wish to obtain dental or eyeglass coverage or to enroll in managed care plans that reduce their out-of-pocket costs.

The legislation stipulated that as of 2005 all newly enrolled Medicare beneficiaries would be covered for a complete physical examination and other preventive services, such as blood tests to screen for diabetes. The new law also aimed to assist Americans in paying out-of-pocket health costs by enabling the creation of health savings accounts, which allow Americans to set aside up to $4,500 per year, tax free, to save for medical expenses.

Regardless, concerns about the solvency of the Medicare program and its capacity to meet the health care needs of growing numbers of Americans aging into eligibility have been increasing in recent years. The media have reported the ill effects of coverage gaps, with multiple stories of older adults opting to forgo prescription medication because they were unable to afford it. The 2010 health care reform legislation not only aims to extend the program's solvency for an additional 10 years but also fills the coverage gap (known as the so-called donut hole) in prescription drug coverage by giving all Medicare beneficiaries who reach the gap a $250 rebate beginning in 2011 and completely closing the gap by 2020. This is an eagerly anticipated benefit for many Medicare beneficiaries because according to the Democratic Policy Committee, in "Strengthening Medicare for Our Nation's Seniors" (April 1, 2010, http://dpc.senate.gov/healthreformbill/healthbill91.pdf), over 8 million older adults reached the gap in 2007.

TABLE 6.4

Percentage of persons under age 65 with private health insurance at the time of interview, by age group and poverty status, 1997–2009

Age group and year	Total	Poor	Near poor	Not poor	Unknown
			Poverty status[a]		
Under 65 years			Percent of persons with private health insurance coverage[b]		
1997	70.8	22.9	53.5	87.6	66.7
1998	72.0	23.1	53.0	88.1	67.1
1999	73.1	26.1	50.9	88.9	68.0
2000	71.8	25.2	49.1	87.4	68.8
2001	71.6	25.5	48.4	87.2	67.8
2002	69.8	26.0	46.5	86.0	63.9
2003	68.2	23.4	42.3	85.8	64.1
2004[c]	68.6	20.0	44.9	85.0	66.3
2005	68.4	22.1	43.2	84.7	66.2
2006[d]	66.5	20.6	40.6	84.1	65.7
2007[e]	66.8	20.1	37.9	83.8	61.7
2008[c]	65.4	17.9	36.3	82.5	60.7
2009[c] (Jan.–Sept.)	63.4	13.7	36.0	81.9	59.0
Under 18 years					
1997	66.2	17.5	55.0	88.9	61.7
1998	68.5	19.3	56.3	89.9	62.1
1999	69.1	20.2	52.1	90.6	63.8
2000	67.1	19.5	48.8	88.4	64.2
2001	66.7	18.1	48.4	88.4	62.2
2002	63.9	17.2	44.9	86.9	56.3
2003	62.6	14.4	39.9	86.5	58.8
2004[c]	63.1	12.6	43.0	86.4	60.0
2005	62.4	15.0	40.0	85.6	59.3
2006[d]	59.7	13.1	36.9	85.9	57.8
2007[e]	59.9	11.9	34.0	85.1	54.8
2008[c]	58.3	10.4	32.9	83.1	54.8
2009[c] (Jan.–Sept.)	56.2	8.2	33.0	82.5	56.2
18–64 years					
1997	72.8	26.8	52.6	87.1	68.6
1998	73.5	25.8	50.9	87.4	69.1
1999	74.7	30.4	50.2	88.2	69.7
2000	73.8	29.2	49.3	87.1	70.6
2001	73.7	31.7	48.4	86.8	69.9
2002	72.3	31.8	47.5	85.7	66.9
2003	70.6	29.0	43.7	85.5	66.0
2004[c]	70.9	24.9	46.0	84.6	68.6
2005	70.9	26.8	45.0	84.4	68.7
2006[d]	69.2	25.5	42.6	83.6	68.6
2007[e]	69.6	25.4	40.4	83.4	64.0
2008[e]	68.1	22.7	38.3	82.4	62.7
2009[e] (Jan.–Sept.)	66.3	17.4	37.7	81.7	59.9

[a]Poverty status is based on family income and family size, using the U.S. Census Bureau's poverty thresholds. "Poor" persons are defined as those below the poverty threshold; "near poor" persons have incomes of 100% to less than 200% of the poverty threshold; and "not poor" persons have incomes of 200% of the poverty threshold or greater. The percentage of respondents with unknown poverty status was 19.1% in 1997, 23.6% in 1998, 26.4% in 1999, 27.0% in 2000, 27.1% in 2001, 28.1% in 2002, 31.5% in 2003, 29.6% in 2004, 28.9% in 2005, 30.7% in 2006, 18.0% in 2007 15.8% in 2008, and 12.5% in the first three quarters of 2009. Estimates may differ from estimates based on both reported and imputed income.
[b]The category "private health insurance" excludes plans that paid for only one type of service, such as accidents or dental care. A small number of persons were covered by both public and private plans and thus were included in both categories.
[c]In 2004, a much larger than expected proportion of respondents reported a family income of "$2." Based on extensive review, these "$2" responses were coded to "not ascertained" for the final 2004 National Health Interview Survey (NHIS) data files. Effective with the March 2006 Early Release report the 2004 estimates were recalculated to reflect this editing decision. The problem with the "$2" income reports was fixed in the 2005 NHIS.
[d]In 2006, NHIS underwent a sample redesign. The impact of the new sample design on estimates presented in this report is minimal.
[e]In 2007, the income section of NHIS was redesigned, and estimates by poverty status may not be directly comparable with earlier years.

SOURCE: Michael E. Martinez and Robin A. Cohen, "Table 6. Percentage of Persons under Age 65 Years with Private Health Insurance Coverage at the Time of Interview, by Age Group and Poverty Status: United States, 1997–September 2009," in *Health Insurance Coverage: Early Release of Estimates from the National Health Interview Survey, January–September 2009*, National Center for Health Statistics, March 2010, http://www.cdc.gov/nchs/data/nhis/earlyrelease/insur201003.pdf (accessed May 29, 2010)

CHILDREN

In 2009, 6.1 million (8.2%) children under the age of 18 were uninsured. (See Figure 6.2.) Thirteen percent had been uninsured for part of the year preceding the interview and 4.9% had been uninsured for more than a year. (See Table 6.5.) In 2009 poor children (12.1%) and near-poor children (12.2%) were much more likely to be uninsured at the time of the interview than not-poor children (4.9%). (See Table 6.1.) The percentage of children without health insurance at the time of the interview declined from 13.9% in 1997 to 8.2% in 2009. (See Figure 6.6.)

Figure 6.7 shows that from 1997 to 2009 the percentage of poor and near-poor children who lacked health insurance coverage decreased. In 2009, 56.2% of American children

TABLE 6.5

Percentage of persons under age 18 who were uninsured at the time of interview, for at least part of the past year, or for more than a year, by age group, 1997–2009

Age group and year	Uninsured[a] at the time of interview	Uninsured[a] for at least part of the past year[b]	Uninsured[a] for more than a year[b]
		Percent	
Under 18 years			
1997	13.9	18.1	8.4
1998	12.7	17.1	7.6
1999	11.8	16.3	7.2
2000	12.3	16.7	7.0
2001	11.0	15.2	6.3
2002	10.5	14.6	5.6
2003	10.1	13.7	5.3
2004 (Method 1)[c]	9.6	12.9	5.4
2004 (Method 2)[c]	9.4	12.7	5.4
2005[c]	8.9	12.6	5.3
2006[c, d]	9.3	13.0	5.2
2007[c]	8.9	12.6	5.0
2008[c]	8.9	13.3	5.6
2009[c] (Jan.–Sept.)	8.2	13.0	4.9

[a]A person was defined as uninsured if he or she did not have any private health insurance, Medicare, Medicaid, Children's Health Insurance Program (CHIP), state-sponsored or other government-sponsored health plan, or military plan. A person was also defined as uninsured if he or she had only Indian Health Service coverage or had only a private plan that paid for one type of service, such as accidents or dental care.
[b]A year is defined as the 12 months prior to interview.
[c]Beginning in the third quarter of 2004, two additional questions were added to the National Health Interview Survey (NHIS) insurance section to reduce potential errors in reporting Medicare and Medicaid status. Persons aged 65 years and over not reporting Medicare coverage were asked explicitly about Medicare coverage, and persons under age 65 with no reported coverage were asked explicitly about Medicaid coverage. Estimates of uninsurance for 2004 were calculated without using the additional information from these questions (noted as Method 1) and with the responses to these questions (noted as Method 2). Respondents who were reclassified as "covered" by the additional questions received the appropriate follow-up questions concerning periods of noncoverage for insured respondents. These reclassified respondents were excluded in the tabulation of "uninsured for more than a year" using Method 1 in 2004. Beginning in 2005, all estimates were calculated using Method 2.
[d]In 2006, NHIS underwent a sample redesign. The impact of the new sample design on estimates presented in this report is minimal.

SOURCE: Michael E. Martinez and Robin A. Cohen, "Table 1. Percentage of Persons Who Lacked Health Insurance Coverage at the Time of Interview, for at Least Part of the Past Year, or for More Than a Year, by Age Group: United States, 1997–September 2009," in *Health Insurance Coverage: Early Release of Estimates from the National Health Interview Survey, January–September 2009*, National Center for Health Statistics, March 2010, http://www.cdc.gov/nchs/data/nhis/earlyrelease/insur201003.pdf (accessed May 29, 2010)

were insured under private health insurance plans, either privately purchased or obtained through their parents' workplace, and 37.4% were covered by public health plans. (See Table 6.3.) The rate of private coverage decreased from 66.2% in 1997 to 56.2% in 2009; during this period public coverage increased from 21.4% to 37.4%. Martinez and Cohen observe that the majority (81.5%) of poor children and more than 50% of near-poor children were covered by a public health plan in 2009. (See Figure 6.8.)

Some health care industry observers believed the 1996 welfare reform law, the Personal Responsibility and Work Opportunity Reconciliation Act, would reduce enrollment in Medicaid. Under the 1996 law, federal money once dispensed through the Aid to Families with Dependent

FIGURE 6.6

Percentage of children under age 18 years without health insurance at the time of interview, for at least part of the past year, or for more than a year, 1997–2009

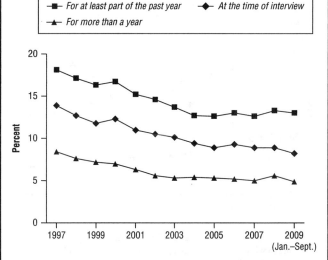

SOURCE: Michael E. Martinez and Robin A. Cohen, "Figure 6. Percentage of Children under Age 18 Years Who Lacked Health Insurance Coverage at the Time of Interview, for at Least Part of the Past Year, or for More Than a Year: United States, 1997–September 2009," in *Health Insurance Coverage: Early Release of Estimates from the National Health Interview Survey, January–September 2009*, National Center for Health Statistics, March 2010, http://www.cdc.gov/nchs/data/nhis/earlyrelease/insur201003.pdf (accessed May 29, 2010)

FIGURE 6.7

Percentage of children under 18 without health insurance, by poverty status, 1997–2009

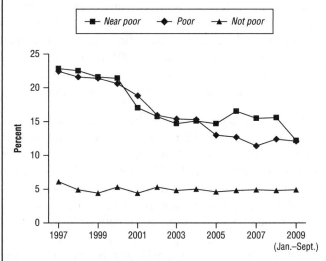

SOURCE: Michael E. Martinez and Robin A. Cohen, "Figure 6. Percentage Uninsured at the Time of Interview, by Poverty Status, for Children under 18 Years: United States, 1997–September 2009," in *Health Insurance Coverage: Early Release of Estimates from the National Health Interview Survey, January–September 2009*, National Center for Health Statistics, March 2010, http://www.cdc.gov/nchs/data/nhis/earlyrelease/insur201003.pdf (accessed May 29, 2010)

FIGURE 6.8

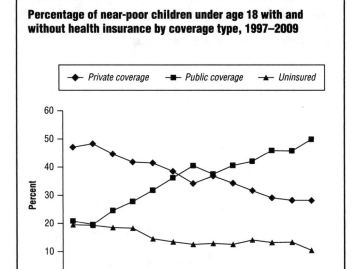

Percentage of near-poor children under age 18 with and without health insurance by coverage type, 1997–2009

SOURCE: Michael E. Martinez and Robin A. Cohen, "Figure 10. Percentage with Health Insurance, by Coverage Type, and Percentage Uninsured at the Time of Interview, for Near-Poor Children under 18 Years: United States, 1997–September 2009," in *Health Insurance Coverage: Early Release of Estimates from the National Health Interview Survey, January–September 2009*, National Center for Health Statistics, March 2010, http://www.cdc.gov/nchs/data/nhis/earlyrelease/insur201003.pdf (accessed May 29, 2010)

Children program was now given as a block grant (a lump sum of money) to states. In addition, the law no longer required that children who received cash assistance were automatically enrolled in the Medicaid program. The law gave states greater leeway in defining their requirements for aid, and in a few states some families were no longer eligible for Medicaid. Regardless, Table 6.6 shows that enrollment in Medicaid actually increased, rather than decreased, from 26.6 million in 1995 to 36.2 million in 2007. During this period the percentage of children covered by Medicaid also rose, from 21.5% to 29.8%.

Some industry analysts attributed the declining proportion of uninsured children and the increasing proportion of children covered by Medicaid during the late 1990s to expansion of the Children's Health Insurance Program, which targeted children from low-income families and was instituted during the late 1990s. Others believed the economic boom of the late 1990s may have played a role in slowing or preventing even greater enrollment growth in Medicaid and predicted that the economic downturn and the uncertainty of the early years of the 21st century would reverse the downward trend in both the share of the population without health insurance and Medicaid enrollment. These industry observations were borne out as the economic downturn spurred growth in the proportion of children covered by Medicaid.

In 2009 many health care advocacy groups, including the American Academy of Pediatrics, continued to agitate for federal legislation such as the MediKids Health Insurance Act to provide health insurance for all children in the United States by 2012 regardless of family income level. The 2010 health care reform legislation responded to this request by approving health insurance coverage for children. More specifically, the Democratic Policy Committee explains in "Health Reform for Children" (April 1, 2010, http://dpc.senate.gov/healthreformbill/healthbill84.pdf) that the legislation eliminates preexisting coverage exclusions for children and maintains funding for the Children's Health Insurance Program for two years through fiscal year 2015. It requires children's health insurance to provide coverage for basic dental and vision care. The legislation also guarantees children access to affordable child-only health insurance policies, regardless of whether their parents change or leave their jobs, relocate, or become ill or disabled.

HEALTH INSURANCE PORTABILITY AND ACCOUNTABILITY ACT

In August 1996 President Bill Clinton (1946–) signed the Health Insurance Portability and Accountability Act (HIPAA). This legislation aimed to provide better portability (transfer) of employer-sponsored insurance from one job to another. HIPAA ensured that people who had employer-sponsored health coverage would be able to maintain their health insurance even if they lost their job or moved to a different company. They would, of course, have to continue to pay for their insurance. However, they no longer had to fear that they would be denied coverage because of preexisting medical conditions or be forced to go without health insurance for prolonged waiting periods.

Industry observers and policy makers viewed HIPAA as an important first step in the federal initiative to significantly reduce the number of uninsured people in the United States. Besides its portability provisions, HIPAA changed tax laws to make it easier for Americans to pay for medical care and initiated a pilot program of MSAs that would grow into a significant new initiative in paying for health care.

HEALTH SAVINGS ACCOUNTS

HIPAA also authorized a pilot program: a five-year demonstration project designed to test the concept of MSAs, which are similar to individual retirement accounts. Beginning on January 1, 1997, approximately 750,000 people with high-deductible health plans (HDHPs; high-deductible plans were defined as those that carried a deductible of $1,600 to $2,400 for an individual or $3,200 to $4,800 for families) could make tax-deductible contributions into interest-bearing savings accounts. The funds deposited into these accounts could be used to purchase health insurance policies and pay co-payments and deductibles. People using MSAs could also

TABLE 6.6

Medicaid coverage of persons under 65, by selected characteristics, selected years 1984–2007

[Data are based on household interviews of a sample of the civilian noninstitutionalized population]

Characteristic	1984[a]	1989[a]	1995[a]	1997	2000[b]	2004(1)[c]	2004(2)[c]	2005[c]	2006[c]	2007[c]
					Number in millions					
Total[d]	14.0	15.4	26.6	22.9	23.2	31.1	31.6	33.2	36.2	36.2
					Percent of population					
Total[d]	6.8	7.2	11.5	9.7	9.5	12.3	12.5	12.9	14.0	13.9
Age										
Under 18 years	11.9	12.6	21.5	18.4	19.6	25.9	26.4	27.2	29.9	29.8
Under 6 years	15.5	15.7	29.3	24.7	24.7	31.8	32.4	34.0	36.6	36.6
6–17 years	10.1	10.9	17.4	15.2	17.2	23.1	23.4	23.9	26.7	26.4
18–44 years	5.1	5.2	7.8	6.6	5.6	7.5	7.7	8.3	8.6	8.7
18–24 years	6.4	6.8	10.4	8.8	8.1	10.3	10.4	11.3	11.4	11.4
25–34 years	5.3	5.2	8.2	6.8	5.5	7.6	7.8	8.0	8.3	8.5
35–44 years	3.5	4.0	5.9	5.2	4.3	5.7	5.8	6.6	7.1	7.0
45–64 years	3.4	4.3	5.6	4.6	4.5	5.4	5.5	5.5	6.3	5.9
45–54 years	3.2	3.8	5.1	4.0	4.2	5.4	5.5	5.2	6.4	6.0
55–64 years	3.6	4.9	6.4	5.6	4.9	5.4	5.5	5.8	6.1	5.7
Sex										
Male	5.4	5.7	9.6	8.4	8.2	10.8	11.0	11.6	12.6	12.5
Female	8.1	8.6	13.4	11.1	10.8	13.7	13.9	14.3	15.5	15.2
Sex and marital status[e]										
Male:										
Married	1.9	1.8	2.9	2.5	2.2	2.9	3.0	3.5	3.7	3.5
Divorced, separated, widowed	4.9	5.4	7.7	5.7	6.1	6.7	6.8	7.0	7.9	7.8
Never married	4.8	5.6	8.1	7.0	7.2	10.2	10.4	10.4	11.6	11.3
Female:										
Married	2.6	3.0	5.2	3.5	3.1	4.2	4.3	4.7	4.6	4.7
Divorced, separated, widowed	16.0	16.1	19.0	14.7	12.7	14.9	15.2	14.6	16.2	16.3
Never married	10.7	11.9	16.5	14.2	13.2	16.9	17.1	17.3	19.0	18.1
Race[f]										
White only	4.6	5.1	8.9	7.4	7.1	10.2	10.4	11.0	11.8	11.4
Black or African American only	20.5	19.0	28.5	22.4	21.2	24.5	24.9	24.9	26.6	27.7
American Indian or Alaska Native only	28.2*	29.7	19.0	19.6	15.1	18.0	18.4	24.2	24.3	21.2
Asian only	8.7*	8.8*	10.5	9.6	7.5	9.6	9.8	8.2	9.7	8.7
Native Hawaiian or other Pacific Islander only	—	—	—	—	*	*	*	*	*	*
2 or more races	—	—	—	—	19.1	19.0	19.3	22.0	24.0	27.9
Hispanic origin and race[f]										
Hispanic or Latino	13.3	13.5	21.9	17.6	15.5	21.9	22.5	22.9	23.1	24.7
Mexican	12.2	12.4	21.6	17.2	14.0	21.9	22.4	23.0	23.0	25.9
Puerto Rican	31.5	27.3	33.4	31.0	29.4	28.5	29.1	31.9	35.7	28.0
Cuban	4.8*	7.7*	13.4	7.3	9.2	17.9	17.9	17.7	11.3*	13.3
Other Hispanic or Latino	7.9	11.1	18.2	15.3	14.5	19.9	20.8	19.7	20.2	21.4
Not Hispanic or Latino	6.2	6.5	10.2	8.7	8.5	10.5	10.7	11.1	12.3	11.7
White only	3.7	4.1	7.1	6.1	6.1	7.8	7.9	8.5	9.5	8.5
Black or African American only	20.7	19.0	28.1	22.1	21.0	24.1	24.6	24.8	26.2	27.3
Age and percent of poverty level[g]										
Under 65 years:										
Below 100%	33.0	37.6	48.4	40.5	38.4	44.2	45.0	45.7	45.8	47.6
100%–less than 150%	7.7	10.9	19.1	17.9	20.7	26.5	27.1	28.7	29.4	31.8
150%–less than 200%	3.2	5.1	8.3	8.3	11.5	16.6	16.9	18.1	18.0	20.3
200% or more	0.6	1.1	1.7	1.8	2.3	3.5	3.5	3.7	4.1	3.8

deduct any employer contributions into the accounts as tax-deductible income. Any unspent money remaining in the MSA at the end of the year was carried over to the next year, thereby allowing the account to grow.

To be eligible to create an MSA, individuals had to be less than 65 years old, self-employed, and uninsured or had to work in firms with 50 or fewer employees that did not offer health care coverage. Withdrawals to cover out-of-pocket medical expenses were tax free and the money invested grew on a tax-deferred basis. Using MSA funds

for any purpose unrelated to medical care or disability resulted in a 15% penalty. However, when MSA users reached age 65, the money could be withdrawn for any purpose and was taxed at the same rate as ordinary income.

Supporters of MSAs believed consumers would be less likely to seek unnecessary or duplicative medical care if they knew they could keep the money left in their accounts for themselves at the end of the year. Experience demonstrated that MSAs could simultaneously help contain health care costs, allow consumers greater control

TABLE 6.6

Medicaid coverage of persons under 65, by selected characteristics, selected years 1984–2007 [CONTINUED]

[Data are based on household interviews of a sample of the civilian noninstitutionalized population]

Characteristic	1984[a]	1989[a]	1995[a]	1997	2000[b]	2004(1)[c]	2004(2)[c]	2005[c]	2006[c]	2007[c]
					Percent of population					
Under 18 years:										
Below 100%	43.2	47.9	66.0	58.0	58.5	69.2	70.7	71.2	72.0	75.0
100%–less than 150%	9.0	12.3	27.2	28.7	35.0	46.6	47.6	49.0	52.1	55.4
150%–less than 200%	4.4	6.1	13.1	13.0	21.3	31.9	32.4	35.3	35.8	39.9
200% or more	0.8	1.8	3.3	3.1	5.1	8.0	8.0	8.3	8.9	8.5

*Estimates are considered unreliable.
—Data not available.
[a]Data prior to 1997 are not strictly comparable with data for later years due to the 1997 questionnaire redesign.
[b]Estimates for 2000–2002 were calculated using 2000-based sample weights and may differ from estimates in other reports that used 1990-based sample weights for 2000–2002 estimates.
[c]Beginning in quarter 3 of the 2004 National Health Interview Survey (NHIS), persons under 65 years with no reported coverage were asked explicitly about Medicaid coverage. Estimates were calculated without and with the additional information from this question in the columns labeled 2004(1) and 2004(2), respectively, and estimates were calculated with the additional information starting with 2005 data.
[d]Includes all other races not shown separately, those with unknown marital status, and, in 1984 and 1989, persons with unknown poverty level.
[e]Includes persons 14–64 years of age.
[f]The race groups, white, black, American Indian or Alaska Native, Asian, Native Hawaiian or other Pacific Islander, and 2 or more races, include persons of Hispanic and non-Hispanic origin. Persons of Hispanic origin may be of any race. Starting with 1999 data, race-specific estimates are tabulated according to the 1997 Revisions to the Standards for the Classification of Federal Data on Race and Ethnicity and are not strictly comparable with estimates for earlier years. The five single-race categories plus multiple-race categories shown in the table conform to the 1997 standards. Starting with 1999 data, race-specific estimates are for persons who reported only one racial group; the category 2 or more races includes persons who reported more than one racial group. Prior to 1999, data were tabulated according to the 1977 standards with four racial groups and the Asian only category included Native Hawaiian or other Pacific Islander. Estimates for single-race categories prior to 1999 included persons who reported one race or, if they reported more than one race, identified one race as best representing their race. Starting with 2003 data, race responses of other race and unspecified multiple race were treated as missing, and then race was imputed if these were the only race responses. Almost all persons with a race response of other race were of Hispanic origin.
[g]Percent of poverty level is based on family income and family size and composition using U.S. Census Bureau poverty thresholds. Poverty level was unknown for 10%–11% of persons under 65 years of age in 1984 and 1989. Missing family income data were imputed for 15%–16% of persons under 65 years of age in 1994–1996, 23% in 1997, and 27%–33% in 1998–2007.
Notes: The category, Medicaid coverage, includes persons who had any of the following at the time of interview: Medicaid, other public assistance through 1996, state-sponsored health plan starting in 1997, or Children's Health Insurance Program (CHIP) starting in 1999; it includes those who also had another type of coverage in addition to one of these. In 2007, 11.2% of persons under 65 years of age reported being covered by Medicaid, 1.2% by state-sponsored health plans, and 1.5% by CHIP. The number of persons with Medicaid coverage was calculated by multiplying the percent with Medicaid coverage by the number of persons under age 65 in the civilian non-institutionalized U.S. population. Percents were calculated with unknown values excluded from denominators.

SOURCE: Adapted from "Table 139. Medicaid Coverage among Persons under 65 Years of Age, by Selected Characteristics: United States, Selected Years 1984–2007," in *Health, United States, 2009: With Special Feature on Medical Technology*, U.S. Department of Health and Human Services, Centers for Disease Control and Prevention, National Center for Health Statistics, 2010, http://www.cdc.gov/nchs/data/hus/hus09.pdf (accessed May 21, 2010)

and freedom of choice of health care providers, enable consumers to save for future medical and long-term care expenses, and improve access to medical care.

In February 2001 President Bush advocated more liberal rules governing MSAs and proposed making them permanently available to all eligible Americans. Congress reviewed the president's proposed reforms and during its 2001–02 session lowered the minimum annual deductible to increase the number of eligible Americans, allowed annual MSA contributions up to 65% of the maximum deductible for individuals and 75% for families, and extended the availability of MSAs through December 31, 2003.

The Medicare Modernization Act of 2003 included provisions to establish health savings accounts (HSAs) for the general population. Like the MSA program it replaced, HSAs offer a variety of benefits, including more choice, greater control, and individual ownership. Specific features of HSAs include:

- Permanence and portability
- Availability to all individuals with a qualified HDHP
- Minimum deductible of $1,000 per individual plan and $2,000 per family plan

- Allowing annual contributions to equal 100% of the deductible
- Allowing both employer and employee contributions
- Not placing a cap on taxpayer participation
- Allowing tax-free rollover of up to $500 in unspent flexible spending accounts

As of 2010, HSAs enabled individuals to deposit up to $3,050 ($6,150 for families) per year in the accounts tax free and the funds were rolled over from one year to the next. Also, funds could be withdrawn to pay for medical bills or saved for future needs, including retirement.

Pros and Cons of HSAs

Catherine Hoffman and Jennifer Tolbert of the Kaiser Family Foundation state in *Health Savings Accounts and High Deductible Health Plans: Are They an Option for Low-Income Families?* (October 2006, http://www.kff.org/uninsured/upload/7568.pdf) that "HSAs and HDHPs are no more affordable for low-income families than existing plans, and the high deductibles associated with these plans may shift even more health care costs onto them." Furthermore, greater cost sharing may reduce health care use among people with low incomes, especially those with chronic conditions or disabilities and others with high-cost medical needs.

Nonetheless, America's Health Insurance Plans, a national association that represents nearly 1,300 companies providing health insurance coverage to more than 200 million Americans, reports in *January 2010 Census Shows 10 Million People Covered by HSA/High-Deductible Health Plans* (May 2010, http://www.ahipresearch.org/pdfs/HSA2010.pdf) that as of January 2010, 10 million people had an HSA. This was an increase of 2 million people since January 2009. HSA plan enrollment varied by geography with the highest percentages in Vermont (13.8%), Minnesota (9.2%), Colorado (9.2%), Arkansas (8.2%) Indiana (8.1%), and Ohio (8%).

Advocates of HSAs believe that by having consumers assume an increasing burden of escalating medical care costs, HSAs will stimulate both comparison shopping for health care providers and competition that will ultimately reduce the rate at which costs are rising. In "HSA Enrollment Grows amid Cost Cuts" (*Business Insurance*, May 24, 2010), Jerry Geisel explains the appeal of HSAs: they impose less cost sharing on employees than traditional health plans and offer tax breaks that are not available with other health plans.

However, other industry analysts question whether employer cost savings are the result of HSA enrollees' decisions to forgo needed medical care. Also, Geisel observes that the emphasis on cost sharing may be a drawback for workers who make frequent use of costly health services.

There is also speculation that the 2010 health care reform legislation will spur consumers to purchase high-deductible, lower premium plans. Ross Kerber reports in "Advocates See Growth for Health Savings Accounts" (Reuters, March 23, 2010) that by 2010 HSAs had grown to $8.6 billion from their inception in 2003, and John Vellines, the president of Health Savings Administrators, opined that there would be "an explosion of these assets"—with HSAs growing to between $50 billion and $100 billion.

HEALTH INSURANCE COSTS CONTINUE TO SKYROCKET

According to the Kaiser Family Foundation, in *Employer Health Benefits: 2009 Annual Survey* (2009, http://ehbs.kff.org/pdf/2009/7936.pdf), health insurance premiums continued to increase much faster than inflation and wages, growing a cumulative 131% between 1999 and 2009 and far outpacing cumulative wage growth of 38% during the same period. Premiums averaged $5,791 for individual coverage and $13,375 for family coverage. Workers paid an average of $779 per year toward the premium for individual coverage and $3,515 per year toward the premium for family coverage.

The Kaiser Family Foundation explains that the percentage of workers with deductibles for individual coverage of $1,000 or more increased, as did the average co-payments for primary or specialty physician office visits. Annual deductibles for individual coverage ranged from $634 for PPO members to $1,838 for those in HDHPs. The majority (77%) of covered workers incurred co-payments for office visits and prescription drugs. More than three-quarters (78%) of workers were enrolled in plans with co-payments or another form of cost sharing for prescription drugs.

The Kaiser Family Foundation finds that 60% of employers offered health benefits in 2009, down just 3% from the previous year. Furthermore, 21% of employers surveyed reported that they had either reduced the scope of their health benefits or increased cost sharing in response to the economic downturn, and 15% said they had increased workers' share of premium costs.

HEALTH INSURERS HAVE NEW AND HEIGHTENED OVERSIGHT

One of the consequences of the 2010 health reform legislation was the establishment of the Office of Consumer Information and Insurance Oversight (OCIIO). The OCIIO is responsible for overseeing many of the provisions of the Health Care and Education Affordability Reconciliation Act, which was signed into law by President Obama in March 2010.

The OCIIO is responsible for ensuring compliance with the new insurance market rules, such as the elimination of the preexisting condition exclusions for children that took effect in 2010 and the development of a federally funded high-risk pool that will temporarily extend health insurance coverage to people with preexisting conditions who are currently uninsured. The high-risk pool program will operate until 2014, when state-based health insurance exchanges become available.

The OCIIO will also assist states to establish insurance rates and will offer guidance and oversight for the state-based insurance exchanges. It will administer several special programs, including temporary insurance options for early retirees, which will reimburse participating employment-based plans for some of the costs of health benefits for early retirees and their families. Furthermore, the OCIIO will create and regularly update an Internet portal that provides information about insurance options.

Health Insurers Lobby to Influence Implementation of Health Reform Law

In "Health Insurance Companies Try to Shape Rules" (*New York Times*, May 15, 2010), Robert Pear reports that in 2010 health insurance companies were lobbying federal and state officials in an effort to protect their ability to increase insurance premiums and spend a minimum percentage of premium dollars collected on direct patient care, as opposed to using it for administrative expenses or keeping it as corporate profits. Of the legislation's 40 provisions affecting insurers, the provision that forbids insurers from an "'unreasonable' premium increase" and another that requires that premiums be used for "health care services and 'activities that improve health care quality' for patients" appear to be the requirements the insurance companies are most eager to redefine to their advantage. For example, insurers that offer coverage to large groups are expected to spend 85% of premiums on "'clinical services' and quality-enhancing activities." For health insurance coverage sold to individuals or small groups, the insurers must devote 80% of premiums to patient care and quality initiatives.

Health Insurers Have to Comply with Many New Regulations

Roni Caryn Rabin reports in "In Health Law, a Clearer View of Coverage" (*New York Times*, May 17, 2010) that even though health insurers are likely to benefit from increasing numbers of subscribers, the new legislation will require them to offer a package of basic health benefits comparable to the coverage offered by employer plans to individuals with preexisting conditions, and they will have to present their plans in standardized formats that enable consumers to compare every aspect of them—coverage, cost sharing, provider networks, deductibles, and co-payments. Consumers will be able to select one of four standardized levels of coverage and benefits, with progressively increasing premiums associated with higher levels of coverage. Also standardized by the PPACA is a cap on out-of-pocket expenses: after patients reach a limit of $5,950 a year for individuals and $11,900 for families, the plans must cover all additional health care costs. Furthermore, the law eliminates lifetime limits, which are commonly between $1 million and $2 million, amounts that are easily exceeded by some people with chronic, serious medical conditions such as acquired immunodeficiency syndrome (AIDS), some cancers, and organ transplants.

MENTAL HEALTH PARITY

In terms of mental health care, parity refers to the premise that the same range and scope of insurance benefits available for other illnesses should be provided for people with mental illness. Historically, private health insurance plans have provided less coverage for mental illness than for other medical conditions. Coverage for mental health was more restricted and often involved more cost sharing (higher co-payments and deductibles) than coverage for medical care. As a result, many patients with severe mental illness, who frequently required hospitalizations and other treatment, quickly depleted their mental health coverage.

During the 1990s there was growing interest in parity of mental health with other health services. The Mental Health Parity Act of 1996 sought to bring mental health benefits closer to other health benefits. The act amended the 1944 Public Health Service Act and the 1974 Employee Retirement Income Security Act by requiring parity for annual and lifetime dollar limits but did not place restrictions on other plan features such as hospital and office visit limits. It also imposed federal standards on the mental health coverage offered by employers through group health plans. By 2007 more than two-thirds of states had laws governing mental health parity that were more comprehensive in scope than the federal legislation, and one-third of the states required full parity.

Legislation Establishes Mental Health Parity

The Paul Wellstone and Pete Domenici Mental Health Parity and Addiction Equity Act of 2008 expands on the Mental Health Parity Act by prohibiting group health plans and group health insurance companies from imposing treatment limitations or financial requirements for coverage of mental health that are different from those used for medical and surgical benefits. In "New Rules Promise Better Mental Health Coverage" (*New York Times*, January 29, 2010), Robert Pear explains that eliminating disparities between physical health care and mental health care will make it easier for people to obtain care for conditions ranging from depression and anxiety to eating disorders and substance abuse. The Obama administration anticipates that the parity requirement will benefit "111 million people in 446,400 group health plans offered by private employers, and 29 million people in 20,000 plans sponsored by state and local governments." The act is projected to increase insurance premiums by 0.4%, which translates into $25.6 billion between 2010 and 2019.

Actual Effects of Federal Mental Health Parity Legislation on Employers

Howard H. Goldman et al. confirm in "Behavioral Health Insurance Parity for Federal Employees" (*New England Journal of Medicine*, vol. 354, no. 13, March 30, 2006) that costs are not likely to increase when workers are given the same coverage for mental health and substance abuse treatment as they are for other medical care. The researchers consider seven Federal Employees Health Benefits plans that offer mental health and substance abuse benefits on a par with medical benefits beginning in January 2001. Among people who used mental health services, spending attributable to parity decreased significantly for three plans and did not change significantly for the four remaining plans. The institution of parity was also associated with significant reductions in out-of-pocket spending in five of the seven plans. Goldman et al. conclude that offering parity "can improve insurance protection without increasing total costs."

Parity May Not Solve All Access Problems

According to Robert Pear, in "Fight Erupts over Rules Issued for 'Mental Health Parity' Insurance Law" (*New*

York Times, May 9, 2010), health insurance companies believe that parity alone will not eliminate all obstacles to gaining access to mental health care. The insurers oppose some of the provisions of the parity legislation, especially the requirement to have a single deductible for all medical and mental health services combined, rather than the traditional practice of separate deductibles. Insurers contend that because the single deductible will be higher than the previous separate mental health deductible, it may serve to impede access to mental health care.

Pear explains that even though "the Obama administration praised the work of [managed behavioral health organizations (MBHOs)], saying they increased the use of mental health care while holding down costs," several of these MBHOs have taken aim at some of the provisions of the parity legislation. In particular, the MBHOs claim that the requirement to use a single deductible and the prohibition of nonquantitative treatment limitations (NQTLs are cost-control strategies that unlike annual and lifetime dollar limits or number of visit limits cannot be measured numerically) for mental health treatment will hinder their ability to offer parity coverage. The law states that NQTLs such as design of prescription drug formularies that limit drug coverage may not be applied to mental health coverage unless they are also used for medical and surgical insurance coverage. The article "APA Supports Provisions Being Challenged in Court" (*Psychiatric News*, vol. 45, no. 10, May 21, 2010) quotes James H. Scully Jr. of the American Psychiatric Association as saying, "NQTLs prevent patients from gaining access to adequate mental health and substance use disorder treatment, which is the very problem [the parity legislation] sought to rectify."

FINANCING THE 2010 HEALTH CARE REFORM LEGISLATION

An analysis of the financial impact of the 2010 health care reform legislation was conducted by the Congressional Budget Office (CBO; http://www.cbo.gov/ftpdocs/113xx/doc11379/AmendReconProp.pdf) in March 2010.

The CBO reveals that from 2010 to 2019 the enactment of major components of the PPACA will cost an estimated $938 billion and reduce the federal deficit by $143 billion. Approximately $124 billion of the savings come from provisions dealing with health care and federal revenues, and the remaining $19 billion come from the education provisions. In "House Leaders Announce $940 Billion Health-Care Compromise Bill" (*Washington Post*, March 19, 2010), Lori Montgomery and Paul Kane report that during the second decade of its implementation, from 2020 to 2029, the bill is anticipated to reduce the deficit by $1.2 trillion.

In May 2010 the CBO (http://www.cbo.gov/ftpdocs/114xx/doc11490/LewisLtr_HR3590.pdf) amended its estimates and identified additional discretionary costs of $115 billion. These discretionary costs include the continuation of recent funding levels for health-related programs that were previously authorized and that the PPACA authorized for future years. Because these are not new costs associated with implementation of the legislation, they were not considered in the March 2010 forecast.

The implementation of the PPACA will be financed by a combination of health care savings resulting from programs that improve efficiency and accountability; incentivize quality and cost-effective care; and reduce waste, fraud, and inefficiencies. Phil Galewitz indicates in "Consumers Guide to Health Reform" (April 13, 2010, http://www.kaiserhealthnews.org/stories/2010/march/22/consumers-guide-health-reform.aspx) that revenues will be generated via taxes on the wealthiest Americans. Beginning in 2013, individuals who earn more than $200,000 per year and couples who earn more than $250,000 per year will pay a Medicare payroll tax of 2.3%. The wealthiest Americans will also pay a 3.8% tax on unearned income such as dividends. Furthermore, in 2018 there will be a 40% excise tax on employers who offer high-end so-called Cadillac insurance plans that cost $10,200 per year for individuals and $27,500 per year for families.

CHAPTER 7
INTERNATIONAL COMPARISONS OF HEALTH CARE

International comparisons are often difficult to interpret because definitions of terms and reliability of data as well as cultures and values differ. What is important in one society may be unimportant or even nonexistent in another. A political or human right that is important in one nation may be meaningless in a neighboring nation. Evaluating the quality of health care systems is an example of the difficulties involved in comparing one culture to another.

Even within the United States there are cultural and regional variations in health care delivery. A visit to a busy urban urgent care center might begin with the patient completing a brief medical history, followed by five or 10 minutes with a nurse who measures and records the patient's vital signs (pulse, respiration, and temperature), and conclude with a 15-minute visit with a physician, who diagnoses the problem and prescribes treatment. In contrast, on the islands of Hawaii a visit with a healer may last several hours and culminate with a prayer, song, or an embrace. Hawaiian healers, called kahunas, are unhurried and offer an array of herbal remedies, bodywork (massage, touch, and manipulative therapies), and talk therapies (counseling and guidance), because they believe that the healing quality of the encounter, independent of any treatment offered, improves health and well-being.

Even though comparing the performance of health care systems and health outcomes (how people fare as a result of receiving health care services) is of benefit to health care planners, administrators, and policy makers, the subjective nature of such assessments should be duly considered.

A COMPARISON OF HEALTH CARE SPENDING, RESOURCES, AND UTILIZATION

The Organisation for Economic Cooperation and Development (OECD) provides information about 32 member countries that are governed democratically and participate in the global market economy. It collects and publishes data about a wide range of economic and social issues including health and health care policy. The OECD member nations are generally considered the wealthier, more developed nations in the world. The OECD (2010, http://www.oecd.org/pages/0,3417,en_36734052_36761800_1_1_1_1_1,00.html) indicates that its member countries are Australia, Austria, Belgium, Canada, Chile, the Czech Republic, Denmark, Finland, France, Germany, Greece, Hungary, Iceland, Ireland, Italy, Japan, Korea, Luxembourg, Mexico, the Netherlands, New Zealand, Norway, Poland, Portugal, the Slovak Republic, Slovenia, Spain, Sweden, Switzerland, Turkey, the United Kingdom, and the United States.

Percentage of Gross Domestic Product Spent on Health Care

Even though health has always been a concern for Americans, the growth in the health care industry since the mid-1970s has made it a major factor in the U.S. economy. For many years the United States has spent a larger proportion of its gross domestic product (GDP; the total market value of final goods and services produced within an economy in a given year) on health care than have other nations with similar economic development. According to the OECD, in *Health at a Glance 2009: OECD Indicators* (December 2009, http://www.oecd-ilibrary.org/content/book/health_glance-2009-en; Chile and Slovenia are not discussed in this report because it was published before they joined the OECD, so the OECD provides data for just the 30 previously mentioned countries), in 2007 U.S. health expenditures were 16% of the GDP, the highest rate in the OECD. (See Figure 7.1.) Other nations that spent large percentages of GDP on health care in 2007 included France (11%), Switzerland (10.8%), Germany (10.4%), Belgium (10.2%), Canada (10.1%), Austria (10.1%), Portugal (9.9%), the Netherlands (9.8%), Denmark (9.8%), and Greece (9.6%). Of the member nations that reported health care expenditure data in 2007, Turkey (5.7%), Mexico (5.9%), and Poland (6.4%) spent the least in the OECD.

FIGURE 7.1

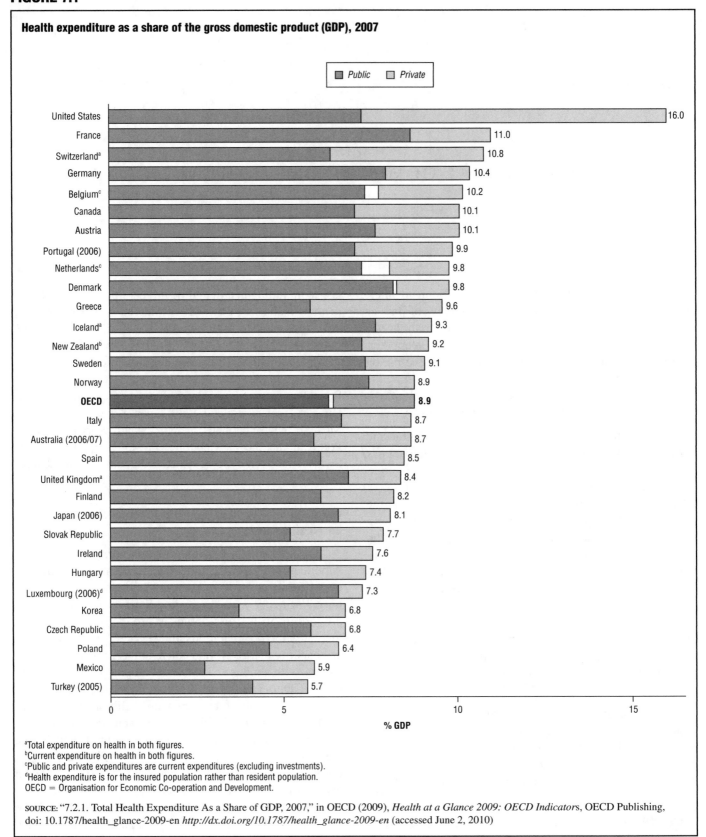

Health expenditure as a share of the gross domestic product (GDP), 2007

Public ☐   Private ☐

Country	% GDP
United States	16.0
France	11.0
Switzerland[a]	10.8
Germany	10.4
Belgium[c]	10.2
Canada	10.1
Austria	10.1
Portugal (2006)	9.9
Netherlands[c]	9.8
Denmark	9.8
Greece	9.6
Iceland[a]	9.3
New Zealand[b]	9.2
Sweden	9.1
Norway	8.9
OECD	**8.9**
Italy	8.7
Australia (2006/07)	8.7
Spain	8.5
United Kingdom[a]	8.4
Finland	8.2
Japan (2006)	8.1
Slovak Republic	7.7
Ireland	7.6
Hungary	7.4
Luxembourg (2006)[d]	7.3
Korea	6.8
Czech Republic	6.8
Poland	6.4
Mexico	5.9
Turkey (2005)	5.7

% GDP

[a]Total expenditure on health in both figures.
[b]Current expenditure on health in both figures.
[c]Public and private expenditures are current expenditures (excluding investments).
[d]Health expenditure is for the insured population rather than resident population.
OECD = Organisation for Economic Co-operation and Development.

SOURCE: "7.2.1. Total Health Expenditure As a Share of GDP, 2007," in OECD (2009), *Health at a Glance 2009: OECD Indicators*, OECD Publishing, doi: 10.1787/health_glance-2009-en *http://dx.doi.org/10.1787/health_glance-2009-en* (accessed June 2, 2010)

Per Capita Spending on Health Care

According to the OECD, in *Health at a Glance 2009*, the United States also experienced the highest per capita spending for health care services in 2007, spending an average of $7,290 per citizen. No other country came close to spending this amount per capita in 2007: Norway spent $4,763 per citizen; Switzerland, $4,417; Luxembourg, $4,162; Canada, $3,895; the Netherlands, $3,837; Austria,

$3,763; France, $3,601; Belgium, $3,595; Germany, $3,588; Denmark, $3,512; Ireland, $3,424; Sweden, $3,323; Iceland, $3,319; and Australia, $3,137. In 2007 Turkey ($618) spent the least per capita of any OECD member nation on health care, followed by Mexico ($823), Poland ($1,035), and Hungary ($1,388).

Who Pays for Health Care?

Public expenditures for health care services as a percentage of GDP vary widely between the OECD member nations. Public spending on health accounted for about 73% of total health spending on average across OECD member countries in 2007, and the remaining 27% of spending was paid by private sources, mainly private insurance and individuals. (See Figure 7.2.) In the United States public funding accounted for 45.4% of total health spending. By contrast, public sources in Luxembourg and the Czech Republic accounted for 90.9% and 85.2%, respectively, of total health spending. Other nations with above-average contributions of public funding to health expenditures included Denmark (84.5%), Norway (84.1%), Iceland (82.5%), Sweden (81.7%), the United Kingdom (81.7%), Japan (81.3%), Ireland (80.7%), New Zealand (80.1%), France (79%), Germany (76.9%), Italy (76.5%), Austria (76.4%), the Netherlands (74.8%), and Finland (74.6%). Public expenditures on health per capita were lowest in Mexico (45.2%), the United States (45.4%), Korea (54.9%), and Switzerland (59.3%).

In terms of out-of-pocket payments as a share of total health expenditures in 2007, the United States was below the OECD average. (See Figure 7.3.) In the Netherlands and France out-of-pocket payments as a share of total health expenditures were very low. In contrast, out-of-pocket spending as a share of total health care spending was highest in Mexico and Greece. Figure 7.3 reveals that out-of-pocket spending as a share of total health care spending was also high in Korea, Switzerland, the Slovak Republic, Hungary, and Poland.

Private health insurance fills the gap between public expenditures and out-of-pocket costs. Among the OECD member countries declaring private insurance as a percentage of total expenditures for health in 2007, the United States' private insurance expenditure far outstripped all other countries. (See Figure 7.3.) Because the United States does not currently have a government-funded national health care program that provides coverage for all of its citizens, U.S. private insurance expenditures cover the costs generally assumed by government programs that finance health care delivery in comparable OECD member nations. The Patient Protection and Affordable Care Act (PPACA) of 2010 promises not only to provide health insurance coverage for 95% of Americans but also to change the ways in which Americans purchase and pay for health care. In 2014, when U.S. citizens will be required to have health care coverage (or pay a penalty), it is anticipated that the mix of payment sources (public, private, and out of pocket) will shift. For example, expanded Medicaid eligibility may increase the share of public expenditures, and establishment of limits on maximum health plan deductibles may reduce out-of-pocket expenditures.

Spending on Public Health and Prevention Programs and Pharmaceutical Drugs

Interestingly, even though the United States spent more on health care than other OECD member nations in 2007, it devoted a smaller percentage of total health expenditures (3.3%) on public health and prevention programs than did Canada (7.3%), Finland (5.8%), the Netherlands (5.1%), the Slovak Republic (5%), New Zealand (4.9%), Hungary (4.1%), Belgium (4.1%), Germany (3.7%), and Sweden (3.6%). (See Figure 7.4.) This percentage is likely to increase in the coming years as the PPACA places increased emphasis on the provision of preventive health services and coverage for health screening and other preventive medical care.

In 2007 the United States spent more per capita ($878) on pharmaceutical drugs than any other OECD member country. (See Figure 7.5.) The average pharmaceutical spending was $461 per capita. The per capita pharmaceutical spending was also high in Canada ($691), Greece ($677), France ($588), Belgium ($566), Spain ($562), and Germany ($542). In contrast, Mexico spent $198 and New Zealand spent $241 per capita on pharmaceuticals.

Hospital Utilization Statistics

The number of acute hospital beds is a gross measure of resource availability; however, it is important to remember that it does not reflect capacity to provide emergency or outpatient hospital care. In general, it also does not measure the number of beds devoted to nonacute or other long-term care, although it is known that in Japan many of the beds designated as acute care are actually used for long-term care. Of the OECD member countries reporting acute care hospital beds per 1,000 population, Japan (8.2), Korea (7.1), Austria (6.1), Germany (5.7), and the Czech Republic (5.2) had the highest number of acute care beds in 2007. (See Figure 7.6.) The United States was among the lowest, at 2.7 beds per 1,000 population in 2007, trailed only by the United Kingdom (2.6), Spain (2.5), Sweden (2.1), and Mexico (1).

Hospital lengths of stay have consistently declined since 1960, in part because increasing numbers of illnesses can be treated as effectively in outpatient settings and because many countries have reduced inpatient hospitalization rates and average length of stay (ALOS) to control health care costs. In 2007 Japan (19 days) had the longest acute care ALOS of the OECD member nations, followed by Germany (7.8 days), Switzerland (7.8 days), and the

FIGURE 7.2

Public share of total health expenditure, 2007

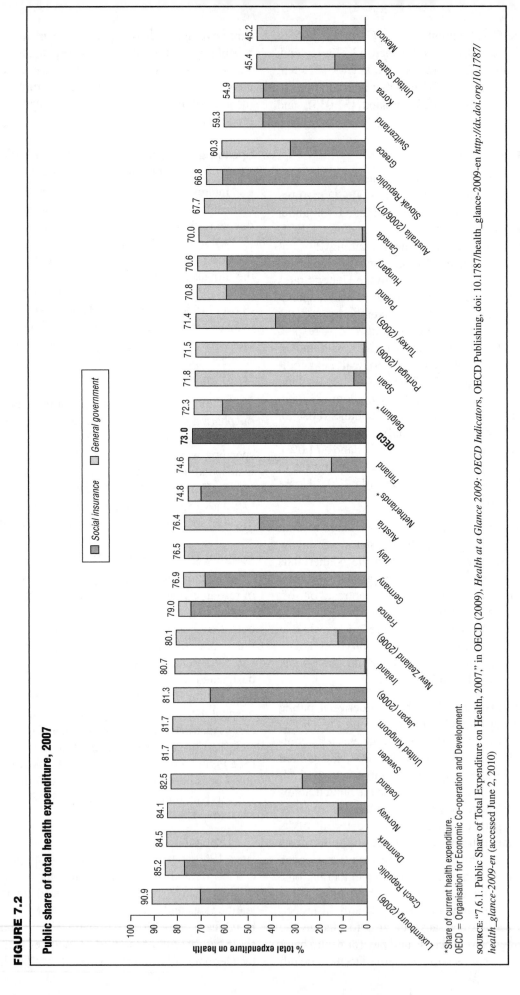

* Share of current health expenditure.

OECD = Organisation for Economic Co-operation and Development.

SOURCE: "7.6.1. Public Share of Total Expenditure on Health, 2007," in OECD (2009), *Health at a Glance 2009: OECD Indicators*, OECD Publishing, doi: 10.1787/health_glance-2009-en http://dx.doi.org/10.1787/health_glance-2009-en (accessed June 2, 2010)

FIGURE 7.3

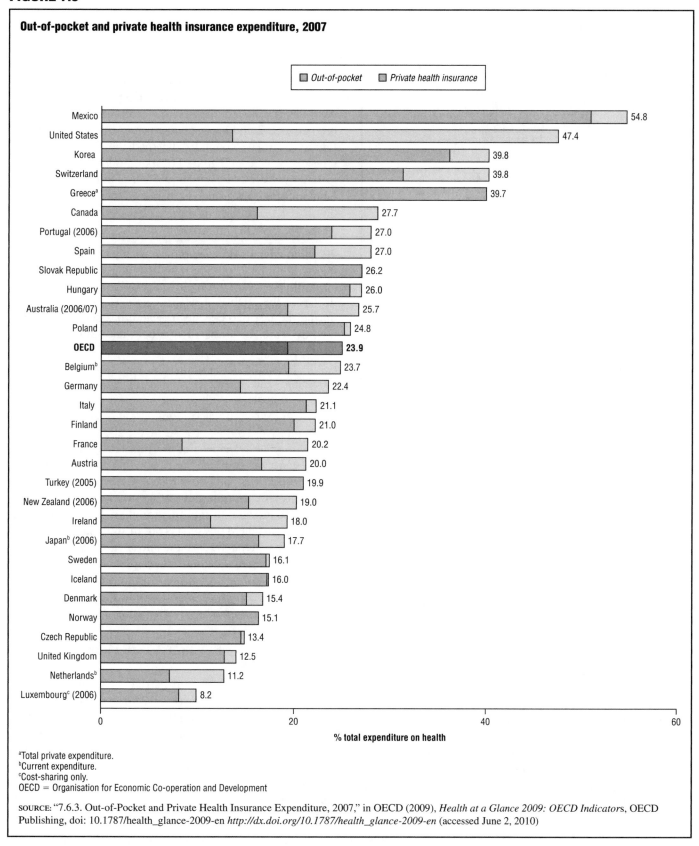

Out-of-pocket and private health insurance expenditure, 2007

Legend: ■ Out-of-pocket ■ Private health insurance

Country	% total expenditure on health
Mexico	54.8
United States	47.4
Korea	39.8
Switzerland	39.8
Greece[a]	39.7
Canada	27.7
Portugal (2006)	27.0
Spain	27.0
Slovak Republic	26.2
Hungary	26.0
Australia (2006/07)	25.7
Poland	24.8
OECD	**23.9**
Belgium[b]	23.7
Germany	22.4
Italy	21.1
Finland	21.0
France	20.2
Austria	20.0
Turkey (2005)	19.9
New Zealand (2006)	19.0
Ireland	18.0
Japan[b] (2006)	17.7
Sweden	16.1
Iceland	16.0
Denmark	15.4
Norway	15.1
Czech Republic	13.4
United Kingdom	12.5
Netherlands[b]	11.2
Luxembourg[c] (2006)	8.2

% total expenditure on health

[a]Total private expenditure.
[b]Current expenditure.
[c]Cost-sharing only.
OECD = Organisation for Economic Co-operation and Development

SOURCE: "7.6.3. Out-of-Pocket and Private Health Insurance Expenditure, 2007," in OECD (2009), *Health at a Glance 2009: OECD Indicators*, OECD Publishing, doi: 10.1787/health_glance-2009-en *http://dx.doi.org/10.1787/health_glance-2009-en* (accessed June 2, 2010)

Czech Republic (7.7 days). (See Figure 7.7.) The shortest hospital stays in 2007 occurred in Denmark (3.5 days), Mexico (3.9 days), Turkey (4.4 days), and Sweden (4.5 days). The United States' ALOS was 5.5 days in 2007, which is on par with Greece and Iceland, at 5.6 and 5.4 days, respectively.

FIGURE 7.4

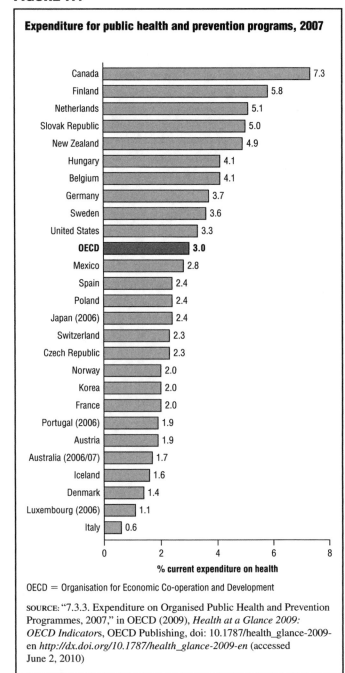

Expenditure for public health and prevention programs, 2007

Country	% current expenditure on health
Canada	7.3
Finland	5.8
Netherlands	5.1
Slovak Republic	5.0
New Zealand	4.9
Hungary	4.1
Belgium	4.1
Germany	3.7
Sweden	3.6
United States	3.3
OECD	**3.0**
Mexico	2.8
Spain	2.4
Poland	2.4
Japan (2006)	2.4
Switzerland	2.3
Czech Republic	2.3
Norway	2.0
Korea	2.0
France	2.0
Portugal (2006)	1.9
Austria	1.9
Australia (2006/07)	1.7
Iceland	1.6
Denmark	1.4
Luxembourg (2006)	1.1
Italy	0.6

OECD = Organisation for Economic Co-operation and Development

SOURCE: "7.3.3. Expenditure on Organised Public Health and Prevention Programmes, 2007," in OECD (2009), *Health at a Glance 2009: OECD Indicators*, OECD Publishing, doi: 10.1787/health_glance-2009-en *http://dx.doi.org/10.1787/health_glance-2009-en* (accessed June 2, 2010)

Medical practice, particularly the types and frequency of procedures performed, also varies from one country to another. The OECD looked at rates of cesarean section (delivery of a baby through an incision in the abdomen as opposed to vaginal delivery) per 100 births and found both growth in the rates of cesarean section (as a percentage of all births) and considerable variation in the rates for this surgical procedure. In 2007 the highest rates for cesarean sections per 100 live births were reported in Mexico (39.9), Italy (39.7), Turkey (36), Korea (32), Portugal (31.2), and the United States (31.1). (See Figure 7.8.) Because cesarean section is performed in the hospital and generally involves at least an overnight stay, the frequency with which it and other surgical procedures are performed contributes to hospitalization rates and expenditures.

Physicians' Numbers Are Increasing

Since 1960 the OECD member nations have all enjoyed growing physician populations. In 2007 Greece and Belgium reported the highest ratio of practicing physicians, 5.4 and 4 per 1,000 population, respectively, with most countries ranging between 2 and 4 physicians per 1,000 population. (See Figure 7.9.) The countries that had the fewest practicing physicians were in Turkey (1.5 per 1,000 population), followed by Korea (1.7), Mexico (2), and Japan (2.1). The United States and the United Kingdom had 2.4 and 2.5 physicians per 1,000 population, respectively.

The ratio of physicians to population is a limited measure of health care quality, because many other factors, such as the availability of other health care providers as well as accessibility and affordability of health care services, also influence the quality of health care systems. Furthermore, during the last two decades research has shown that more medical care, in terms of numbers and concentration of health care providers, is not necessarily linked to better health status for the population. For example, David C. Goodman and Elliott S. Fisher of Dartmouth Medical School indicate in "Physician Workforce Crisis? Wrong Diagnosis, Wrong Prescription" (*New England Journal of Medicine*, vol. 358, no. 16, April 17, 2008) that "the presence of more physicians doesn't translate into better care." The researchers find that the regions with higher physician supplies are more likely to report issues such as suboptimal continuity of care, communication problems among physicians, and greater difficulty providing high-quality care than in areas where physicians are in short supply. Furthermore, how patients fare as a result of care and treatment is no better in regions with a large supply of physicians than in areas with lower physician concentrations. Goodman and Fisher reconfirm the observation that more care does not necessarily ensure better outcomes.

OVERVIEWS OF SELECTED HEALTH CARE SYSTEMS

Gerard F. Anderson and Patricia Markovich of Johns Hopkins University observe in *Multinational Comparisons of Health Systems Data, 2008* (April 15, 2010, http://www.commonwealthfund.org/Content/Publications/Chartbooks/2010/Apr/Multinational-Comparisonsof-Health-Systems-Data-2008.aspx) that despite having the most costly health system in the world, the United States does not compare favorably to other industrialized countries on most dimensions of performance.

Anderson and Markovich look at OECD data for several industrialized countries: Australia, Canada, France, Germany, the Netherlands, New Zealand, Switzerland, the United Kingdom, and the United States. The most significant difference between the United States and the other countries is the lack of universal health insurance coverage.

FIGURE 7.5

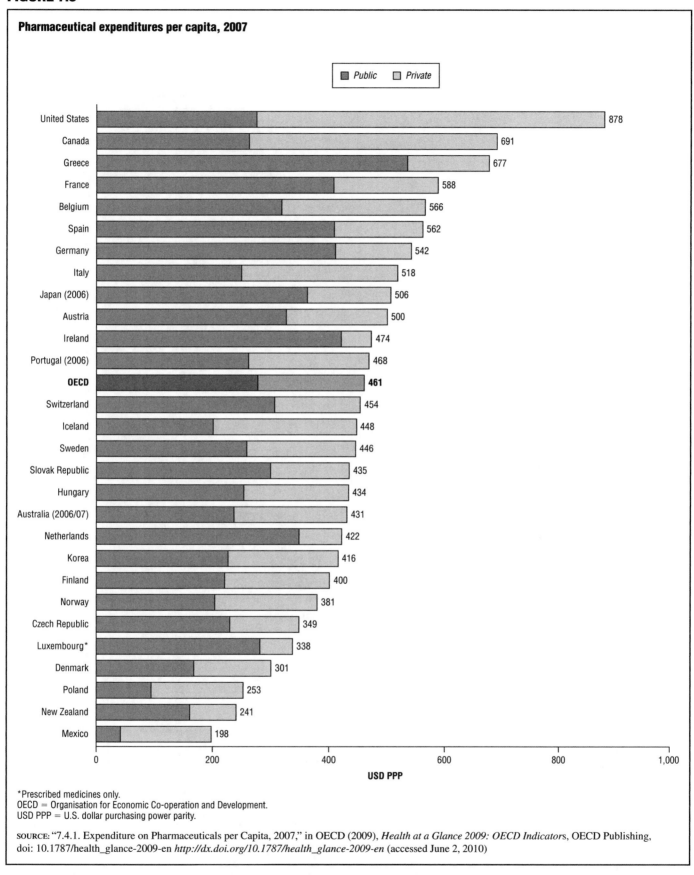

Pharmaceutical expenditures per capita, 2007

Public   *Private*

Country	Value
United States	878
Canada	691
Greece	677
France	588
Belgium	566
Spain	562
Germany	542
Italy	518
Japan (2006)	506
Austria	500
Ireland	474
Portugal (2006)	468
OECD	**461**
Switzerland	454
Iceland	448
Sweden	446
Slovak Republic	435
Hungary	434
Australia (2006/07)	431
Netherlands	422
Korea	416
Finland	400
Norway	381
Czech Republic	349
Luxembourg*	338
Denmark	301
Poland	253
New Zealand	241
Mexico	198

USD PPP

*Prescribed medicines only.
OECD = Organisation for Economic Co-operation and Development.
USD PPP = U.S. dollar purchasing power parity.

SOURCE: "7.4.1. Expenditure on Pharmaceuticals per Capita, 2007," in OECD (2009), *Health at a Glance 2009: OECD Indicators*, OECD Publishing, doi: 10.1787/health_glance-2009-en *http://dx.doi.org/10.1787/health_glance-2009-en* (accessed June 2, 2010)

This gap in coverage explains why Americans go without needed health care because of cost more often than people in other OECD countries and why, in comparison to the other countries, the United States does not fare well in

FIGURE 7.6

Acute care hospital beds, 1995 and 2007

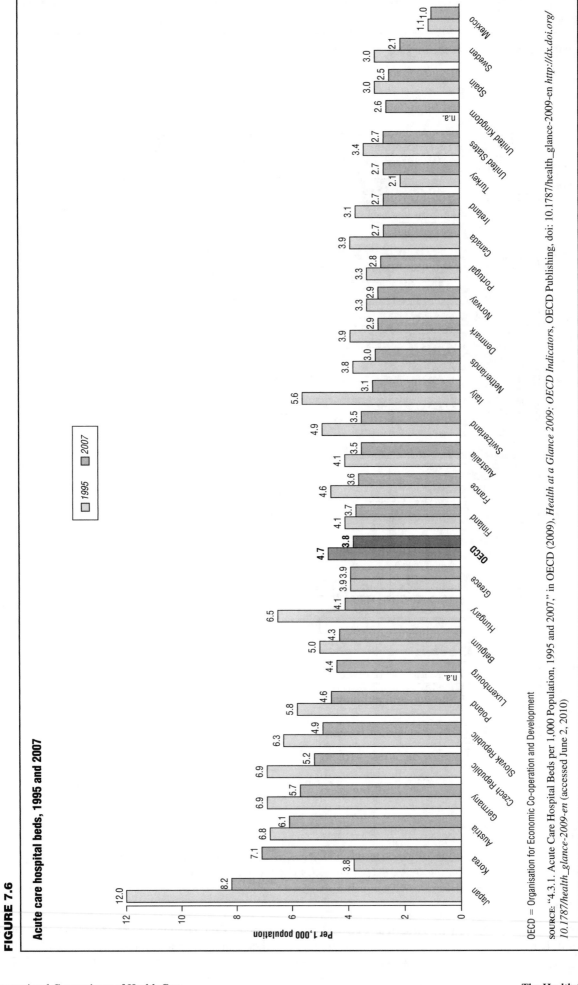

OECD = Organisation for Economic Co-operation and Development

SOURCE: "4.3.1. Acute Care Hospital Beds per 1,000 Population, 1995 and 2007," in OECD (2009), *Health at a Glance 2009: OECD Indicators*, OECD Publishing, doi: 10.1787/health_glance-2009-en *http://dx.doi.org/ 10.1787/health_glance-2009-en* (accessed June 2, 2010)

FIGURE 7.7

Average length of stay for acute care, 1995 and 2007

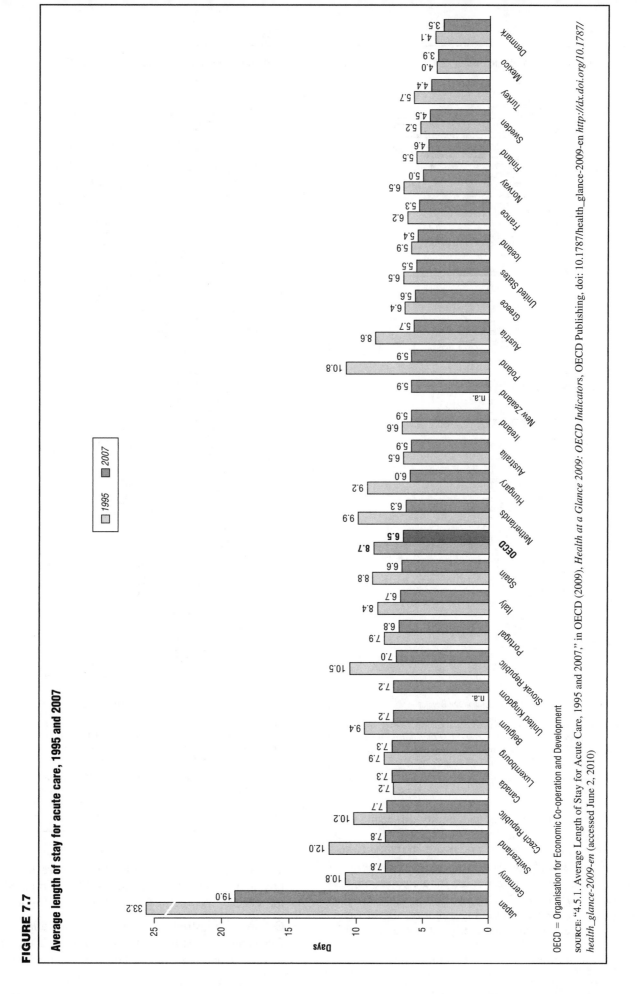

OECD = Organisation for Economic Co-operation and Development

SOURCE: "4.5.1. Average Length of Stay for Acute Care, 1995 and 2007," in OECD (2009), *Health at a Glance 2009: OECD Indicators*, OECD Publishing, doi: 10.1787/health_glance-2009-en *http://dx.doi.org/10.1787/health_glance-2009-en* (accessed June 2, 2010)

FIGURE 7.8

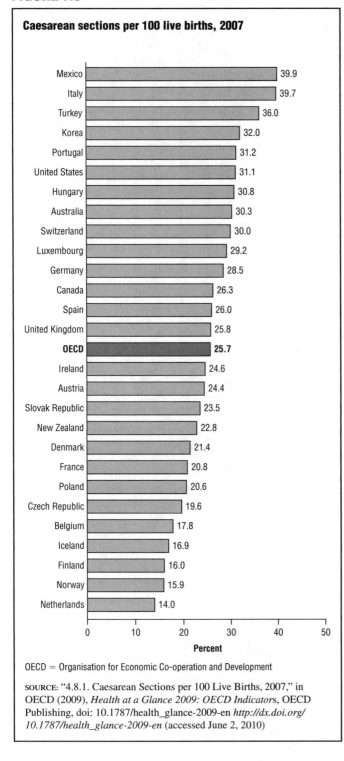

Caesarean sections per 100 live births, 2007

Country	Value
Mexico	39.9
Italy	39.7
Turkey	36.0
Korea	32.0
Portugal	31.2
United States	31.1
Hungary	30.8
Australia	30.3
Switzerland	30.0
Luxembourg	29.2
Germany	28.5
Canada	26.3
Spain	26.0
United Kingdom	25.8
OECD	**25.7**
Ireland	24.6
Austria	24.4
Slovak Republic	23.5
New Zealand	22.8
Denmark	21.4
France	20.8
Poland	20.6
Czech Republic	19.6
Belgium	17.8
Iceland	16.9
Finland	16.0
Norway	15.9
Netherlands	14.0

Percent

OECD = Organisation for Economic Co-operation and Development

SOURCE: "4.8.1. Caesarean Sections per 100 Live Births, 2007," in OECD (2009), *Health at a Glance 2009: OECD Indicators*, OECD Publishing, doi: 10.1787/health_glance-2009-en *http://dx.doi.org/10.1787/health_glance-2009-en* (accessed June 2, 2010)

FIGURE 7.9

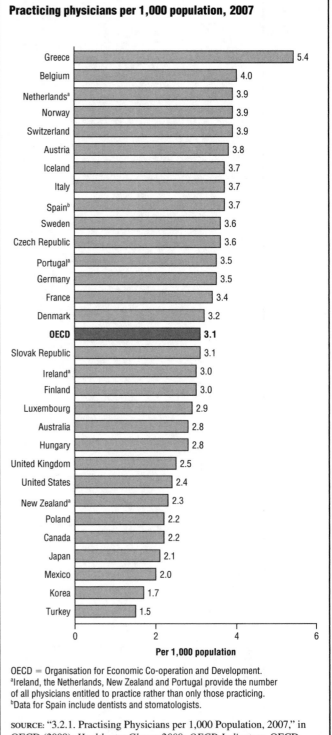

Practicing physicians per 1,000 population, 2007

Country	Value
Greece	5.4
Belgium	4.0
Netherlands[a]	3.9
Norway	3.9
Switzerland	3.9
Austria	3.8
Iceland	3.7
Italy	3.7
Spain[b]	3.7
Sweden	3.6
Czech Republic	3.6
Portugal[a]	3.5
Germany	3.5
France	3.4
Denmark	3.2
OECD	**3.1**
Slovak Republic	3.1
Ireland[a]	3.0
Finland	3.0
Luxembourg	2.9
Australia	2.8
Hungary	2.8
United Kingdom	2.5
United States	2.4
New Zealand[a]	2.3
Poland	2.2
Canada	2.2
Japan	2.1
Mexico	2.0
Korea	1.7
Turkey	1.5

Per 1,000 population

OECD = Organisation for Economic Co-operation and Development.
[a]Ireland, the Netherlands, New Zealand and Portugal provide the number of all physicians entitled to practice rather than only those practicing.
[b]Data for Spain include dentists and stomatologists.

SOURCE: "3.2.1. Practising Physicians per 1,000 Population, 2007," in OECD (2009), *Health at a Glance 2009: OECD Indicators*, OECD Publishing, doi: 10.1787/health_glance-2009-en *http://dx.doi.org/10.1787/health_glance-2009-en* (accessed June 2, 2010)

measures of access to care and equity in health care between high- and low-income populations. The OECD reports in *Health at a Glance 2009* that in 2007 the United States was trailed only by Turkey and Mexico in terms of providing health insurance coverage for a core set of services. (See Figure 7.10.) As the provisions of the PPACA take effect, and the overwhelming majority of Americans have health care coverage, these disparities may diminish.

Other key findings by the OECD include:

- The United States had the third-lowest number of physician contacts per person—3.8—compared with the OECD average of 6.8 in 2007. (See Figure 7.11.)

- Of seven industrialized countries—Australia, Canada, Germany, the Netherlands, New Zealand, the United Kingdom, and the United States—the United Kingdom

FIGURE 7.10

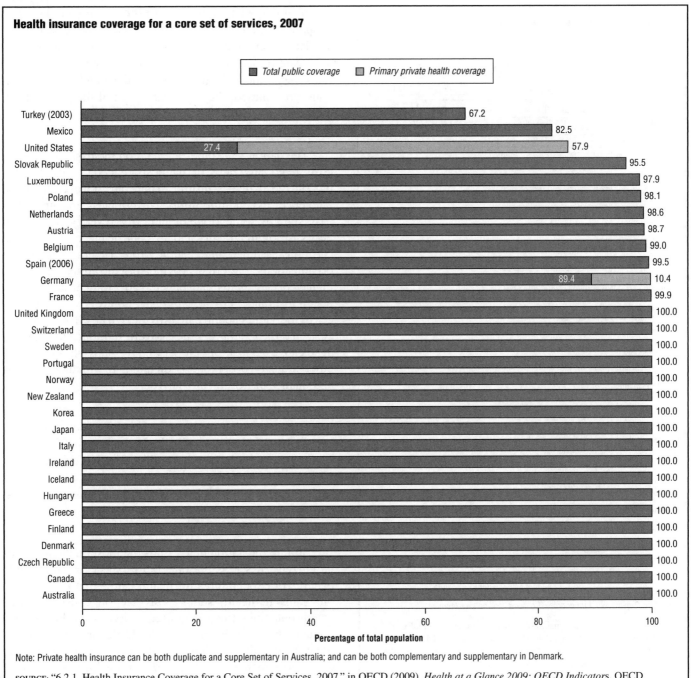

Health insurance coverage for a core set of services, 2007

Note: Private health insurance can be both duplicate and supplementary in Australia; and can be both complementary and supplementary in Denmark.

SOURCE: "6.2.1. Health Insurance Coverage for a Core Set of Services, 2007," in OECD (2009), *Health at a Glance 2009: OECD Indicators*, OECD Publishing, doi: 10.1787/health_glance-2009-en *http://dx.doi.org/10.1787/health_glance-2009-en* (accessed June 2, 2010)

boasted the highest percentage of adults (52%) with no out-of-pocket medical expenses in 2007.

- Of all the OECD member countries, the United States ranked near the bottom of the list in terms of death rates from ischemic heart disease. For example, the OECD average for males was 126 deaths per 100,000 population in 2006, whereas for males in the United States the rate was 145 deaths per 100,000 population. By comparison, males in Japan had just 41 deaths per 100,000 population; in Korea, 47 deaths; in France, 54 deaths; in the Netherlands, 76 deaths; and in Spain, 78 deaths.

- The United States reported the second-highest prevalence of diabetes among adults aged 20 to 79 years in 2010, at 10.3%.

- The United States performed more imaging studies in 2007 than all the other OECD member nations. For example, in Australia there were 20.2 magnetic resonance imaging exams performed per 1,000 population, compared with the U.S. rate of 91.2. Similarly, in 2007 there were 227.8 computed axial tomography scans performed per 1,000 population in the United States, compared with just 45.1 per 1,000 population in France.

FIGURE 7.11

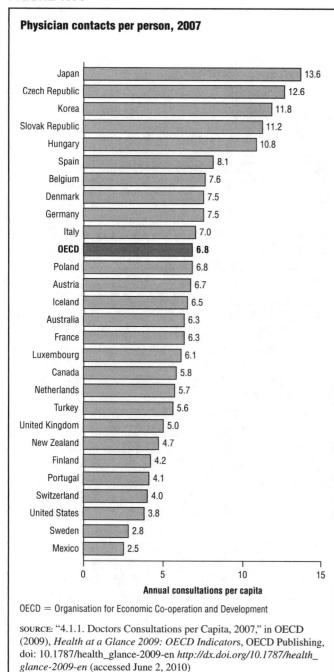

Physician contacts per person, 2007

Country	Annual consultations per capita
Japan	13.6
Czech Republic	12.6
Korea	11.8
Slovak Republic	11.2
Hungary	10.8
Spain	8.1
Belgium	7.6
Denmark	7.5
Germany	7.5
Italy	7.0
OECD	6.8
Poland	6.8
Austria	6.7
Iceland	6.5
Australia	6.3
France	6.3
Luxembourg	6.1
Canada	5.8
Netherlands	5.7
Turkey	5.6
United Kingdom	5.0
New Zealand	4.7
Finland	4.2
Portugal	4.1
Switzerland	4.0
United States	3.8
Sweden	2.8
Mexico	2.5

Annual consultations per capita

OECD = Organisation for Economic Co-operation and Development

SOURCE: "4.1.1. Doctors Consultations per Capita, 2007," in OECD (2009), *Health at a Glance 2009: OECD Indicators*, OECD Publishing, doi: 10.1787/health_glance-2009-en *http://dx.doi.org/10.1787/health_glance-2009-en* (accessed June 2, 2010)

The United States

The U.S. health care financing system is based on the consumer sovereignty, or private insurance, model. Employer-based health insurance is tax subsidized—that is, health insurance premiums are a tax-deductible business expense and are not generally taxed as employee compensation. The premiums for individual policies purchased by self-employed Americans became fully tax deductible in 2003. Benefits, premiums, and provider reimbursement methods differ among private insurance plans and among public programs as well.

Most physicians who provide both ambulatory care (hospital outpatient service and office visits) and inpatient hospital care are generally reimbursed on either a fee-for-service or per capita basis (literally, per head, but in managed care frequently per member per month), and payment rates vary among insurers. Increasing numbers of physicians are salaried; they are employees of the government, hospital, and health care delivery systems, universities, and private industry.

The nation's hospitals are paid on the basis of charges, costs, negotiated rates, or diagnosis-related groups, depending on the patient's insurer. There are no overall global budgets or expenditure limits. Nevertheless, managed care (oversight by some group or authority to verify the medical necessity of treatments and to control the cost of health care) has assumed an expanding role. Health maintenance organizations, preferred provider organizations, and other managed care plans and payers (government and private health insurance) now exert greater control over the practices of individual health care providers in an effort to control costs. To the extent that they govern reimbursement, managed care organizations are viewed by many physicians and other industry observers as dictating the methods, terms, and quality of health care delivery.

IS THE UNITED STATES SPENDING MORE AND GETTING LESS? A primary indicator of the quality of health care delivery in any nation is the health status of its people. Many factors can affect the health of individuals and populations: heredity, race and ethnicity, gender, income, education, geography, violent crime, environmental agents, and exposure to infectious diseases, as well as access to and availability of health care services.

Still, in the nation that spends the most on the health of its citizens, it seems reasonable to expect to see tangible benefits of expenditures for health care—that is, measurable gains in health status. This section considers three health outcomes (measures used to assess the health of a population)—life expectancy at birth, infant mortality (death), and the incidence of cancer—to determine the extent to which U.S. citizens derive health benefits from record-high outlays for medical care.

Overall, life expectancy at birth consistently increased in all the OECD member countries since 1960; however, historically, U.S. life expectancy has remained slightly below the OECD average. (See Figure 7.12.) Infant mortality also declined sharply during this period, but the United States fared far worse than most OECD member countries—in 2007 the United States had the third-highest infant mortality rate. (See Figure 7.13.) Despite the well-funded U.S. battle against cancer, in 2006 the United States came in seventh for its cancer mortality rates (134 deaths of females and 191 deaths of males per 100,000 population). (See Figure 7.14.) Interestingly, the OECD finds in *Health at a Glance 2009* that given the low rank of the United States on many measures and indicators of health status, the United

FIGURE 7.12

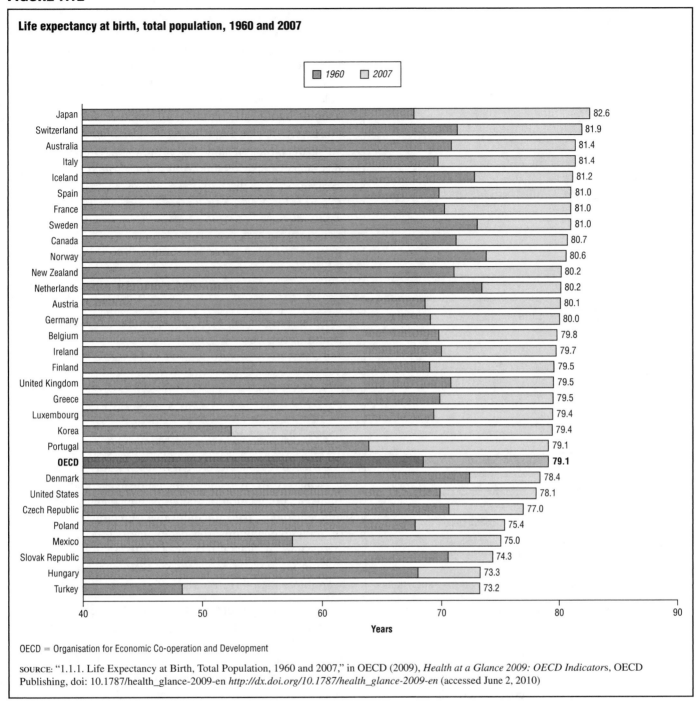

Life expectancy at birth, total population, 1960 and 2007

■ 1960   □ 2007

Country	Value
Japan	82.6
Switzerland	81.9
Australia	81.4
Italy	81.4
Iceland	81.2
Spain	81.0
France	81.0
Sweden	81.0
Canada	80.7
Norway	80.6
New Zealand	80.2
Netherlands	80.2
Austria	80.1
Germany	80.0
Belgium	79.8
Ireland	79.7
Finland	79.5
United Kingdom	79.5
Greece	79.5
Luxembourg	79.4
Korea	79.4
Portugal	79.1
OECD	**79.1**
Denmark	78.4
United States	78.1
Czech Republic	77.0
Poland	75.4
Mexico	75.0
Slovak Republic	74.3
Hungary	73.3
Turkey	73.2

Years

OECD = Organisation for Economic Co-operation and Development

SOURCE: "1.1.1. Life Expectancy at Birth, Total Population, 1960 and 2007," in OECD (2009), *Health at a Glance 2009: OECD Indicators*, OECD Publishing, doi: 10.1787/health_glance-2009-en *http://dx.doi.org/10.1787/health_glance-2009-en* (accessed June 2, 2010)

States boasted the third-highest percentage of adults (88.1%) who considered themselves to be in good health in 2007.

Cathy Schoen et al. find in "Toward Higher-Performance Health Systems: Adults' Health Care Experiences in Seven Countries, 2007" (*Health Affairs*, vol. 26, no. 6, November–December 2007), a seven-nation survey of Australia, Canada, Germany, the Netherlands, New Zealand, the United Kingdom, and the United States, wide-ranging differences in access, after-hours care, and coordination but also common concerns.

In 2007 U.S. health care consumers faced the highest out-of-pocket costs, were the least able to schedule timely appointments with their physicians, and along with Canadians were the most likely to seek nonemergency care in emergency departments. They reported the highest rates of safety issues including lab test errors, medical or medication errors, medical record and test delays, perceptions of waste, and excessive time devoted to administrative paperwork. There were also many examples of inefficiencies and uncoordinated, fragmented care including:

FIGURE 7.13

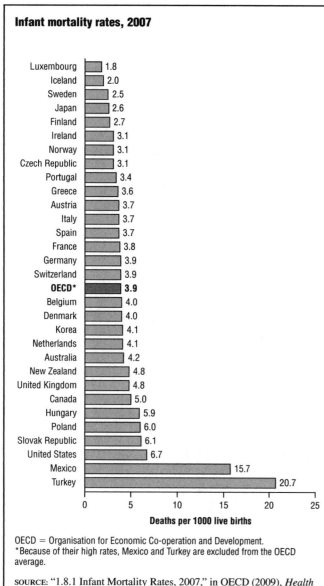

Infant mortality rates, 2007

Country	Deaths per 1000 live births
Luxembourg	1.8
Iceland	2.0
Sweden	2.5
Japan	2.6
Finland	2.7
Ireland	3.1
Norway	3.1
Czech Republic	3.1
Portugal	3.4
Greece	3.6
Austria	3.7
Italy	3.7
Spain	3.7
France	3.8
Germany	3.9
Switzerland	3.9
OECD*	3.9
Belgium	4.0
Denmark	4.0
Korea	4.1
Netherlands	4.1
Australia	4.2
New Zealand	4.8
United Kingdom	4.8
Canada	5.0
Hungary	5.9
Poland	6.0
Slovak Republic	6.1
United States	6.7
Mexico	15.7
Turkey	20.7

Deaths per 1000 live births

OECD = Organisation for Economic Co-operation and Development.
*Because of their high rates, Mexico and Turkey are excluded from the OECD average.

SOURCE: "1.8.1 Infant Mortality Rates, 2007," in OECD (2009), *Health at a Glance 2009: OECD Indicators*, OECD Publishing, doi: 10.1787/ health_glance-2009-en *http://dx.doi.org/10.1787/health_glance-2009-en* (accessed June 2, 2010)

experiences, including spending more time with their physicians, greater involvement in health care decision making, and better coordination of care. These patients were also much less likely to have experienced medical errors, received conflicting information from different doctors, or found that diagnostic tests or medical records were unavailable at the time of care.

Germany

The German health care system is based on the social insurance model. Statutory sickness funds and private insurance cover the entire population. In "Health Care in Germany" (2005, http://www.civitas.org.uk/pubs/bb3Germany.php), David G. Green, Ben Irvine, and Ben Cackett state that 90% of the population receives health care through the country's statutory health insurance program. Employees and employers finance these sickness funds through payroll contributions. Nearly all employers, including small businesses and low-wage industries, must participate. The remainder of the population is covered by private health insurance.

During the late 1990s Germany was the second highest among all the OECD member countries in health expenditures per capita, but Mark Pearson of the OECD notes in "Disparities in Health Expenditure across OECD Countries: Why Does the United States Spend So Much More Than Other Countries?" (September 30, 2009, http:// www.oecd.org/dataoecd/5/34/43800977.pdf) that by 2007 it ranked 10th in health expenditures per capita. Public funds, a combination of social insurance and general government funds, paid for more than three-quarters (76.9%) of total expenditures for health care. (See Figure 7.2.) According to the OECD, in *Health at a Glance 2009*, 79% of all medical care services were publicly funded, as were more than three-quarters of pharmaceuticals.

Ambulatory (outpatient) and inpatient care operate in completely separate spheres in the German health care system. German hospitals are public and private, operate for profit and not for profit, and generally do not have outpatient departments. Ambulatory care physicians are paid on the basis of fee schedules that are negotiated between the organizations of sickness funds and the organizations of physicians. A separate fee schedule for private patients uses a similar scale.

In 1993 Germany's Health Care Reform Law went into effect. Among its many provisions, the law tied increases in physician, dental, and hospital expenditures to the income growth rate of members of the sickness funds. It also limited the licensing of new ambulatory care physicians (based on the number of physicians already in an area) and set a cap for overall pharmaceutical outlays. Still, in 2007 Germany boasted 3.5 practicing physicians per 1,000 population, a ratio that was higher than well over half the OECD member countries. (See Figure 7.9.) The 1993

- 23% of Americans—the highest rate of any country in the survey—said they experienced coordination problems, either unavailability of medical records during physician office visits or duplication of tests

- 20% of Americans recounted instances when physicians recommended a treatment they thought had little or no benefit; this rate was also high in Germany

- Only the Netherlands (31%) surpassed the United States (24%) for patient reports of time spent on paperwork or resolving disputes related to medical bills or insurance; in the other countries, fewer than 15% of patients expressed this concern

In all the countries surveyed, patients with a primary source of medical care reported significantly more favorable

FIGURE 7.14

Cancer mortality rates for males and females, 2006

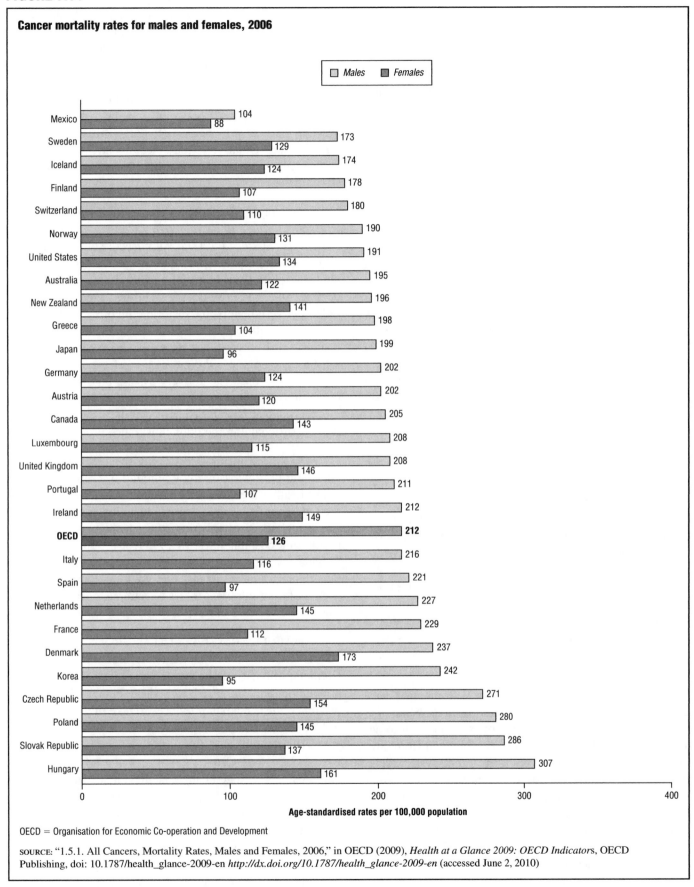

OECD = Organisation for Economic Co-operation and Development

SOURCE: "1.5.1. All Cancers, Mortality Rates, Males and Females, 2006," in OECD (2009), *Health at a Glance 2009: OECD Indicators*, OECD Publishing, doi: 10.1787/health_glance-2009-en *http://dx.doi.org/10.1787/health_glance-2009-en* (accessed June 2, 2010)

legislation also changed the hospital compensation system from per diem (per day) payments to specific fees for individual procedures and conditions.

Other German health care reform measures instituted during the 1990s also served to stimulate competition between sickness funds and improved coordination of inpatient and ambulatory care. During the mid-1990s the government also attempted to control health care costs by reducing health benefits, such as limiting how often patients could visit health spas to recuperate.

The health care reforms were not, however, successful at containing health care costs. Growth in health care spending was attributed to the comparatively high level of health care activity and resources, along with rising pharmaceutical expenditures and efforts to meet the health care needs of an aging population. According to Ulrike Siewert et al., in "Health Care Consequences of Demographic Changes in Mecklenburg-West Pomerania: Projected Case Numbers for Age-Related Diseases up to the Year 2020, Based on the Study of Health in Pomerania (SHIP)" (*Deutsches Ärzteblatt International*, vol. 107, no. 18, May 2010), the German health care system is not adequately prepared to meet the challenges of providing medical care for an aging population. The researchers also observe that decreasing numbers of physicians in rural areas may exacerbate the challenge of delivering needed services.

Canada

The Canadian system has been characterized as a provincial government health insurance model, in which each of the 10 provinces operates its own health system under general federal rules and with a fixed federal contribution. All provinces are required to offer insurance coverage for all medically necessary services, including hospital care and physician services. However, additional services and benefits may be offered at the discretion of each province. Most provinces cover preventive services, routine dental care for children, and outpatient drugs for older adults (with a co-payment) and the poor. No restrictions are placed on a patient's choice of physicians.

Canadian citizens have equal access to medical care, regardless of their ability to pay. Entitlement to benefits is linked to residency, and the system is financed through general taxation. Private insurance is prohibited from covering the same benefits covered by the public system, yet a majority of Canadians are covered by private supplemental insurance policies. These policies generally cover services such as adult dental care, cosmetic surgery, and private or semiprivate hospital rooms. In 2007, 70% of all health expenditures were public and 27.7% were funded by private health insurance and out-of-pocket expenditures. (See Figure 7.2 and Figure 7.3.)

Most hospitals are not for profit and are funded on the basis of global institution-specific or regional budgets.

(A global institution-specific budget allocates a lump sum of money to a large department or area; then all the groups in that department or area must negotiate to see how much of the total money each group receives.) Physicians in both inpatient and outpatient settings are paid on a negotiated, fee-for-service basis. The systems vary somewhat from province to province, and certain provinces, such as Quebec, have also established global budgets for physician services. Some provinces, including British Columbia, Alberta, and Ontario, require health care premiums for services; however, the Canada Health Act prohibits denial of health services on the basis of inability to pay premiums.

The Canadian Institute for Health Information explains in *Exploring the 70/30 Split: How Canada's Health Care System Is Financed* (2005, http://secure.cihi.ca/cihiweb/products/FundRep_EN.pdf) that the federal government's contribution to Canada's health care bill has progressively declined in the past two decades. During the early 1980s the federal government paid a historic high of 50% of the total health care bill, but by 1998 it paid less than 20%. The resulting shift in costs has increased the expenditures paid by the provinces and the out-of-pocket expenses paid by Canadian citizens. The delivery system consists mostly of community hospitals and self-employed physicians. Nearly all of Canadian hospital beds are public; private hospitals do not participate in the public insurance program.

FINANCIAL PROBLEMS. During the 1990s public revenues did not increase rapidly enough in Canada to cover rising health care costs. The Canadian government attributed many of the financial problems to lower revenue from taxes, higher prices for biomedical technology, and relatively long hospital stays. In 1993, for the first time since Canada instituted universal health insurance 27 years earlier, Canadians were required to pay for common services, such as throat cultures to test for streptococcal infections (the bacterial cause of strep throat).

CONTROLLING COSTS. Claire Sibonney reports in "Soaring Costs Force Canada to Reassess Health Model" (Reuters, May 31, 2010) that the combination of an aging population and the need to reduce budget deficits has prompted the Canadian provinces to take measures to control health care costs, which have been rising about 6% per year. The consensus is that no one wants to disassemble what has become Canada's most popular social program, but most agree that change is inevitable. In "Factbox: Canada's Universal Healthcare System" (Reuters, May 31, 2010), Sibonney notes that according to a 2009 poll, 86% of Canadians support "public solutions to make our public healthcare stronger." Given the popularity of the Canadian health care system, the provincial governments have endeavored to cut costs in several ways, such as:

- Ontario has taken steps to reduce the costs of pharmaceutical drugs

- British Columbia has moved to reimburse hospitals using a fee-for-service model rather than block grants

- Quebec has instituted a health tax and proposed a fee, not unlike the co-payments many U.S. health plans use, for each visit to a health care practitioner

- Ontario has proposed tying hospital executives' compensation to the quality of care delivered by hospitals and plans to increase the number of salaried physicians

Other initiatives under consideration in 2010 to keep Canada's current health care system affordable and sustainable included reimbursing physicians based on the quality and efficiency of the care they deliver, reducing prescription drug coverage for the country's wealthier older adults, and controlling the use of expensive medical technology.

The United Kingdom

The United Kingdom employs the National Health Service (NHS), or Beveridge, model to finance and deliver health care. The entire population is covered under a system that is financed primarily from general taxation. There is minimal cost sharing. In 2007, 81.7% of all health spending was from public funds. (See Figure 7.2.) Michael Ybarra notes in "Healthcare around the World" (*American Academy of Emergency Medicine*, vol. 16, no. 6, 2009) that in 2010 the NHS was the world's "largest provider of medical care services and the world's fourth largest employer."

Of the United Kingdom's hospital beds, 90% are public and generally owned by the NHS. In 2007 there were 2.6 beds per 1,000 population, which was comparable to the United States (2.7 beds per 1,000 population) but fewer than other European nations, such as France (3.6) and Italy (3.1). (See Figure 7.6.) Laura Donnelly reports in "NHS Hospitals Lose 32,000 Beds in a Decade" (*Telegraph* [London, England], May 24, 2008) that the number of NHS hospital beds declined from 198,848 in 1997 to 167,019 in 2007.

Services are organized and managed by regional and local public authorities. General practitioners serve as primary care physicians and are reimbursed on the basis of a combination of capitation payments (payments for each person served), fee for service, and other allowances. Hospitals receive overall budget allotments from district health authorities, and hospital-based physicians are salaried. Private insurance reimburses both physicians and hospitals on a fee-for-service basis.

Self-employed general practitioners are considered independent contractors, and salaried hospital-based physicians are public employees. The United Kingdom continues to face acute physician shortages: in 2007 there were fewer physicians per capita (2.5 per 1,000 population) than in most other OECD member countries. (See Figure 7.9.) After 1991 it became possible for large physician practices to become "budget holders" and receive larger capitation

payments. Similarly, individual hospitals could become "self-governing trust hospitals," enabling them to compete for patients and market their services. Even though emergency health services are available immediately, people requiring elective surgery, such as hip replacement, may end up on waiting lists for months or even years.

Since 2000 the NHS has experienced considerable change. The private sector has assumed a role in funding both buildings and services within the NHS. The authority to make decisions about local health care needs, priorities, and budgets has been delegated to local communities in some areas.

The NHS pioneered many cost-containment measures that are currently used by the United States and other countries seeking to slow escalating health care expenditures. These approaches to evaluating and managing health care costs include:

- Cost-effective analysis: calculated as a ratio, and often expressed as the cost per year per life saved, the cost-effectiveness analysis of a drug or procedure relates the cost of the drug or procedure to the health benefits it produces. This analysis enables delivery of clinically efficient, cost-effective care.

- Cost-minimization analysis: primarily applied to the pharmaceutical industry, this technique identifies the lowest cost among pharmaceutical alternatives that provide clinically comparable health outcomes.

- Cost-utility analysis: this measures the costs of therapy or treatment. Economists use the term *utility* to describe the amount of satisfaction a consumer receives from a given product or service. This analysis measures outcomes in terms of patient preference and is generally expressed as quality-adjusted life years. For example, an analysis of cancer chemotherapy drugs considers the various adverse side effects of these drugs because some patients may prefer a shorter duration of symptom-free survival rather than a longer life span marked by pain, suffering, and dependence on others for care.

According to Ybarra, the NHS has experienced relatively modest increases in health care costs—approximately 3% per year since its inception during the 1940s. In 2008 the NHS had a budget of approximately $200 billion. Ybarra asserts that even though the United Kingdom boasts higher life expectancy than the United States and generally good clinical outcomes, because newer therapies are not adopted as quickly as they are in the United States (at least in part because they may be more costly than conventional treatment) and are not widely available, the country has less favorable survival rates for certain types of cancers.

France

The French health care system is based on the social insurance, or Bismarck, model. Virtually the entire population is covered by a legislated, compulsory health insurance plan that is financed through the social security system. Three major programs, and several smaller ones, are quasi-autonomous, nongovernmental bodies. Ybarra explains that the system is financed through employee and employer payroll tax contributions and that individuals pay 5.3% of their income toward the health care system. In *Health at a Glance 2009*, the OECD notes that the total expenditure for health in France was 11% in 2007.

The public share of total health spending in 2007 was 79%, and 7% of expenditures represented direct, out-of-pocket payments. (See Figure 7.2 and Figure 7.3.) Physicians practicing in municipal health centers and in public hospitals are salaried, but physicians in private hospitals and in ambulatory care settings are typically paid on a negotiated, fee-for-service basis. The government establishes the reimbursement schedule for physicians and for other health care goods and services including pharmaceutical drugs. Public hospitals are granted lump-sum budgets, and private hospitals are paid on the basis of negotiated per diem payment rates. According to Ybarra, many employers offer their workers supplemental insurance as a benefit, and individuals can purchase private supplemental insurance to pay for pharmaceutical drugs, prostheses, dental care, and health care at private for-profit hospitals. The OECD reports that the number of hospital beds per 1,000 population declined from 4.6 in 1995 to 3.6 in 2007. (See Figure 7.6.)

In April 1996 the French government announced major reforms aimed at containing rising costs in the national health care system. The new system monitored each patient's total health costs and penalized physicians if they overran their budgets for specific types of care and prescriptions. In addition, French citizens were required to consult general practitioners before going to specialists. Initially, physicians—specialists, in particular—denounced the reforms and warned that they could lead to rationing and compromise the quality of health care. Over time, however, these cost-containment efforts met with less resistance from physicians and consumers. By 2010 physicians and hospitals were generally accepting of moderate fee schedules, cost-sharing arrangements, and global budgeting to control costs.

Japan

Japan's health care financing is also based on the social insurance model and, in particular, on the German health care system. Approximately 81.3% of health expenditures are from public funds. (See Figure 7.2.) Three general programs cover the entire population: Employee Health Insurance, Community Health Insurance, and Health and Medical Services for the Aged. Adam Dougherty of the Insure the Uninsured Project states in "Japan: The Health Care System" (July 9, 2008, http://www.itup.org/Reports/ Fresh%20Thinking/Japan.pdf) that 63% of the population obtains coverage through 1,800 not-for-profit, nongovernmental, employer-sponsored plans. Small businesses, the self-employed, and farmers are covered through Community Health Insurance, which is administered by a conglomeration of local governmental and private bodies. Older adults are covered by a separate plan that largely pools funds from the other plans. The Japanese health expenditure is below the expected level for a country with Japan's standard of living, and its emphasis is on the government, as opposed to business, bearing the major financial burden for the nation's health care.

The health care system, which cost 8.1% of Japan's GDP in 2006, is financed through employer and employee income-related premiums. (See Figure 7.1.) There are different levels of public subsidization of the three general programs. Limited private insurance exists for supplemental coverage and is purchased by about one-third of the population. In 2006 it accounted for 1.7% of health expenditures, whereas out-of-pocket expenses accounted for 16%. (See Figure 7.3.)

Physicians and hospitals are paid on the basis of national, negotiated fee schedules. Japan manages with fewer physicians per capita than most OECD member countries—just 2.1 physicians per 1,000 population. (See Figure 7.9.) Physicians practicing in public hospitals are salaried, whereas those practicing in physician-owned clinics and private hospitals are reimbursed on a fee-for-service basis. The amount paid for each medical procedure is rigidly controlled. Physicians not only diagnose, treat, and manage illnesses but also prescribe and dispense pharmaceuticals, and a considerable portion of a physician's income is derived from dispensing prescription drugs.

A close physician-patient relationship is unusual in Japan; the typical physician tries to see as many patients as possible in a day to earn a living. A patient going to a clinic for treatment may have to wait many hours in a crowded facility. As a result, health care is rarely a joint physician-patient effort. Instead, physicians tend to dictate treatment without fully informing patients about their conditions or the tests, pharmaceutical drugs, and therapies that have been ordered or prescribed. In 2007 Japan boasted the highest number of physician contacts per person out of all the OECD member countries, at 13.6. (See Figure 7.11.)

According to Dougherty, about 80% of Japan's hospitals are privately operated (and often physician owned) and the remaining 20% are public. Hospitals are paid according to a uniform fee schedule, and for-profit hospitals are prohibited. Even though hospital admissions are less frequent, hospital stays in Japan are typically far longer than in the United States or in any other OECD member nation, allowing hospitals and physicians to overcome the limitations of the fee schedules. (See Figure 7.7.)

The health status of the Japanese is one of the best in the world. Japanese men and women are among the longest living in all of the OECD member countries. In 2007 life expectancy was 82.6 years. (See Figure 7.12.) The Japanese infant mortality rate in 2007, at 2.6 deaths per 1,000 live births, was bested only by Luxembourg (1.8), Iceland (2), and Sweden (2.5). (See Figure 7.13.) These two statistics are usually considered reliable indicators of a successful health care system. It should be noted, though, that Japan does not have a large impoverished class, as the United States does, and its diet is considered to be among the healthiest in the world.

Ybarra explains that Japan's health care system has no doubt contributed to the country's preeminent health status, but the current health economics research has not yet determined the extent to which Japan's health care system contributes to its health status. Even though the Japanese system, which is based on social insurance, provides basic medical care, comprehensive preventive services, and free choice of doctors to every citizen at affordable costs, not all of its health outcomes are ideal. For example, rates of heart disease are lower in Japan than in the United States, but the chances of surviving a heart attack are significantly better in the United States.

CHAPTER 8
CHANGE, CHALLENGES, AND INNOVATION IN HEALTH CARE DELIVERY

Since the 1970s the U.S. health care system has experienced rapid and unprecedented change. The sites where health care is delivered have shifted from acute inpatient hospitals to outpatient settings, such as ambulatory care and surgical centers, clinics, physicians' offices, and long-term care and rehabilitation facilities. Patterns of disease have changed from acute infectious diseases that require episodic care to chronic conditions that require ongoing care. Even threats to U.S. public health have changed—for example, epidemics of infectious diseases have largely been replaced by epidemics of chronic conditions such as obesity, diabetes, and mental illness. At the end of 2001 the threat of bioterrorism became an urgent concern of health care planners, providers, policy makers, and the American public; between 2009 and 2010 the nation was mobilized to mitigate the effects of the H1N1 pandemic influenza; and in 2010 the government took historic action by passing the Patient Protection and Affordable Care Act (PPACA), which aims to provide health care coverage to nearly all of the nation's people.

There are new health care providers—midlevel practitioners (advanced practice nurses, certified nurse midwives, physician assistants, and medical technologists)—and new modes of diagnosis such as genetic testing. Furthermore, the rise of managed care, the explosion of biotechnology, and the availability of information on the Internet have dramatically changed how health care is delivered.

The PPACA emphasizes the use of health information technology (IT), especially the adoption of electronic health records (EHRs). The act promotes the use of EHRs and other IT not only to help achieve the objectives of health care reform, including intensifying efforts to assess, monitor, and improve patient safety and quality of service delivery, but also to ensure cost-effective health service delivery and reduce the growth of health care expenditures.

Some health care industry observers suggest the speed at which these changes have occurred has further harmed an already complicated and uncoordinated health care system. There is concern that the present health care system cannot keep pace with scientific and technological advances. Many worry that the health care system is already unable to deliver quality care to all Americans and that it is so disorganized that it will be unable to meet the needs of the growing population of older Americans and the estimated 32 million Americans who will have health care coverage by 2014, or to respond to the threat of another pandemic or an act of bioterrorism.

This chapter considers several of the most pressing challenges and opportunities faced by the U.S. health care system. These include:

- Safety: ensuring safety by protecting patients from harm or injury inflicted by the health care system (e.g., preventing medical errors, reducing hospital-acquired infections, and safeguarding consumers from medical fraud). Besides actions to reduce problems caused by the health care system, safety and quality may be ensured by providers' use of clinical practice guidelines (e.g., standardized plans for diagnosis and treatment of disease and the effective application of technology to information and communication systems).

- Information management: IT, including the Internet, can provide health care providers and consumers with timely access to medical data, patient information, and the clinical expertise of specialists. For example, Gerard F. Anderson et al. discuss in "Health Care Spending and Use of Information Technology in OECD Countries" (*Health Affairs*, vol. 25, no. 3, May–June 2006) that effective deployment of IT can also reduce health care expenditures. The Organisation for Economic Cooperation and Development (OECD) reports in "Information and Communication Technologies" (*Health Update*, no. 7, July 2009) that "many OECD governments have developed nation-wide strategies, set targets, allocated significant resources and established coordination bodies to promote widespread use of [information and communication technologies]." OECD member nations are employing IT solutions to manage patients with chronic diseases, improve access to care for people living in rural or remote locations, improve patient safety, and enhance overall quality of care, principally by improving the coordination and documentation of care.

- Innovation: widespread use of innovations in health care delivery should be recommended only after objective analysis has demonstrated that the innovation will measurably benefit the safety, effectiveness, efficiency, or timeliness of health service delivery. Innovations should also be considered if they have the potential to reduce waste of equipment, supplies, or personnel time or if they have the capacity to allocate or distribute health care more equitably. Equitable distribution refers to access to care that does not vary in quality based on the characteristics (e.g., race, gender, ethnicity, or socioeconomic status) of the population served.

SAFETY

Even though the United States is generally viewed as providing quality health care services to its citizens, the Institute of Medicine (IOM) estimates in the landmark report *To Err Is Human: Building a Safer Health System* (1999, http://www.nap.edu/books/0309068371/html/) that as many as 98,000 American deaths per year are the result of preventable medical errors. More than 7,000 of these deaths are estimated to be due to preventable medication errors.

In 2010 HealthGrades, Inc., an independent health care quality research organization that grades hospitals based on a range of criteria and provides hospital ratings to health plans and other payers, issued its seventh update of the 1999 IOM report. In *HealthGrades Seventh Annual Patient Safety in American Hospitals Study* (March 2010, http://www.healthgrades.com/media/DMS/pdf/PatientSafetyIn AmericanHospitalsStudy2010.pdf), HealthGrades finds that even though participation in patient safety initiatives to reduce the frequency of medical errors has increased, there is still considerable variation in patient safety in U.S. hospitals.

HealthGrades looks at Medicare patient records and nearly every one of the nation's 5,000 hospitals to assess the mortality (death) and economic impact of medical errors and injuries that occurred during hospital admissions nationwide from 2006 to 2008. The organization finds that close to 1 million patient safety incidents occurred in nearly 40 million Medicare hospitalizations.

Some of the most significant patient safety findings are:

- From 2006 to 2008 a total of 958,202 patient safety events affecting 908,401 Medicare beneficiaries were identified. An estimated 218,572 events and 22,590

deaths could have been prevented and saved $2.1 billion during this three-year period.

- Medicare patients hospitalized from 2006 to 2008 who experienced at least one safety event had a one in 10 chance of dying as a result of the event.

- Patient-safety incidents with the highest rates per 1,000 hospitalizations were failure to rescue (this indicator identifies patients who die following the development of a complication and assumes that quality hospitals identify these complications promptly and treat them aggressively), decubitus ulcer (bedsores), postoperative respiratory failure (failure of lung function following surgical procedures), and postoperative sepsis (bacterial infection in the bloodstream following surgical procedures).

- Over the course of the study, the rates of eight out of 15 key patient safety indicators worsened. For example, the rate of postoperative sepsis increased from 14.6 cases per 1,000 at-risk hospitalizations in 2006 to 18.4 cases per 1,000 at-risk hospitalizations in 2008, an increase of 26%.

Strengthening Safety Measures

In response to a request from the U.S. Department of Health and Human Services (HHS), the IOM's Committee on Data Standards for Patient Safety created a detailed plan to develop standards for the collection, coding, and classification of patient safety information. The 550-page plan, *Patient Safety: Achieving a New Standard for Care* (2004), called on the HHS to assume the lead in establishing a national health information infrastructure that would provide immediate access to complete patient information and decision support tools, such as clinical practice guidelines, and capture patient safety data for use in designing constantly improving and safer health care delivery systems.

The IOM plan exhorted all health care settings to develop and implement comprehensive patient safety programs and recommended that the federal government launch patient safety research initiatives aimed at increasing knowledge, developing tools, and disseminating results to maximize the effectiveness of patient safety systems. The plan also advised the designation of a standardized format and terminology for identifying and reporting data related to medical errors.

In July 2005 President George W. Bush (1946–) signed into law the Patient Safety and Quality Improvement (PSQI) Act. Angela S. Mattie and Rosalyn Ben-Chitrit surmise in "Patient Safety Legislation: A Look at Health Policy Development" (*Policy, Politics, and Nursing Practice*, vol. 8, no. 4, November 2007) that the IOM calls for action to improve patient safety in *To Err Is Human* are credited with heightening awareness of this issue and prompting Congress to pass legislation.

In "No Mention of Patient Safety Legislation" (*Health Affairs*, vol. 29, no. 2, June 2010), William Riley of the University of Minnesota, Minneapolis, observes that the PSQI Act created a voluntary error reporting system. This system, called a patient safety organization network, offers the opportunity to "prospectively prevent injury through analysis of mistakes and close calls that have been voluntarily reported by providers." It also protects providers from legal recourse when they report lapses in safety or instances of errors.

Who Is Responsible for Patient Safety?

Many federal, state, and private-sector organizations work together to reduce medical errors and improve patient safety. The Centers for Disease Control and Prevention (CDC) and the U.S. Food and Drug Administration (FDA) are the leading federal agencies that conduct surveillance and collect information about adverse events resulting from treatment or the use of medical devices, drugs, or other products. Michael R. Eber et al. report in "Clinical and Economic Outcomes Attributable to Health Care–Associated Sepsis and Pneumonia" (*Archives of Internal Medicine*, vol. 170, no. 4, February 22, 2010) that every year 1.7 million patients are diagnosed with hospital- and health care–acquired infections and that in 2006 two hospital-acquired infections—sepsis and pneumonia—claimed 48,000 lives, resulted in 2.3 million extra patient-days in the hospital, and cost $8.1 billion. These two infections account for nearly half of the 99,000 deaths per year from hospital-acquired infections reported by the CDC.

The Centers for Medicare and Medicaid Services acts to reduce medical errors for Medicare, Medicaid, and State Children's Health Insurance Program beneficiaries through its peer review organizations. Peer review organizations concentrate on preventing delays in diagnosis and treatment that have adverse effects on health.

The U.S. Departments of Defense and of Veterans Affairs (VA), which is responsible for health care services for U.S. military personnel, their families, and veterans, have instituted computerized systems that have reduced medical errors. The VA established the Centers of Inquiry for Patient Safety, and its hospitals also use bar-code technology and computerized medical records to prevent medical errors.

Safe medical care is also a top priority of the states and the private sector. In 2000 some of the nation's largest corporations, including General Motors and General Electric, joined together to address health care safety and efficacy (the ability of an intervention to produce the intended diagnostic or therapeutic effect in optimal circumstances) and to help direct their workers to health care providers (hospitals and physicians) with the best performance records. Called the Leapfrog Group (http://www.leapfrog

group.org/), this business coalition was founded by the Business Roundtable, a national association of Fortune 500 chief executive officers, to leverage employer purchasing power that initiates innovation and improves the safety of health care.

The Leapfrog Group publishes hospital quality and safety data to assist consumers in making informed hospital choices. Hospitals provide information to the Leapfrog Group through a voluntary survey that requests information about hospital performance across four quality and safety practices with the potential to reduce preventable medical mistakes and improve health care quality. In 2009 the Leapfrog Hospital Survey was completed by 1,244 hospitals in 48 states. Leah F. Binder, the chief executive officer of the Leapfrog Group, explains in *2009 Select Leapfrog Hospital Survey Results: Hospital Quality and Resource Use and What Hospitals Are Doing to Improve* (April 13, 2010, http://www.leapfroggroup.org/media/file/Binder_Presentation_412310.pdf) that studies reveal that a hospital's performance on Leapfrog is "a good indicator of a hospital's overall quality."

IMPROVING TEAMWORK TO PREVENT MEDICAL ERRORS AND IMPROVE PATIENT SAFETY. In November 2007 the Agency for Healthcare Research and Quality (AHRQ) and the Department of Defense launched TeamSTEPPS (http://teamstepps.ahrq.gov/abouttoolsmaterials.htm), a program that aims to optimize patient outcomes by improving communication and other teamwork skills among health care professionals. TeamSTEPPS applies team training principles that were developed in military aviation and in private industry to health care delivery. Carolyn M. Clancy, the director of the AHRQ, asserts in "Physicians and Nurses Together Can Improve Patient Safety" (*Medscape Journal of Medicine*, vol. 10, no. 2, February 11, 2008), that "nurses are trained to manage a variety of patient care situations, while physicians regard their role as having ultimate responsibility for the patients. In few instances do both nurses and physicians train together, a disconnect that can be counterproductive to high-quality healthcare.... In the new culture of medicine, teamwork should be the standard, not the ideal. As physicians, we can be leaders in the effort to instill teamwork where we practice and do right by our patients."

Professional societies are also concerned with patient safety. Over half of all the Joint Commission on Accreditation of Healthcare Organizations' (JCAHO) hospital standards pertain to patient safety. Since 2002 hospitals seeking accreditation from the JCAHO have been required to adhere to stringent patient safety standards to prevent medical errors. The JCAHO standards also require hospitals and individual health care providers to inform patients when they have been harmed in the course of treatment. The aim of these standards is to prevent medical errors by identifying actions and systems likely to produce problems before they occur. An example of this type of preventive measure, which is called prospective review, is close scrutiny of hospital pharmacies to be certain that the ordering, preparation, and dispensing of medications is accurate. Similar standards have been developed for JCAHO-accredited nursing homes, outpatient clinics, laboratories, and managed care organizations.

On January 1, 2004, the JCAHO began surveying and evaluating health care organizations using new medication management standards. The new standards revise and consolidate existing standards and place even greater emphasis on medication safety. The revised standards increase the role of pharmacists in managing appropriate and safe medication use and strengthen their authority to implement organization-wide improvements in medication safety.

In 2010 the JCAHO's (http://www.premierinc.com/quality-safety/tools-services/safety/topics/) national patient safety goals included improving:

- The accuracy of patient identification to ensure that treatment is administered to the correct patient

- The effectiveness of communication between caregivers to ensure timely reporting of critical test results and prompt treatment

- The safety of medication use

- Hand hygiene of health care workers to reduce the spread of health care–associated infections

- Efforts to reduce the risk of acquiring multidrug-resistant health care–associated infections and prevent surgical site infections

- Hospitals' ability to identify safety risks such as risk for suicide in their patient populations

HOSPITALS DESIGNED FOR SAFETY. HealthGrades observes in *Seventh Annual Patient Safety in American Hospitals Study* that many hospitals are taking steps to improve patient safety and that a growing number of states—including California, Minnesota, New York, Ohio, Oregon, Pennsylvania, Washington, and Wisconsin—publish hospital patient safety information on their websites. Gautam Naik reports in "Ounce of Prevention to Reduce Errors, Hospitals Prescribe Innovative Designs" (*Wall Street Journal*, May 8, 2006) other novel approaches, such as hotlines to enable staff to anonymously report medical errors and architectural innovations such as slip-proof floors, special lighting to aid in diagnosis, round rather than sharp interior wall corners, and standardized layout of equipment enabling staff to quickly and easily access needed equipment and supplies. Some hospitals have chosen to abandon the practice of recycling the air in their buildings to reduce the risk of spreading infections. Others have chosen to forgo vinyl coverings on external walls because it attracts infection-causing mold.

In "Effect of Bar-Code Technology on the Safety of Medication Administration" (*New England Journal of Medicine*, vol. 362, no. 18, May 6, 2010), Eric G. Poon et al. look at the frequency of medication errors before and after the implementation of bar-code technology to verify a patient's identity and the medication to be administered. The researchers find that the bar-code technology significantly reduced the rate of medication errors—errors in administering medication were reduced by 41% and there was a 51% reduction in potential adverse effects resulting from these errors. Poon et al. conclude that because the hospital where they conducted the study administers about 5.9 million doses of medication per year, the use of bar-code technology is anticipated to prevent 95,000 potential adverse drug events.

CLINICAL PRACTICE GUIDELINES

Clinical practice guidelines (CPGs) are evidence-based protocols—documents that advise health care providers about how to diagnose and treat specific medical conditions and diseases. CPGs offer physicians, nurses, other health care practitioners, health plans, and institutions objective, detailed, and condition- or disease-specific action plans.

Widespread dissemination and use of CPGs began during the 1990s in an effort to improve the quality of health care delivery by giving health care professionals access to current scientific information on which to base clinical decisions. The use of guidelines also aimed to enhance quality by standardizing care and treatment throughout a health care delivery system such as a managed care plan or hospital and throughout the nation.

Early attempts to encourage physicians and other health professionals to use CPGs was met with resistance, because many physicians rejected CPGs as formulaic "cookbook medicine" and believed they interfered with physician-patient relationships. Over time, however, physicians were educated about the quality problems that resulted from variations in medical practice, and opinions about CPGs gradually changed. Physician willingness to use CPGs also increased when they learned that adherence to CPGs offered some protection from medical malpractice and other liability. Nurses and other health professionals more readily adopted CPGs, presumably because their training and practice was oriented more toward following instructions than physicians' practices had been.

The National Guideline Clearinghouse (http://www.guideline.gov/) is a database of CPGs that have been produced by the AHRQ in conjunction with the American Medical Association and the American Association of Health Plans. The clearinghouse offers guideline summaries and comparisons of guidelines covering the same disease or condition prepared by different sources and serves as a resource for the exchange of guidelines between practitioners and health care organizations.

CPGs vary depending on their source. All recovery and treatment plans, however, are intended to generate the most favorable health outcomes. Federal agencies such as the U.S. Public Health Service and the CDC, as well as professional societies, managed care plans, hospitals, academic medical centers, and health care consulting firms, have produced their own versions of CPGs.

Practically all guidelines assume that treatment and healing will occur without complications. Because CPGs represent an optimistic approach to treatment, they are not used as the sole resource for development or evaluation of treatment plans for specific patients. CPGs are intended for use in conjunction with evaluation by qualified health professionals able to determine the applicability of a specific CPG to the specific circumstances involved. Modification of the CPGs is often required and advisable to meet specific, organizational objectives of health care providers and payers.

It is unrealistic to expect that all patients will obtain ideal health outcomes as a result of health care providers' use of CPGs. Guidelines may have greater utility as quality indicators. Evaluating health care delivery against CPGs enables providers, payers, and policy makers to identify and evaluate care that deviates from CPGs as part of a concerted program of continuous improvement of health care quality.

COMMUNICATION AND INFORMATION MANAGEMENT TECHNOLOGIES

The explosion of communication and information management technologies has already revolutionized health care delivery and holds great promise for the future. Health care data can be easily and securely collected, shared, stored, and used to promote research and development over great geographic distances and across traditionally isolated industries. Online distance learning programs for health professionals and the widespread availability of reliable consumer health information on the Internet have increased understanding and awareness of the causes and treatment of illness. This section describes several recent applications of technology to the health care system.

Telemedicine

The term *telemedicine* describes a variety of interactions that occur by way of telephone lines. Telemedicine may be as simple and commonplace as a conversation between a patient and a health professional in the same town or as sophisticated as surgery directed via satellite and video technology from one continent to another.

Anita Majerowicz and Susan Tracy describe in "Bridging Gaps in Healthcare Delivery" (*Journal of the American Health Information Management Association*, vol. 81, no. 5, May 2010) the benefits of telemedicine, including:

- Reduced healthcare costs
- Increased patient access to providers, especially in medically underserved areas
- Improved quality and continuity of care
- Faster and more convenient treatment resulting in reduction of lost work time and travel costs for patients

In "The Doctor Will See You Now. Please Log On" (*New York Times*, May 28, 2010), Milt Freudenheim reports that in North America the interactive telemedicine market has grown about 10% each year; in 2010 alone it generated an estimated $500 million in revenue. An example of interactive telemedicine is Internet or telephone-enabled video-teleconferencing, which creates a meeting between a patient and primary care physician in one location and a physician specialist elsewhere when a face-to-face consultation is not feasible because of time or distance. Peripheral equipment even enables the physician specialist to perform a virtual physical examination and hear the patient's heart sounds through a stethoscope. The availability of desktop videoconferencing has expanded this form of telemedicine from a novelty found exclusively in urban, university teaching hospitals to a valuable tool for patients and physicians in rural areas who were previously underserved and unable to access specialists readily.

Another application of telemedicine is transtelephonic pacemaker monitoring. (Cardiac pacemakers are battery-operated implanted devices that maintain normal heart rhythm.) Cardiac technicians at the device monitoring company are able to check the implanted cardiac pacemaker's functions, including the status of its battery. Transtelephonic pacemaker monitoring is able to identify early signs of possible pacemaker failure and detect potential pacemaker system abnormalities, thereby reducing the number of emergency replacements. It can also send an electrocardiogram rhythm strip to the patient's cardiologist (physician specialist in heart diseases).

Freudenheim notes that the entire telemedicine market, which includes health care applications for smart phones and in-home monitoring devices that relay patient data using telephone lines, is about $3.9 billion. Medicare and Medicaid reimburse physicians and hospitals that provide remote care to patients in rural, underserved regions, and some private insurers offer coverage of interactive video technologies. Because the PPACA allocates about $1 billion annually for research into telemedicine and other health care innovations, industry observers predict continuing growth in the development and utilization of this technology.

Despite the promise and growing popularity of telemedicine, Freudenheim observes that several groups, including state regulators at the Texas Medical Board, caution that physicians who conduct remote consultations might miss subtle medical indicators. The American

Academy of Family Physicians is not opposed to telemedicine; however, the professional society encourages patients to maintain a direct relationship with a physician who can monitor their health and treatment.

Sanjiv N. Singh and Robert M. Wachter of the University of California, San Francisco, observe in "Perspectives on Medical Outsourcing and Telemedicine—Rough Edges in a Flat World?" (*New England Journal of Medicine*, vol. 358, no. 15, April 10, 2008) increasing use of telemedicine, with particularly strong growth in the fields of radiology, dermatology, mental health consultation, and home care. The researchers report that as many as 300 U.S. hospitals and two-thirds of radiology practices use some form of teleradiology and that the VA conducts nearly a quarter of a million teleconsultations per year.

Telemedicine appears to improve patient outcomes. For example, Andreas S. Morguet et al. find in "Impact of Telemedical Care and Monitoring on Morbidity in Mild to Moderate Chronic Heart Failure" (*Cardiology*, vol. 111, no. 2, 2008) that telemedical care and monitoring may reduce the frequency and severity of illness in patients with chronic heart failure (a condition in which the heart is unable to supply the body with enough blood). In "Telemedicine Facilitates CHF Home Health Care for Those with Systolic Dysfunction" (*International Journal of Telemedicine and Applications*, 2008), Pennie S. Seibert et al. find improved control of congestive heart failure when telemedicine was implemented.

Telemedicine has been used in schools to improve access to care, treat middle ear infections, and increase appropriate referral to specialists. It has also proven beneficial in helping to manage asthma in school-aged children. David A. Bergman et al. note in "The Use of Telemedicine Access to Schools to Facilitate Expert Assessment of Children with Asthma" (*International Journal of Telemedicine and Applications*, 2008) that asthma care was improved through a telemedicine link between an asthma specialist and a school-based asthma program, which involved real-time video and audio conferencing between the patient and school nurse on-site at the school and the asthma specialist at San Francisco General Hospital. The researchers conducted the program in three urban schools to determine the feasibility of asthma-focused telemedicine. They find that the program produced significant improvements in health status outcomes and note that the use of telemedicine ensured that children identified with asthma received comprehensive assessments, action plans, and asthma education. Bergman et al. conclude that telemedicine "allowed for a more efficient use of the asthma subspecialist's time when contrasted with hospital-based asthma clinics."

Telemedicine has also proven to be a cost-effective alternative to emergency department visits. Kevin McKeever reports in "Telemedicine a Cost-Effective Alternative to ER Visits" (*HealthDay News*, May 9, 2008) on two presentations that were made at the May 2008 Pediatrics Annual Societies meeting in Honolulu, Hawaii. The first presentation was by researchers from the University of Rochester Medical Center, which operates a Rochester-based telemedicine program that provides an interactive online pediatric health care service. McKeever asserts that "telemedicine is a cost-effective way to replace more than a quarter of all visits to the pediatric emergency department." The second presentation noted that telemedicine has the capacity to provide quality care at a lower cost—saving payers more than $14 per child per year.

Wireless Technology in the Hospital

According to Alden Solovy, Suzanna Hoppszallern, and Sarah B. Brown, in "100 Most Wired: Being Most Wired in a Down Economy" (*Hospitals and Health Networks*, vol. 83, no. 7, July 2009), the economic recession forced many hospitals to slow their IT installation and implementation plans. The researchers' assertion is based on the results of the 2009 Most Wired Survey and Benchmarking Study, which revealed that the most wired hospitals continue to demonstrate increased efficiency, quality, safety, and cost containment. The survey asked hospitals how they use IT to address business processes, safety and quality, workforce, customer service, and public health and safety.

Several hospitals employed IT to improve patient flow and to improve workflow by, for example, providing a central location for the nursing task list, so that all of a nurse's activities for an upcoming shift, including physician orders, reminders, and nursing interventions, are in one convenient place. IT was also employed to measure and analyze process improvements such as "time to care"—the time between order placement and delivery of care. The most wired hospitals used IT to facilitate electronic ordering and bedside medication matching to reduce the number of potential medication errors. They also used "smart alerts"—real-time monitors that use information in the medical record to identify patients with potentially deteriorating conditions. Other uses of IT include disseminating digital images, such as radiological images, to multiple sites, such as clinics and physicians' offices, and automating processes in the operating room.

However, industry observers caution that IT is not itself a solution to the many problems plaguing the U.S. health care system. It is one of many tools for achieving process improvements that lead to better outcomes, and it must be used in combination with other tools and techniques to affect care.

Eric J. Thomas et al. of the University of Texas Health Science Center in Houston, Texas, find in "Association of Telemedicine for Remote Monitoring of Intensive Care Patients with Mortality, Complications, and Length of Stay" (*Journal of the American Medical Association*, vol. 302, no. 24, December 2009) that even though tele-medicine is increasingly common, at least one study finds that telemedicine enabling physician specialists to simul-taneously monitor several intensive care units (ICUs) from a single location does not improve specific measures of quality of care—specifically the length of stay or the over-all mortality. The researchers conclude, "Given the expense of tele-ICU technology, the conflicting evidence about its effectiveness, and the existence of other effective quality improvement interventions for ICUs, further use of this technology should proceed in the context of careful monitoring of patient outcomes and costs."

A TELEMEDICINE PARTNERSHIP. During the late 1990s the National Cancer Institute (NCI) developed TELESY-NERGY, a video conferencing system that enables health care professionals to collaborate with one another on cancer research and treatment, independent of their geographic locations. The NCI (May 7, 2010, http://telesynergy.nih.gov/overview.html) notes that as of 2010, more than 20 facilities around the world were using the TELESY-NERGY system. Twelve facilities were awarded grant funding to help disparate populations access cancer treat-ment and to advance distance-learning programs in cancer research.

Online Patient-Physician Consultations

In "How to Get Paid for Online Consults" (*American Medical News*, March 22, 2010), Pamela Lewis Dolan reports that "a growing number of insurers are paying for online communication between physicians and patients. And when insurers don't cover it, many patients are willing to pay out of pocket for the convenience." Dolan explains that e-mail exchanges between patients and their physicians are considered billable when they address "a specific prob-lem not associated with a prior visit, online or in-office, within the previous seven days." E-mail that is sent as follow-up to a visit that occurred within the past seven days, such as an e-mail that details laboratory test results or requests a prescription refill, cannot be billed separately.

Gil C. Grimes et al. find in "Patient Preferences and Physician Practices for Laboratory Test Results Notifica-tion" (*Journal of the American Board of Family Medicine*, vol. 22, no. 6, November–December 2009) that both patients and physicians prefer the U.S. mail to communi-cate normal laboratory and other test results and that phone calls and e-mail were their second and third choices. The researchers also observe that a written and printed letter automatically documents the communication of the test results in the medical record, and this may not be the case when results are delivered via telephone or e-mail.

One important advantage of electronic encounters (e-encounters) over telephone conversations is the patient's ability to communicate home monitoring results such as blood pressure or blood glucose levels in a format that is easily included as documentation in the patient's perma-nent (paper or electronic) medical record. Another advant-age is that less time devoted to telephone calls improves the efficiency of the physician's office, thereby boosting pro-ductivity and potentially reducing practice expenses.

Concerns about e-encounters center on privacy and security of patient information exchanged and physician reimbursement for the time spent in electronic correspond-ence with patients. Besides legal and privacy issues, some industry observers suggest that guidelines should be devel-oped for e-encounters to ensure that they are clinically appropriate and are not used as substitutes for needed, but more costly, face-to-face office visits.

Despite promising research findings about the benefits of e-mail correspondence between patients and physicians and increasing consumer demand for e-mail, instant mes-saging, and texting, industry observers caution that the shift toward e-encounters could create additional expectations for physicians. For example, in "The Future of Your Med-ical Data" (*Scientific American*, April 12, 2010), Katherine Harmon asserts that physicians could face liability chal-lenges if they fail to address certain information contained in an e-mail. Experts also note that e-encounters could raise new reimbursement issues and introduce time pressures that interrupt physicians' already busy work schedules.

Richard J. Baron of Greenhouse Internists in Philadel-phia, Pennsylvania, asserts in "What's Keeping Us So Busy in Primary Care? A Snapshot from One Practice" (*New England Journal of Medicine*, vol. 362, no. 17, April 29, 2010) that he and his colleagues respond to nearly 17 e-mails per day. More than half (59.3%) were for the interpretation of test results, 21.7% were for responding to patients, 9.3% were for administrative problems, 5% were for acute problems, 2.8% were for proactive outreach to patients, and 1.9% were for discussions with consultants.

Is Applied Technology the Solution to the Nursing Shortage?

In "What Nurses Want" (*Government Health IT*, vol. 3, no. 2, March 31, 2008), John Pulley explains that many efforts are being made to address the current nursing short-age in the United States. Instead of trying to recruit more nurses and nursing students, the American Academy of Nurses (AAN) is endeavoring to make better use of nurses, in large measure by using IT to improve their efficiency. With the assistance of the Robert Wood Johnson Founda-tion, the AAN Workforce Commission examined the work processes and environments of nurses at 25 sites throughout the United States.

The commission found that nurses want IT solutions to assist with coordination and delivery of care, communica-tion, discharge planning, documentation, patient transport, and supplies and equipment. Nurses also want electronic medical records, computerized order entry systems to eliminate problems that arise from illegible handwriting, touch-screen or voice-activated technology for documentation, and automated networks to collect and download patient data. They are especially enthusiastic about hands-free tools and wireless technology. Other needs identified by the commission include nurses' desire for increased use of radio frequency identification technology to track people, supplies, and equipment, and greater use of robotics to deliver supplies. Nurses also endorse the use of smart beds that monitor patient movements and pressure sensors to help reduce the frequency of bedsores.

TECHNOLOGY MAY HELP EDUCATE MORE NURSES. One key factor limiting the supply of nurses is a shortage of nursing faculty, which restricts class size and ultimately the numbers of nurses graduating each year. According to Jennifer M. Sims of the Veterans' Affairs Medical Center in Louisville, Kentucky, in "Nursing Faculty Shortage in 2009" (*Dimensions of Critical Care Nursing*, vol. 28, no. 5, September–October 2009), in 2005 more than 1,300 full-time nursing faculty positions were vacant and approximately 147,000 applicants were turned away from nursing schools because of a lack of qualified faculty. Sims asserts that one way to remedy this situation may be to offer some nursing courses online. In "Making Time: Moving the Faculty Dossier to an Electronic Format" (*Mosby's Nursing Consult*, vol. 26, no. 2, March 2010), Martha Kelly and Sandra B. Lewenson of Pace University suggest that technology can help nursing faculty find the time needed to prepare the documentation that is required by academic institutions for annual reviews, promotion, and tenure. Kelly and Lewenson created an ongoing electronic repository of faculty data and documentation that includes a faculty electronic dossier (a collection of articles and other information about a specific topic) in place of the traditional paper dossier.

Patricia Allen, Yvonne VanDyke, and Myrna L. Armstrong describe in "'Growing Your Own' Nursing Staff with a Collaborative Accelerated Second-Degree, Web-Based Program" (*Journal of Continuing Education in Nursing*, vol. 41, no. 3, March 2010) the success of an online accelerated degree program that is designed to produce new baccalaureate-prepared nurses. The researchers report that graduates of the program feel well prepared and have excellent career prospects following graduation.

MORE STAFF, RATHER THAN TECHNOLOGY, IS KEY TO IMPROVING PATIENT SAFETY AND QUALITY OF CARE. Despite rapid advances in technology, many industry observers feel that it is not sufficient to solve the nursing shortage that the Bureau of Labor Statistics projects in the press release "Employment Projections: 2008–18" (December 10, 2009, http://www.bls.gov/news.release/pdf/ecopro.pdf) will require over 1 million replacement nurses by 2018. In "The Recent Surge in Nurse Employment: Causes and Implications" (*Health Affairs*, vol. 28, no. 4,

July–August 2009), Peter I. Buerhaus, David I. Auerbach, and Douglas O. Staiger observe that even though the nursing shortage slowed as a result of the economic recession, it is still forecast to reach 260,000 registered nurses by 2025—twice as large as any U.S. nursing shortage since the mid-1960s. The researchers identify the retirement of older nurses as the key contributor to the anticipated shortfall.

According to Annette Richardson and Julie Storr, in "Patient Safety: A Literative Review on the Impact of Nursing Empowerment, Leadership, and Collaboration" (*International Nursing Review*, vol. 57, no. 1, March 2010), because of their proximity to patients, nurses are in an ideal position to drive safety and quality initiatives. The researchers conducted a comprehensive review of the relevant literature and conclude that nursing leadership, collaboration, and empowerment can exert a demonstrable impact on patient safety.

Promise of Robotics

One technological advance that promises to reduce hospital operating costs and enable hospital workers to spend more time caring for patients is the use of robots. Once relegated to the realm of science fiction, the 21st century has seen a resurgence of interest in automated machines such as self-guided robots to perform many routine hospital functions.

In "Hospital Robots of the Future" (Hospitalmanagement.net, April 29, 2010), Chris Lo describes several novel uses of robotics in hospitals: self-guiding robots that deliver and dispense medication; robots that enable physicians to perform remote, real-time consultations and communicate with patients at a distance; and robots that monitor critically ill patients in the ICU. According to Kawanza Newson, in "Robot Now Makes Tracks through Hospital" (*Journal Sentinel* [Milwaukee, Wisconsin], March 31, 2008), a robotic cart that looks like a train warns onlookers to "pardon my caboose" when it backs up and makes deliveries of oxygen monitors and feeding pumps.

Some robots are involved in more than simply routine, menial tasks. Barnaby J. Feder explains in "Prepping Robots to Perform Surgery" (*New York Times*, May 4, 2008) that a growing number of surgeons delegate much of their work to medical robots controlled from computer consoles. The robotic system allows a cardiovascular surgeon to perform heart surgery without touching the patient, or a urologist to ensure precise, tremor-free incisions to prevent damage to delicate nerves during prostate surgery. Seated at a console with a computer and video monitor, the surgeon uses handgrips and foot pedals to manipulate robotic arms that hold scalpels, sutures, and other surgical instruments to perform the operation. These robotic systems have been approved for use by the FDA, and in 2008 they represented a $1 billion segment of the medical device industry.

The newest surgical robots are miniature versions that can be inserted through a laparoscope. Bhavin C. Shah et al. describe in "Miniature in Vivo Robotics and Novel Robotic Surgical Platforms" (*Urology Clinics of North America*, vol. 36, no. 2, May 2009) miniature robots that are equipped with cameras and guided by a joystick. These miniature robots can be inserted into the abdominal cavity or peritoneal cavity to perform diagnostic imaging and assist with surgical tasks. They can also be inserted through small orifices or swallowed and can remain implanted for months to perform specific tasks. Shah et al. explain that "small fully implantable robots can be manipulated from the outside with much less force and trauma to the tissues, allowing for more precision and delicate handling of surgical fields."

Robots do not, however, trump humans in all aspects of health care delivery. In "Enhanced Gait-Related Improvements after Therapist- versus Robotic-Assisted Locomotor Training in Subjects with Chronic Stroke: A Randomized Controlled Study" (*Stroke*, vol. 39, no. 6, June 2008), T. George Hornby et al. compare the results of physical therapist–assisted training and rehabilitation of stroke patients with training provided by a robotic device. The researchers find that physical therapist–assisted training produced greater improvement in walking speed and symmetry as well as in overall walking ability than did training provided by a robotic device. At the end of treatment, the increase in gait speed and the ability to stand using one limb was twice as high in the group of patients receiving services from physical therapists than in the group treated by robots.

INNOVATION SUPPORTS QUALITY HEALTH CARE DELIVERY

The health care industry is awash in wave after wave of new technologies, models of service delivery, reimbursement formulae, legislative and regulatory changes, and increasingly specialized personnel ranks. Creating change in hospitals and in other health care organizations requires an understanding of diffusion—the process and channels by which new ideas are communicated, spread, and adopted throughout institutions and organizations. Diffusion of technology involves all the stakeholders in the health care system: policy makers and regulatory agencies establish safety and efficacy, government and private payers determine reimbursement, vendors of the technology are compared and one is selected, hospitals and health professionals adopt the technology and are trained in its use, and consumers are informed about the benefits of the new technology.

The decision to adopt new technology involves a five-stage process beginning with knowledge about the innovation. The second stage is persuasion, the period when decision makers form opinions based on experience and knowledge. Decision is the third phase, when commitment is made to a trial or pilot program, and is followed by implementation, the stage during which the new technology is put in place. The process concludes with the confirmation stage, the period during which the decision makers seek reinforcement for their decision to adopt and implement the new technology.

Communicating Quality

In "Evidence That Consumers Are Skeptical about Evidence-Based Health Care" (*Health Affairs*, vol. 29, no. 7, June 2010), Kristin L. Carman et al. considered how consumers define and characterize quality care. The researchers were especially interested in finding out the extent to which consumers understand and appreciate evidence-based health care, which encompasses a range of actions including use of evidence-based practice guidelines, shared decision making, comparative effectiveness research, and transparency of cost and quality information. Consumer attitudes and beliefs about evidence-based health care is of increasing importance because the PPACA emphasizes its use. Carman et al. assert that if consumers do not understand evidence-based care or do not view it as a useful way to inform their decisions about providers and treatments, the move to incorporate it in the emerging health care delivery system will not be successful.

Carman et al. report that consumers' beliefs, values, and knowledge were not consistent with what policy makers prescribe as evidence-based health care. There was little understanding and considerable confusion about the meaning of terms such as *medical evidence* and *quality guidelines*. Most consumers continued to believe that when it comes to health care, more care, more costly care, and newer treatments are always better. These gaps in knowledge and misconceptions about the characteristics of quality care may mean that considerable consumer education will be required before consumers can become fully engaged in evidence-based decision making.

In response to these findings, Carman et al. developed a communication toolkit that aims to "enable employers and unions to communicate with consumers about evidence-based health care and help them become active participants in their care through customizable materials that translate these concepts into clear, simple, and relevant language." The researchers report that the toolkit was favorably received by employers and other health care purchasers, health plans, and provider organizations and that in 2010 efforts were under way to help bridge "the gap between the need for evidence-based health care and the consumers' current perceptions of it."

MAKING THE GRADE: HEALTH CARE REPORT CARDS. The publication of medical outcomes report cards and disease- and procedure-specific morbidity rates (the degree of disability caused by disease) and mortality rates (the number of deaths caused by disease) has attracted widespread media attention and sparked controversy. Advocates for the public release of clinical outcomes and other performance measures contend that despite some essential limitations, these studies offer consumers, employers, and payers the means for comparing health care providers.

Some skeptics question the clinical credibility of scales such as surgical mortality, which they claim are incomplete indicators of quality. Others cite problems with data collection or speculate that data are readily manipulated by providers to enhance marketing opportunities sufficient to compromise the utility and validity of published reports. Long term, the effects of published comparative evaluation of health care providers on network establishment, contracting, and exclusion from existing health plans are uncertain and in many instances may be punitive (damaging). Hospitals and medical groups may be forced to compete for network inclusion on the basis of standardized performance measures.

The number of websites that rate physicians and hospitals continues to grow, with Angie's List and Vitals.com joining more established sites such as Health.org and HealthGrades.com. The sites describe physicians' training, experience, certification, and any disciplinary actions taken against them, as well as patient ratings. They also encourage physicians to respond to patient comments. Some industry observers contend that the sites, especially those that use anonymous ratings, have the potential to further erode patient-physician relationships by prompting physicians to behave defensively. Tara Lagu et al. find in "Patients' Evaluations of Health Care Providers in the Era of Social Networking: An Analysis of Physician-Rating Websites" (*Journal of General Internal Medicine*, May 13,

2010) that despite the proliferation of these websites, consumers are not flocking to them. The researchers scrutinized 33 physician rating websites and find that the overwhelming majority (88%) of reviews were positive. Just 6% were negative and an additional 6% were neutral.

Interestingly, Lagu et al. find that consumers seem to be more interested in rating commercial venues such as restaurants than their physicians. The researchers report that while there were relatively few reviews of physicians, a search of restaurants in Boston's Beacon Hill area "turned up 38 narrative reviews for a single Lebanese restaurant."

Despite legitimate concern about the objectivity, reliability, validity, and the potential for manipulating data, there is consensus that scrutiny and dissemination of quality data will escalate. Business groups and employers continue to request physician, hospital, and health plan data to design their health benefit programs. When choosing between health plans involving the same group of participating hospitals and physicians, employers request plan-specific information to guide their decisions. Companies and employer-driven health care coalitions seeking to assemble their own provider networks rely on physician- and hospital-specific data, such as the quality data provided by HealthGrades, during the selection process.

The most beneficial use of the data is not to be punitive, but to be inspiring to improve health care delivery systematically. When evidence of quality problems is identified, health plans and providers must be prepared to launch a variety of interventions to address and promptly resolve problems.

CHAPTER 9
PUBLIC OPINION ABOUT THE HEALTH CARE SYSTEM

As with many other social issues, public opinion about health care systems, providers, plans, coverage, and benefits varies in response to a variety of personal, political, and economic forces. Personal experience and the experience of friends, family, and community opinion leaders (trusted sources of information such as members of the clergy, prominent physicians, and local business and civic leaders) exert powerful influences on public opinion. Health care marketing executives have known for years that the most potent advertising any hospital, medical group, or managed care plan can have is not a full-page newspaper advertisement or prime-time television ad campaign. It is positive word-of-mouth publicity.

The influence of the news media, advertising, and other attempts to sway health care consumers' attitudes and purchasing behaviors cannot be overlooked. A single story about a miraculous medical breakthrough or lifesaving procedure can reflect favorably on an entire hospital or health care delivery system. Similarly, a lone mistake, an adverse reaction to a drug, or a misstep by a single health care practitioner can impugn (attack as lacking integrity) a hospital, managed care plan, or pharmaceutical company for months or even years, prompting intense media scrutiny of every action taken by the practitioner, facility, or organization.

Political events, the economy, and pending legislation can focus public attention on a particular health care concern, supplant one health-related issue with another, or eclipse health care from public view altogether. In 2005 Hurricanes Katrina and Rita focused attention on the U.S. public health and federal emergency management systems' capacities to effectively respond to disasters. In 2009 and 2010 federal, state, and local government officials implemented successful plans to contain the H1N1 influenza pandemic in the United States. During the same period there was heated debate about the scope and provisions of health care reform legislation, which did not subside even after the March 2010 passage of the Patient Protection and Affordable Care Act (PPACA).

In addition, some industry observers believe health care providers, policy makers, biomedical technology and research firms, and academic medical centers have fanned the flames of consumer dissatisfaction with the U.S. health care system by overselling the promise and the progress of modern medicine. They fear that the overzealous promotion of every scientific discovery with a potential clinical application has created unrealistic expectations of modern medicine. Health care consumers who believe there should be "one pill for every ill" or feel all technology should be made widely available even before its efficacy (the ability of an intervention to produce the intended diagnostic or therapeutic effect in optimal circumstances) has been demonstrated are more likely to be dissatisfied with the present health care system.

AMERICANS' CHANGING VIEWS ON THE ROAD TO HEALTH CARE REFORM

In *More Americans Reliant on Government Healthcare in 2009* (January 28, 2010, http://www.gallup.com/poll/125417/Americans-Reliant-Government-Healthcare-2009.aspx), Elizabeth Mendes of the Gallup Organization observes that there was a slight increase in Americans relying on government-sponsored health care (Medicare, Medicaid, or military/veterans' benefits) between 2008 and 2009. In contrast, during this same period there was a slight decrease in Americans receiving coverage from their employers. (See Figure 9.1.) There were also more uninsured Americans in 2009 than in 2008.

Interestingly, Americans' belief that it is the federal government's responsibility to provide health care coverage to all of its citizens declined from a high of 69% in 2006 to a low of 47% in 2009. (See Figure 9.2.) Views about federal government responsibility for health care coverage fall predictably along political party lines. In

November 2009 roughly three-quarters (77%) of Republicans felt it is not the responsibility of the federal government to provide coverage, whereas the same proportion of Democrats (74%) felt that it is the government's responsibility. (See Figure 9.3.)

In November 2009 Americans were divided about the potential impact of health care reform legislation. Frank Newport of the Gallup Organization reports in *No Clear Mandate from Americans on Healthcare Reform* (November 9, 2009, http://www.gallup.com/poll/124202/No-Clear-Mandate-Americans-Healthcare-Reform.aspx) that 41% thought reform legislation would improve the health care system and 40% felt it would only make things worse. (See Figure 9.4.) Americans were even less optimistic about the impact of health care legislation on their own personal health care situation. According to Newport, just 26% of those surveyed thought their own situation would improve, whereas 36% felt their personal health care would be worse and 31% thought there would be no change. (See Figure 9.5.)

As discussion and debate about the reform legislation progressed, from October to November 2009, Americans' support for the bill waned. In October 40% of survey respondents said they would advise their member of Congress to vote for the bill, but by November just 29% wanted their congressional representative to support it. (See Figure 9.6.) Not unexpectedly, Newport notes that support was divided along party lines, with more than two-thirds (68%) of Republicans opposing the legislation and more than half (55%) of Democrats favoring it. Newport also notes that more Democrats than Republicans or Independents remained undecided about the legislation.

As the health care reform bill made its way through the legislative process, Americans' support for President Barack Obama's (1961–) ability to change the health care system was higher than their support for congressional efforts to advance health care reform. In October 2009, 55% of survey respondents expressed trust in President Obama on health care, compared with just 48% who felt the Democrats in Congress and 37% who felt the Republicans in Congress could be trusted to create change.

FIGURE 9.1

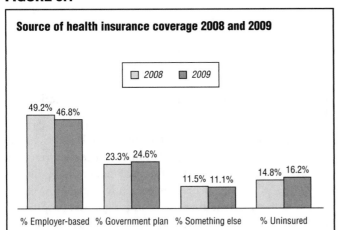

Source of health insurance coverage 2008 and 2009

source: Elizabeth Mendes, "Health Insurance Coverage in the United States, 2008 vs. 2009," in *More Americans Reliant on Government Healthcare in 2009*, The Gallup Organization, January 28, 2010, http://www.gallup.com/poll/125417/Americans-Reliant-Government-Healthcare-2009.aspx (accessed June 16, 2010). Copyright © 2010 by The Gallup Organization. Reproduced by permission of The Gallup Organization.

FIGURE 9.2

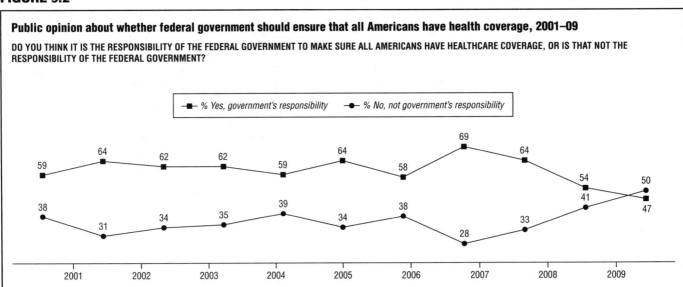

Public opinion about whether federal government should ensure that all Americans have health coverage, 2001–09

DO YOU THINK IT IS THE RESPONSIBILITY OF THE FEDERAL GOVERNMENT TO MAKE SURE ALL AMERICANS HAVE HEALTHCARE COVERAGE, OR IS THAT NOT THE RESPONSIBILITY OF THE FEDERAL GOVERNMENT?

source: Frank Newport, "Do You Think It Is the Responsibility of the Federal Government to Make Sure All Americans Have Healthcare Coverage, or Is That Not the Responsibility of the Federal Government?" in *More in U.S. Say Health Coverage Is Not Gov't. Responsibility*, The Gallup Organization, November 13, 2009, http://www.gallup.com/poll/124253/Say-Health-Coverage-Not-Gov-Responsibility.aspx (accessed June 16, 2010). Copyright © 2010 by The Gallup Organization. Reproduced by permission of The Gallup Organization.

FIGURE 9.3

Public opinion about whether federal government should ensure that all Americans have health coverage, by political party affiliation, November 2009

DO YOU THINK IT IS THE RESPONSIBILITY OF THE FEDERAL GOVERNMENT TO MAKE SURE ALL AMERICANS HAVE HEALTHCARE COVERAGE, OR IS THAT NOT THE RESPONSIBILITY OF THE FEDERAL GOVERNMENT?

By party ID

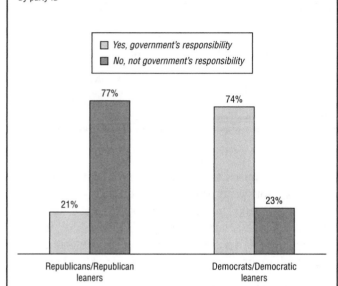

SOURCE: Frank Newport, "Do You Think It Is the Responsibility of the Federal Government to Make Sure All Americans Have Healthcare Coverage, or Is That Not the Responsibility of the Federal Government? By Party ID," in *More in U.S. Say Health Coverage Is Not Gov't. Responsibility*, The Gallup Organization, November 13, 2009, http://www.gallup.com/poll/124253/Say-Health-Coverage-Not-Gov-Responsibility.aspx (accessed June 16, 2010). Copyright © 2010 by The Gallup Organization. Reproduced by permission of The Gallup Organization.

FIGURE 9.4

Public opinion about whether health reform legislation will make the health care system better or worse, November 2009

TAKING EVERYTHING INTO ACCOUNT, IF A NEW HEALTHCARE BILL BECOMES LAW, DO YOU THINK IN THE LONG RUN IT WILL MAKE THE U.S. HEALTHCARE SYSTEM—[ROTATED: BETTER, WOULD IT NOT MAKE MUCH DIFFERENCE, (OR MAKE IT) WORSE]—THAN IT IS NOW?

Asked of a half sample

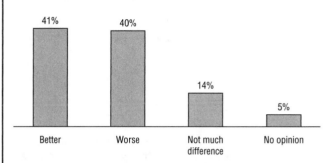

SOURCE: Frank Newport, "Taking Everything into Account, If a New Healthcare Bill Becomes Law, Do You Think in the Long Run It Will Make the U.S. Healthcare System—[ROTATED: Better, Would It Not Make Much Difference, (or Make It) Worse]—Than It is Now?" in *No Clear Mandate from Americans on Healthcare Reform*, The Gallup Organization, November 9, 2009, http://www.gallup.com/poll/124202/No-Clear-Mandate-Americans-Healthcare-Reform.aspx (accessed June 16, 2010). Copyright © 2010 by The Gallup Organization. Reproduced by permission of The Gallup Organization.

(See Figure 9.7.) Even though Democrats and Republicans expressed support for their own party's elected representatives, fewer Republicans (8%) said they felt confident that Republicans in Congress could be trusted to advance health care reform. (See Table 9.1.) By contrast, 55% of Democrats believed Democrats in Congress could be trusted with reforming the health care system.

AMERICANS ARE CONCERNED ABOUT HEALTH CARE COSTS

In view of escalating health care costs and increasing out-of-pocket expenses, it is understandable that Americans are extremely concerned about health care costs. Gallup surveys have repeatedly found that health care costs, which continue to rise much faster than inflation, top the list of health problems Americans believe beset the nation and are perceived as more urgent than threats of specific diseases.

The Gallup Organization notes that in May 2010, two months after passage of the landmark health care reform legislation, Americans continued to worry about health care costs. In fact, Americans were more concerned about their

FIGURE 9.5

Public opinion about whether health reform legislation will make their personal health situation better or worse, November 2009

TAKING EVERYTHING INTO ACCOUNT, IF A NEW HEALTHCARE BILL BECOMES LAW, DO YOU THINK IN THE LONG RUN IT WILL MAKE YOUR OWN HEALTHCARE SITUATION—[ROTATED: BETTER, WOULD IT NOT MAKE MUCH DIFFERENCE, (OR MAKE IT) WORSE]—THAN IT IS NOW?

Asked of a half sample

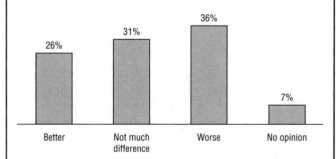

SOURCE: Frank Newport, "Taking Everything into Account, If a New Healthcare Bill Becomes Law, Do You Think in the Long Run It Will Make Your Own Healthcare Situation—[ROTATED: Better, Would It Not Make Much Difference, (or Make It) Worse]—Than It is Now?" in *No Clear Mandate from Americans on Healthcare Reform*, The Gallup Organization, November 9, 2009, http://www.gallup.com/poll/124202/No-Clear-Mandate-Americans-Healthcare-Reform.aspx (accessed June 16, 2010). Copyright © 2010 by The Gallup Organization. Reproduced by permission of The Gallup Organization.

FIGURE 9.6

Public opinion about whether elected officials should vote for or against the health reform bill, October–November 2009

WOULD YOU ADVISE YOUR MEMBER OF CONGRESS TO VOTE FOR OR AGAINST A HEALTHCARE BILL THIS YEAR, OR DO YOU NOT HAVE AN OPINION?

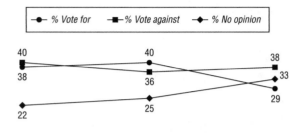

SOURCE: Frank Newport, "Would You Advise Your Member of Congress to Vote for or against a Healthcare Bill This Year, or Do You Not Have an Opinion?" in *No Clear Mandate from Americans on Healthcare Reform*, The Gallup Organization, November 9, 2009, http://www .gallup.com/poll/124202/No-Clear-Mandate-Americans-Healthcare-Reform.aspx (accessed June 16, 2010). Copyright © 2010 by The Gallup Organization. Reproduced by permission of The Gallup Organization.

FIGURE 9.7

Public opinion about whether elected officials can be trusted to change the health care system, October 2009

WHEN IT COMES TO MAKING CHANGES TO THE HEALTHCARE SYSTEM, HOW MUCH TRUST DO YOU HAVE IN EACH OF THE FOLLOWING—A GREAT DEAL, A FAIR AMOUNT, NOT MUCH, OR NONE AT ALL?

Trust in Washington leaders on healthcare reform

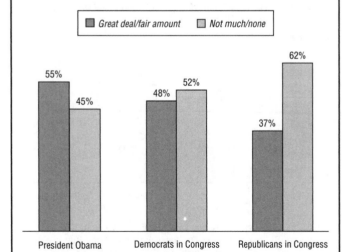

SOURCE: Lydia Saad, "Trust in Washington on Healthcare Reform," in *On Healthcare, Americans Trust Obama More Than Congress*, The Gallup Organization, October 28, 2009, http://www.gallup.com/poll/ 123917/On-Healthcare-Americans-Trust-Obama-More-Than-Congress .aspx (accessed June 16, 2010). Copyright © 2010 by The Gallup Organization. Reproduced by permission of The Gallup Organization.

TABLE 9.1

Public opinion about whether elected officials can be trusted to change the health care system, by political party affiliation, October 2009

WOULD YOU ADVISE YOUR MEMBER OF CONGRESS TO VOTE FOR OR AGAINST A HEALTHCARE BILL THIS YEAR, OR DO YOU NOT HAVE AN OPINION?

	% Vote for	% Vote against	% No opinion
Republicans	8	68	23
Independents	22	44	33
Democrats	55	8	37

SOURCE: Lydia Saad, "Trust in Washington on Healthcare Reform—by Party ID," in *On Healthcare, Americans Trust Obama More Than Congress*, The Gallup Organization, October 28, 2009, http://www.gallup.com/poll/123917/ On-Healthcare-Americans-Trust-Obama-More-Than-Congress.aspx (accessed June 16, 2010). Copyright © 2010 by The Gallup Organization. Reproduced by permission of The Gallup Organization.

ability to pay for routine care or a serious illness than they were in previous years. (See Figure 9.8.) Sixty-one percent of survey respondents worried about not being able to pay the medical costs associated with a serious illness or accident, and another 48% were concerned about not being able to pay for normal, routine health care services. (See Table 9.2.)

The Deloitte Center for Health Solutions indicates in *2010 Survey of Health Care Consumers: Key Findings, Strategic Implications* (2010, http://www.deloitte.com/ assets/Dcom-UnitedStates/Local%20Assets/Documents/ US_CHS_2010SurveyofHealthCareConsumers_050610 .pdf) that consumer anxiety about health care costs appears to be stabilizing. In 2009, 47% of survey respondents said their health care costs increased, compared with 43% of survey respondents in 2010. Likewise, 42% said costs stayed the same in 2009, compared with 46% in 2010. The proportion of consumers—just one out of four—that felt confident about their ability to pay for future medical expenses was unchanged from 2009.

Lydia Saad of the Gallup Organization observes in *"Jobs" Drops to No. 2 on Americans' List of Top Problems* (May 12, 2010, http://www.gallup.com/poll/127949/Jobs-Drops-No-Americans-List-Top-Problems.aspx) that even though the economy (26%) and unemployment (22%) took the top two spots on the list of "most important problems" named by survey respondents in May 2010, health care quality and the high cost of health care was the third-most frequently named problem, garnering 15%. (See Table 9.3.) According to Saad, this percentage was down from 26% in the summer of 2009 and 23% in February 2010.

The national economy and the rate of increase of health care costs, especially out-of-pocket expenses, also play important roles in shaping public opinion. Many surveys show a direct relationship between rising out-of-pocket expenses and dissatisfaction with the health care system.

FIGURE 9.8

Public opinion about worrying about ability to pay for health care, 2001–10

HOW CONCERNED ARE YOU RIGHT NOW ABOUT EACH OF THE FOLLOWING FINANCIAL MATTERS, BASED ON YOUR CURRENT FINANCIAL SITUATION—ARE YOU VERY WORRIED, MODERATELY WORRIED, NOT TOO WORRIED, OR NOT WORRIED AT ALL?

% Very/moderately worried

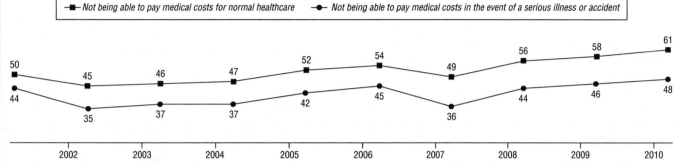

SOURCE: Frank Newport, "How Concerned Are You Right Now about Each of the Following Financial Matters, Based on Your Current Financial Situation—Are You Very Worried, Moderately Worried, Not Too Worried, or Not Worried At All?" in *Americans No Less Worried about Healthcare Costs*, The Gallup Organization, May 7, 2010, http://www.gallup.com/poll/127727/Americans-No-Less-Worried-Healthcare-Costs.aspx (accessed June 16, 2010). Copyright © 2010 by The Gallup Organization. Reproduced by permission of The Gallup Organization.

TABLE 9.2

Public opinion about financial situation and ability to pay for health care, 2010

PLEASE TELL ME HOW CONCERNED YOU ARE RIGHT NOW ABOUT EACH OF THE FOLLOWING FINANCIAL MATTERS, BASED ON YOUR CURRENT FINANCIAL SITUATION—ARE YOU VERY WORRIED, MODERATELY WORRIED, NOT TOO WORRIED, OR NOT WORRIED AT ALL?

	% Worried	% Not worried
Not having enough money for retirement	66	32
Not being able to pay medical costs of a serious illness/accident	61	37
Not being able to maintain the standard of living you enjoy	54	45
Not being able to pay medical costs for normal healthcare	48	48
Not having enough to pay your normal monthly bills	44	54
Not being able to pay your rent, mortgage, or other housing costs	38	56
Not having enough money to pay for your children's college	36	25
Not being able to make the minimum payments on your credit cards	24	58

SOURCE: Frank Newport, "Please Tell Me How Concerned You Are Right Now about Each of the Following Financial Matters, Based on Your Current Financial Situation—Are You Very Worried, Moderately Worried, Not Too Worried, or Not Worried At All?" in *Americans No Less Worried about Healthcare Costs*, The Gallup Organization, May 7, 2010, http://www.gallup.com/poll/127727/Americans-No-Less-Worried-Healthcare-Costs.aspx (accessed June 16, 2010). Copyright © 2010 by The Gallup Organization. Reproduced by permission of The Gallup Organization.

How the Health Care Reform Legislation Will Affect Them

In "Opinion Polls: Obama's Health Care Reform Law Not a Winner So Far" (*Christian Science Monitor*, March 30, 2010), Mark Trumbull reports that a variety of public opinion polls indicate that Americans are concerned about

TABLE 9.3

Public opinion about the top 10 problems facing the country, 2010

	%
Economy in general	26
Unemployment/jobs	22
Poor healthcare/hospitals; high cost of healthcare	15
Government/Congress/politicians; poor leadership; corruption; abuse of power	12
Immigration/illegal aliens	10
Federal budget deficit/federal debt	9
Lack of money	4
Terrorism	4
Ethics/moral/religious/family decline; dishonesty	4
National security	3
Environment/pollution	3
Situation/war in Iraq	3

SOURCE: Lydia Saad, "Top 10 Problems Named As Most Important Facing the U.S.," in *"Jobs" Drops to No. 2 on Americans' List of Top Problems*, The Gallup Organization, May 12, 2010, http://www.gallup.com/poll/127949/Jobs-Drops-No-Americans-List-Top-Problems.aspx (accessed June 17, 2010). Copyright © 2010 by The Gallup Organization. Reproduced by permission of The Gallup Organization.

the PPACA and how it will affect them. Trumbull notes that "voters worry the new law will erode the quality of care and jack up costs, even while it helps reduce the number of people unable to get health insurance." More than half (55%) of Americans think their own health care costs will rise as a result of the legislation and 60% predict that overall health care costs will escalate. Furthermore, nearly half of Americans fear that the PPACA will create too much government involvement in the delivery of health care. One survey even finds that more than half of Americans favor repealing the reform legislation.

In June 2010 Americans were equally divided about the health care reform legislation. A poll conducted by GfK Roper Public Affairs and Media (http://www.pollingreport.com/health.htm) finds that 45% of Americans said they support the legislation passed in March 2010, whereas 42% opposed it. An additional 13% neither supported nor opposed the PPACA.

Opinions about the PPACA were consistent with political party affiliation. For example, the Kaiser Family Foundation (http://www.pollingreport.com/health.htm) conducted a poll in May 2010. The foundation reports that 72% of Democrats favored the legislation and just 14% had an unfavorable opinion of it. The situation was reversed among Republicans: only 8% felt favorable about the reform law and 85% felt unfavorable. The foundation also notes that 35% of respondents did not understand how the health care reform law will affect them or their families.

In *2010 Survey of Health Care Consumers*, the Deloitte Center for Health Solutions notes that in 2010 more respondents favored (42%) than opposed (38%) the government requirement for health insurance coverage. The majority (69%) felt that a government-sponsored plan comparable to Medicare for people under the age of 65 years would stimulate better competition among private health plans. In general, respondents preferred an employer-sponsored health plan (42%) than a government-sponsored plan (25%); however, 38% of the uninsured favored a government-sponsored plan. About half (48%) of the respondents opined that in the current health care delivery system, 50% or more of health care dollars are wasted.

Most American Physicians Favor Health Care Reform

John Aloysius Farrell notes in "The Obama Healthcare Bill Explained: Why the Doctors Like It" (*U.S. News & World Report*, March 22, 2010) that physicians support the PPACA because it does not fundamentally change the way medicine is practiced. Farrell asserts that when all of the provisions of the legislation go into effect, the resulting health care delivery system will be relatively unchanged, "based on people buying health insurance from private insurance companies. A few million working families will qualify for federal tax breaks, or government aid—but only to buy more private insurance."

In "Health Care Reform and the AMA" (*New England Journal of Medicine*, vol. 362, no. 23, June 10, 2010), Salomeh Keyhani and Alex Federman assert that "even though a majority of physicians and AMA [American Medical Association] members supported the public insurance option and the expansion of Medicare, the AMA opposed Medicare expansions and proposed coverage of the uninsured primarily through private means." Keyhani and Federman surveyed physician members of the AMA to determine whether the AMA represented the views of physicians in the insurance expansion debate and to better understand and characterize the physicians the AMA represented. They find that the majority of physicians supported proposals for health insurance expansion that were opposed by the AMA. The physicians whose opinions were consistent with those of the AMA were more likely to be young, male, practice owners, and working in medical specialties such as anesthesiology, pathology, or radiology. Keyhani and Federman conclude that "although the AMA is the most visible organization representing physicians, it did not represent the majority of physicians' views on coverage expansions in recent reform efforts."

Peter R. Orszag and Ezekiel J. Emanuel of the White House Office of Management and Budget opine in "Health Care Reform and Cost Control" (*New England Journal of Medicine*, June 16, 2010) about the PPACA. They state, "In attempting to modernize and improve a large part of the health care system, it may be one of the most ambitious and consequential pieces of legislation in U.S. history." Orszag and Emanuel observe that the bill will significantly reduce health care costs. Total health care expenditures as a percentage of the gross domestic product (the total market value of final goods and services produced within an economy in a given year) are forecast as 0.5% lower in 2030 than they would have been without the provisions of the legislation. The PPACA will reduce the federal budget deficit by more than $100 billion over the first decade and by more than $1 trillion between 2020 and 2030. It will eliminate unnecessary costs by reducing fraud and abuse in the Medicare and Medicaid programs, reducing unnecessary paperwork, and instituting electronic standards and operating rules to be used by all private insurers, Medicare, and Medicaid. According to Orszag and Emanuel, these administrative measures alone are projected to save the federal government an estimated $20 billion over 10 years. The legislation also clears a pathway for the approval of generic biologic drugs (drugs derived from living organisms that are used to prevent, diagnose, or treat diseases) that are expected to save the government more than $7 billion and consumers and insurers additional billions.

CONSUMER SATISFACTION WITH HEALTH CARE FACILITIES

Despite the problems that continue to plague hospitals, such as shortages of nurses and other key personnel, diminished reimbursement, shorter inpatient lengths of stay, sicker patients, and excessively long waiting times for patients in emergency and other hospital departments, consumer satisfaction with hospital services has remained relatively high. In fact, Press Ganey Associates Inc. reports in *Hospital Pulse Report 2009: Patient Perspectives on American Health Care* (2009, http://www.pressganey.com/galleries/default-file/Hospital_Pulse_Report_2009.pdf), which considers the experiences of nearly 3 million patients treated at more than 2,000 hospitals nationwide, that overall patient satisfaction with inpatient hospital care steadily increased between 2003 and 2008. Press Ganey Associates also finds that more patients than ever before—up nearly 2% in 2008 from the previous year—said they would recommend the facility where they had received care to a friend.

Patient satisfaction with hospital care was linked to the hospital's success in communicating and meeting patients' spiritual and emotional needs. This finding, that satisfaction is associated with patient-centered care and intangible qualities of the hospital experience such as sensitivity, attention, and responsiveness to emotional needs, concerns, and complaints, underscores the fact that many health care consumers assess the quality of service they receive in terms of the care and compassion displayed by hospital personnel.

Consistent with the findings that personal care and attention strongly influence satisfaction with hospital care, Press Ganey Associates finds that as the hospital size increases (in terms of number of beds) patient satisfaction decreases. Patient satisfaction was highest, at 87.8%, in hospitals with 50 or fewer beds, and satisfaction declined steadily to 83.7% in hospitals with 600 or more beds. Presumably, this is because larger hospitals, and the health care workers they employ, find it more challenging to deliver the individual care and attention patients have come to associate with quality.

Other patient-related variables and hospital characteristics also influence satisfaction with care. Fewer patients admitted through the emergency department (82.6%) were satisfied, compared with those who did not have emergency admissions (85.6%). This difference may be attributed to the understandable stress and discomfort surrounding an emergency hospital admission, but it may also reflect dissatisfaction with specific hospital qualities such as long waits for admission.

Sarah Morgan asserts in "Patient Satisfaction Declines at Hospitals" (*Smart Money*, May 18, 2010) that consumer satisfaction with hospitals is declining. Morgan reports that the quarterly American Customer Satisfaction Index, which considers customer satisfaction for businesses, including cable and satellite television, wireless and fixed-line phone services, utilities, computer software, and health care, revealed a 5% decrease in satisfaction with hospitals and a 1.9% drop in satisfaction with the health care sector from the previous year. Morgan observes that the six-year low in patient satisfaction with hospitals does not translate into less spending on inpatient hospital care because people will continue to get sick and require hospitalization. Interestingly, Morgan notes that the American Customer Satisfaction Index found patient satisfaction with outpatient hospital care unchanged from the prior quarter; however, satisfaction with emergency departments dropped 12%. In "Higher Hospital Margins Distinguished by Higher Patient Satisfaction" (June 2010, http://www.ahd.com/HFM-DataTrends_JUN10.pdf), a 2010 analysis of Medicare cost data, William Shoemaker of the Healthcare Financial Management

Association identifies a direct relationship between a hospital's profitability and its level of patient satisfaction.

Gienna Shaw explains in "Time to Put Patients First" (*HealthLeaders Magazine*, May 12, 2010) some of the origins of patient dissatisfaction. She notes that "Americans can't understand why they must wait months for an appointment with a specialist. They continually hear horror stories about wrong-site surgeries and hospital-acquired infections. They have trouble getting their physicians, specialists, and alternative providers to talk to each other—let alone communicate effectively with them. And then they get a bill for it all that they can't understand." Shaw asserts that hospitals have lost sight of their mission—caring for patients—and lauds efforts to promote patient-centered care, which is defined as "compassionate care delivered with the highest quality and level of patient safety."

Government Website Posts Patient Satisfaction Survey Data

Amid multiple reports of patient dissatisfaction with selected aspects of health care delivery, there are some hopeful signs, such as improving levels of satisfaction with inpatient hospital care. In *Hospital Pulse Report 2009*, Press Ganey Associates attributes some of the improvement in inpatient hospital care satisfaction to the fact that the federal government posted in March 2008 the results of the Hospital Consumer Assessment of Healthcare Providers and Systems survey on the website "Hospital Compare" (http://www.hospitalcompare.hhs.gov/), which enables consumers to compare up to three hospitals. The site aims to help consumers choose the best hospital for selected medical conditions or surgical procedures such as heart attack, pneumonia, and asthma by detailing how often hospitals give recommended treatments that are known to get the best results for patients with certain medical conditions or surgical procedures. The website includes mortality rates and hospital readmission rates for each hospital as well as other information such as whether the hospital uses electronic health records. It also provides information about a hospital's quality of care, as measured by patient surveys.

In the policy brief "Critical Access Hospital Year 5 Hospital Compare Participation and Quality Measure Results" (March 2010, http://flexmonitoring.org/documents/PolicyBrief15-Hospital-Compare-Yr5.pdf), Michelle Casey, Michele Burlew, and Ira Moscovice of the University of Minnesota Rural Health Research Center consider the reporting of quality and patient satisfaction by critical access hospitals (CAHs)—hospitals that are certified to receive cost-based reimbursement from Medicare, which is intended to improve their financial performance and thereby reduce hospital closures in rural areas, where they are most needed. The researchers report that in 2008 "the percent of CAH patients receiving recommended care has increased for nearly all measures." Casey, Burlew, and

Moscovice also observe that in response to the enactment of the PPACA, which intensified rewards for the provision of quality health care services, CAHs and all other health care providers will face increasing demand for quality data. Health care providers will "be required to demonstrate the quality of the care they are providing to qualify for reimbursement incentives and avoid penalties for poor care."

Consumer groups, employers, labor unions, and other government agencies applaud the dissemination of these data, asserting that it helps promote transparency and accountability. Diana Manos reports in "CMS Adds Mortality, Readmission Data to Its Online Hospital Rating Site" (*Healthcare IT News*, July 9, 2009) that the Centers for Medicare and Medicaid Services (CMS) considers the "Hospital Compare" website to be a vital resource for consumers and notes that in 2008 the site had more than 18 million page views. In 2009 the CMS added mortality and readmission data to the website. According to Manos, Kathleen Sebelius (1948–), the secretary of health and human services, explained that the government is particularly focused on preventing readmissions: "When we reduce readmissions, we improve the quality of care patients receive and cut health care costs." Manos quotes Barry M. Straube, the chief medical officer and director of the CMS's Office of Clinical Standards and Quality, as saying, "More data gives a clearer picture of the quality of care delivered at different hospitals over time, which ultimately increases the value of our mortality information to hospital patients, health care payers, employers, policymakers, and other health care stakeholders."

A GROWING NUMBER LOOK FOR HEALTH INFORMATION ONLINE

Even though public trust in hospitals and personal physicians remains relatively high, and many people seek and receive health education from physicians, nurses, and other health professionals, a growing number of Americans are seeking health information online. Harris Poll researchers dub the millions of adults who seek information on the Internet about specific diseases or tips about how to maintain health "cyberchondriacs."

According to Harris Interactive, in "'Cyberchondriacs' on the Rise?" (August 4, 2010, http://www.harrisinteractive.com/vault/HI-Harris-Poll-Cyberchondriacs-2010-08-04.pdf), the number of people going online to seek health information rose from 154 million in 2009 to 175 million in 2010. The frequency of seeking health information online also grew— 32% of adults in 2010 reported that they "often" look online for health information, up from 22% in 2009.

Harris Interactive notes that cyberchondriacs typically searched the Internet for health information six times per month, up from 5.4 times per month in 2009. The vast majority of cyberchondriacs said they found the information they were seeking (86%) and believe the information

they found on the Internet was reliable (85%). About half (51%) reported using the Internet to obtain information following discussions with their physicians.

Rachael King explains in "Here Come the Cyberchondriacs" (*BusinessWeek*, August 2, 2007) that some industry analysts posit that the growing number of consumers choosing to research medical conditions online is in part motivated by escalating health care costs and the proliferation of high-deductible health plans, which motivate consumers to assume greater responsibility for their care. Cyberchondriacs not only seek information about medical problems but also want to know how much treatment should cost and whether their physician has a good track record treating specific conditions or performing specific procedures. Furthermore, industry observers feel online consumers are seeking greater control over health care decisions, which will serve to incrementally change the nature of relationships between patients and physicians.

In "Consumers Increasingly Turning to Internet, Social Media for Health Care Information" (*iHealthBeat*, April 15, 2010), Mina Kim reports that adults are increasingly looking for health information online. She notes that "in addition to health care websites, such as WebMD, consumers are turning to user-generated health content, such as physician and hospital rankings, blogs and chat groups." Robin A. Cohen and Barbara Stussman of the National Center for Health Statistics confirm in *Health Information Technology Use among Men and Women Aged 18–64: Early Release of Estimates from the National Health Interview Survey, January–June 2009* (February 2010, http://www.cdc.gov/nchs/data/hestat/healthinfo2009/healthinfo2009.htm) that 50.8% of all adults aged 18 to 64 years had used the Internet to look up health information from January to June 2009. (See Figure 9.9.) During this period 6% of adults aged 18 to 64 years refilled a prescription online, 4.9% contacted a health care provider via e-mail, and 2.7% scheduled an appointment with a health care provider using the Internet. (See Figure 9.10.)

According to the Deloitte Center for Health Solutions, in *2010 Survey of Health Care Consumers*, 22% of Generation X (people born between 1965 and 1979) and 23% of Generation Y (people born in 1980 and after) were very interested in using a mobile device to maintain their personal health records in 2010, compared with just 15% of baby boomers (people born between 1946 and 1964) and 17% of older adults. Just 5% of respondents used social networking sites to find information about prescription drugs, 3% communicated with a physician, and 3% corresponded with their health plans. Thirty-three percent of survey respondents expressed privacy and security concerns about online personal health records in 2010, which was down from 38% in 2009.

Reliable public sources of consumer and provider health information on the Internet include the National Institutes of

FIGURE 9.9

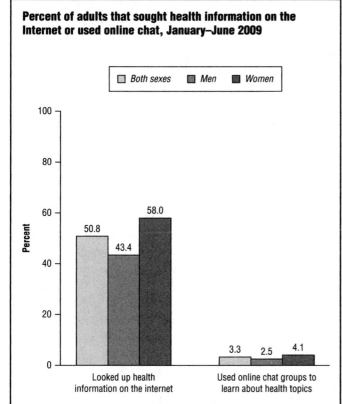

Percent of adults that sought health information on the Internet or used online chat, January–June 2009

SOURCE: Robin A. Cohen and Barbara Stussman, "Figure 1. Percentages of Adults Aged 18–64 Who in the Past 12 Months Looked up Health Information on the Internet or Used Online Chat Groups to Learn about Health Topics, by Sex: United States, January–June 2009," in *Health Information Technology Use among Men and Women Aged 18–64: Early Release of Estimates from the National Health Interview Survey, January–June 2009*, Centers for Disease Control and Prevention, February 2010, http://www.cdc.gov/nchs/data/hestat/healthinfo2009/ healthinfo2009.htm#fig1 (accessed June 19, 2010)

FIGURE 9.10

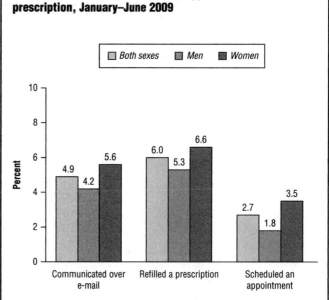

Percent of adults that used the Internet to communicate with a health professional, schedule an appointment or refill a prescription, January–June 2009

SOURCE: Robin A. Cohen and Barbara Stussman, "Figure 2. Percentages of Adults Aged 18–64 Who in the Past 12 Months Used the Internet to Communicate with a Health Care Provider over E-Mail, Refill a Prescription, or Schedule an Appointment with a Health Care Provider, by Sex: United States, January–June 2009," in *Health Information Technology Use among Men and Women Aged 18–64: Early Release of Estimates from the National Health Interview Survey, January–June 2009*, Centers for Disease Control and Prevention, February 2010, http://www.cdc.gov/nchs/data/hestat/healthinfo2009/healthinfo2009 .htm#fig2 (accessed June 19, 2010)

Health, the Centers for Disease Control and Prevention, and MEDLINE. Using this technology effectively is a health system challenge, especially in terms of protecting patient privacy and confidentiality and ensuring that consumers have access to accurate and reliable health information.

MARKETING PRESCRIPTION DRUGS TO CONSUMERS

Even though health care consumers continue to receive much of their information from physicians, nurses, other health professionals, and the Internet, many also learn about health care services and products from reports in the news media and from advertising. Media advertising (the promotion of hospitals, health insurance, managed care plans, medical groups, and related health services and products) has been a mainstay of health care marketing efforts since the 1970s. During the early 1990s pharmaceutical companies made their first forays into advertising of prescription drugs directly to consumers. Before the 1990s pharmaceutical companies' promotion efforts had

focused almost exclusively on physicians, the health professionals who prescribe their products.

Since the mid-1990s spending on prescription drugs has escalated and has become the fastest-growing segment of U.S. health care expenditures. In 1997 the U.S. Food and Drug Administration released guidelines governing direct-to-consumer advertising and seemingly opened a floodgate of print, radio, and television advertisements promoting prescription drugs. Industry observers wondered if this upsurge of direct-to-consumer advertising had resulted in more, and possibly inappropriate, prescribing and higher costs.

Is Direct-to-Consumer Advertising Effective?

It stands to reason that pharmaceutical companies must be receiving significant returns on their direct-to-consumer advertising investments to justify increasing budgets for consumer advertising, but it is difficult to measure the precise impact of consumer advertising on drug sales. Bill Berkrot reports in "US Prescription Drug Sales Hit $300 Billion in 2009" (Reuters, April 1, 2010) that prescription drug sales grew by 5.1% to more than $300 billion in 2009. In "Direct-to-Consumer Advertising in Pharmaceutical Markets: Effects on Demand and Prices" (*Vox*, June 3,

2010), Dhaval Dave of Bentley University notes that spending on direct-to-consumer prescription drug advertising was responsible for 18% of the total increase in prescription drug sales from 1993 to 2005. Of this 18%, about 12% was attributable to more sales and 6% to higher prices. Dave asserts that media promotion may affect price by increasing demand and/or reducing the price-sensitivity of purchasers (individual consumers and group purchasers), which may raise the price of pharmaceuticals. In addition, spending for media advertising may be passed along to consumers in the form of higher prescription drug prices.

According to William E. Boden and George A. Diamond, in "DTCA for PTCA—Crossing the Line in Consumer Health Education?" (*New England Journal of Medicine*, vol. 358, no. 21, May 22, 2008), direct-to-consumer advertising resulted in a favorable return on investment for over 90% of brand-name drugs in 2004, and 10 of the leading 12 brand-name drugs with direct-to-consumer advertising campaigns had sales of more than $1 billion annually. Nearly three-quarters of the brand-name drugs advertised generated "returns in excess of $1.50 for every $1.00 invested and 35% of which had returns in excess of $2.50 for every $1.00 invested."

Is Direct-to-Consumer Advertising of Psychoactive Drugs Helpful or Harmful?

At what point does an understandable response to distressing life events become an indication for drug treatment— and a market opportunity?

—Barbara Mintzes, "Direct to Consumer Advertising Is Medicalising Normal Human Experience" (April 13, 2002)

In *The Numbers Count: Mental Disorders in America* (2010, http://www.nimh.nih.gov/health/publications/the-numbers-count-mental-disorders-in-america/index.shtml), the National Institute of Mental Health estimates that 26.2% of Americans aged 18 years and older are affected by a mental disorder and that 6% suffer from serious mental illness. Other surveys find that as many as 30% of the adults in the United States suffer from mental disorders. The Harvard School of Medicine's National Comorbidity Survey (July 2007, http://www.hcp.med.harvard.edu/ncs/) finds that in any given year 32.4% of all Americans meet the criteria for having a mental illness and that the lifetime prevalence of any diagnosable mental disorder is 57.4%.

Even though these studies rely primarily on self-reporting, they do suggest that the United States is in the throes of an epidemic of mental illness. However, some researchers argue that Americans' mental health is no worse than it was in past decades. They contend that the availability and aggressive marketing of psychopharmacological agents (prescription drugs aimed at mental health problems such as nervousness, anxiety, panic, and shyness) have prompted the overdiagnosis of mental health problems and conditions motivated primarily by the desire to increase drug sales.

Dominick L. Frosch and David Grande explain in "Direct-to-Consumer Advertising of Prescription Drugs" (*LDI Issue Brief*, vol. 15, no. 3, March–April 2010) that there have been advocates and opponents of direct-to-consumer prescription drug advertising since its inception. Advocates contend that it educates consumers, promotes patient participation in clinical decision making, and improves patient adherence to medication and other treatment. Critics argue that it is intended to persuade, not educate, and that it promotes inappropriate use of prescription drugs or diverts consumers from safer, less costly alternatives.

Health care consumers favor advertisements for prescription drugs to treat mental health conditions. According to *The Public on Prescription Drugs and Pharmaceutical Companies* (March 2008, http://kff.org/kaiserpolls/upload/7748.pdf), a *USA Today*/Kaiser Family Foundation/Harvard School of Public Health survey that was conducted in January 2008, 60% of adults feel such advertisements "are mostly good because they improve understanding of these conditions and encourage people to seek treatment, while about a third (36%) think these ads are mostly bad because they encourage people without serious mental health conditions to think they need treatment."

Opponents usually contend that direct-to-consumer advertising is primarily intended to drive sales and that it:

- Increases prescription drug costs

- Does not provide the impartial, objective information that would enable consumers to make informed health choices

- Increases risk because, unlike other consumer goods, prescription drugs, even when administered properly, may cause serious adverse reactions

- Takes unfair advantage of vulnerable people facing difficult treatment choices, especially people who suffer from mental illness

- Aims to increase awareness and utilization of newer products to gain market share and recoup development costs (new drugs are not necessarily safer or more effective but are usually costlier, and often little is known about long-term risks)

- Does not enhance consumer awareness or public health because there is no evidence that advertising helps patients to make better choices about prescription drug use

- May unduly influence physician-prescribing practices; physicians often rely on manufacturers for information about drugs, rather than on independent sources, and many studies show that the physicians most influenced by pharmaceutical advertising tend to prescribe less judiciously

Dominick L. Frosch et al. contend in "A Decade of Controversy: Balancing Policy with Evidence in the

Regulation of Prescription Drug Advertising" (*American Journal of Public Health*, vol. 100, no. 1, January 2010) that such advertising may mislead consumers or prompt them to consider drug treatment for a condition that does not warrant it. The researchers cite the example of advertising campaigns for drugs to treat various anxiety disorders that emphasized feelings of social discomfort with slogans such as "imagine being allergic to people." Similarly, antidepressant print advertisements were found to mislead consumers to believe that their emotional symptoms are best treated with prescription medications. An analysis of advertisements found that direct-to-consumer advertising frequently identifies conditions that may not be recognized by consumers as problems in need of treatment or as treatable. Frosch et al. recommend that "to minimize potential harm and maximize the benefits of DTCA [direct-to-consumer advertising] for population health, the quality and quantity of information should be improved to enable consumers to better self-identify whether treatment is indicated, more realistically appraise the benefits, and better attend to the risks associated with prescription drugs."

Other critics of direct-to-consumer advertising, such as Elizabeth A. Almasi et al., in "What Are the Public Health Effects of Direct-to-Consumer Drug Advertising?" (*PLoS Medicine*, vol. 3, no. 3, March 2006), contend that the information in these advertisements is frequently biased and misleading and that direct-to-consumer advertising increases prescribing costs and has not demonstrated any evidence of health benefits. They also worry that the emphasis on advertisements for new drugs overshadows other vital public health messages about diet, exercise, addictions, social involvement, equity, pollution, climate change, and appropriate use of older drugs.

Regardless, many mental health professionals and consumers favor direct-to-consumer advertising because they believe it informs consumers that there is effective treatment for potentially debilitating mental disorders and helps them to overcome reluctance to seek needed treat-

ment. Nile M. Khanfar, Hyla H. Polen, and Kevin A Clauson observe in "Influence on Consumer Behavior: The Impact of Direct-to-Consumer Advertising on Medication Requests for Gastroesophageal Reflux Disease and Social Anxiety Disorder" (*Journal of Health Communications*, vol. 14, no. 5, July–August 2009) that 40% of people with a social anxiety disorder reported that direct-to-consumer advertising helped them to initiate conversations with their physicians that led to a change of therapy.

According to the Kaiser Family Foundation, in *Public and Physician Views of Direct-to-Consumer Prescription Drug Advertising* (April 2008, http://www.kff.org/spotlight/rxdrugsconsumer/upload/Rx_Drugs_DTC_Ads.pdf), many U.S. physicians suggest that pharmaceutical advertisements are a mixed blessing, in that they simultaneously enhance patient-physician communication and prompt patients to seek unnecessary treatment. In 2006, 80% of physicians said patients sometimes inquire about specific drugs or treatments they see advertised and 28% said patients frequently ask about drugs they see advertised. Forty-two percent of physicians felt these patient inquiries have a positive effect on patient-physician interactions, whereas 21% of physicians felt the inquiries have a negative effect and 35% said they have no impact.

More than half (57%) of the physicians said that when patients ask them about an advertised prescription drug, they prescribe the drug. However, over three-quarters (76%) said they "sometimes" recommend a different prescription drug. Just 5% of physicians said they frequently prescribe the drug that the patients ask for.

The Kaiser Family Foundation also finds that consumers generally favor advertisements of prescription drugs for mental health conditions such as depression and anxiety. Sixty percent "think such ads are mostly good because they improve understanding of these conditions and encourage people to seek treatment." By contrast, 36% "think these ads are mostly bad because they encourage people without serious mental health conditions to think they need treatment."

IMPORTANT NAMES
AND ADDRESSES

Accreditation Association for Ambulatory Health Care
5250 Old Orchard Rd., Ste. 200
Skokie, IL 60077
(847) 853-6060
FAX: (847) 853-9028
E-mail: info@aaahc.org
URL: http://www.aaahc.org/

Administration on Aging
One Massachusetts Ave. NW
Washington, DC 20001
(202) 619-0724
FAX: (202) 357-3555
E-mail: aoainfo@aoa.hhs.gov
URL: http://www.aoa.gov/

Agency for Healthcare Research and Quality
540 Gaither Rd., Ste. 2000
Rockville, MD 20850
(301) 427-1104
URL: http://www.ahrq.gov/

American Academy of Child and Adolescent Psychiatry
3615 Wisconsin Ave. NW
Washington, DC 20016-3007
(202) 966-7300
FAX: (202) 966-2891
URL: http://www.aacap.org/

American Academy of Family Physicians
11400 Tomahawk Creek Pkwy.
Leawood, KS 66211-2680
(913) 906-6000
1-800-274-2237
FAX: (913) 906-6075
URL: http://www.aafp.org/

American Academy of Physician Assistants
950 N. Washington St.
Alexandria, VA 22314-1552
(703) 836-2272

FAX: (703) 684-1924
E-mail: aapa@aapa.org
URL: http://www.aapa.org/

American Association for Geriatric Psychiatry
7910 Woodmont Ave., Ste. 1050
Bethesda, MD 20814-3004
(301) 654-7850
FAX: (301) 654-4137
E-mail: main@aagponline.org
URL: http://www.aagpgpa.org/

American Association for Marriage and Family Therapy
112 S. Alfred St.
Alexandria, VA 22314-3061
(703) 838-9808
FAX: (703) 838-9805
URL: http://www.aamft.org/

American Association of Pastoral Counselors
9504A Lee Hwy.
Fairfax, VA 22031-2303
(703) 385-6967
FAX: (703) 352-7725
E-mail: info@aapc.org
URL: http://www.aapc.org/

American Cancer Society
250 Williams St. NW, Ste. 6000
Atlanta, GA 30303
(404) 320-3333
FAX: (404) 982-3677
URL: http://www.cancer.org/

American Chiropractic Association
1701 Clarendon Blvd.
Arlington, VA 22209
(703) 276-8800
FAX: (703) 243-2593
E-mail: memberinfo@acatoday.org
URL: http://www.acatoday.org/index.cfm

American College of Nurse Practitioners
1501 Wilson Blvd., Ste. 509
Arlington, VA 22209
(703) 740-2529
FAX: (703) 740-2533
E-mail: acnp@acnpweb.org
URL: http://www.acnpweb.org/

American Counseling Association
5999 Stevenson Ave.
Alexandria, VA 22304
1-800-347-6647
FAX: 1-800-473-2329
URL: http://www.counseling.org/

American Dental Association
211 E. Chicago Ave.
Chicago, IL 60611-2678
(312) 440-2500
E-mail: membership@ada.org
URL: http://www.ada.org/

American Diabetes Association
1701 N. Beauregard St.
Alexandria, VA 22311
1-800-342-2383
URL: http://www.diabetes.org/

American Geriatrics Society
Empire State Building
350 Fifth Ave., Ste. 801
New York, NY 10118
(212) 308-1414
FAX: (212) 832-8646
E-mail: info@americangeriatrics.org
URL: http://www.americangeriatrics.org/

American Heart Association
7272 Greenville Ave.
Dallas, TX 75231
1-800-242-8721
URL: http://www.americanheart.org/

American Hospital Association
155 N. Wacker Dr.
Chicago, IL 60606

(312) 422-3000
URL: http://www.aha.org/

American Medical Association
515 N. State St.
Chicago, IL 60654
1-800-621-8335
URL: http://www.ama-assn.org/

American Osteopathic Association
142 E. Ontario St.
Chicago, IL 60611
(312) 202-8000
1-800-621-1773
FAX: (312) 202-8200
E-mail: info@osteotech.org
URL: http://www.osteopathic.org/

American Pharmacists Association
2215 Constitution Avenue NW
Washington, DC 20037
(202) 628-4410
1-800-237-2742
FAX: (202) 783-2351
URL: http://www.aphanet.org/

American Physical Therapy Association
1111 N. Fairfax St.
Alexandria, VA 22314-1488
(703) 684-2782
1-800-999-2782
FAX: (703) 684-7343
URL: http://www.apta.org/

American Psychiatric Association
1000 Wilson Blvd., Ste. 1825
Arlington, VA 22209-3901
(703) 907-7300
E-mail: apa@psych.org
URL: http://www.psych.org/

American Psychiatric Nurses Association
1555 Wilson Blvd., Ste. 530
Arlington, VA 22209
1-866-243-2443
FAX: (703) 243-3390
URL: http://www.apna.org/

American Psychological Association
750 First St. NE
Washington, DC 20002-4242
(202) 336-5500
1-800-374-2721
URL: http://www.apa.org/

American Psychological Society
1133 15th St. NW, Ste. 1000
Washington, DC 20005
(202) 293-9300
FAX: (202) 293-9350
URL: http://www.psychologicalscience.org/

Association of American Medical Colleges
2450 North St. NW
Washington, DC 20037-1126
(202) 828-0400
FAX: (202) 828-1125
URL: http://www.aamc.org/

Center for Mental Health Services
Substance Abuse and Mental Health
Services Administration
PO Box 2345
Rockville, MD 20847
1-800-789-2647
FAX: (240) 221-4295
URL: http://www.mentalhealth.samhsa.gov/

Center for Studying Health System
Change
600 Maryland Ave. SW, Ste. 550
Washington, DC 20024
(202) 484-5261
FAX: (202) 484-9258
URL: http://www.hschange.org/

Centers for Disease Control and
Prevention
1600 Clifton Rd.
Atlanta, GA 30333
1-800-232-4636
E-mail: cdcinfo@cdc.gov
URL: http://www.cdc.gov/

Centers for Medicare and Medicaid
Services
7500 Security Blvd.
Baltimore, MD 21244-1849
(410) 786-3000
1-877-267-2323
URL: http://www.cms.gov/

Children's Defense Fund
25 E St. NW
Washington, DC 20001
(202) 628-8787
1-800-233-1200
E-mail: cdfinfo@childrensdefense.org
URL: http://www.childrensdefense.org/

Families USA
1201 New York Ave. NW, Ste. 1100
Washington, DC 20005
(202) 628-3030
FAX: (202) 347-2417
E-mail: info@familiesusa.org
URL: http://www.familiesusa.org/

Health Coalition on Liability
and Access
PO Box 78096
Washington, DC 20013-8096
E-mail: info@hcla.org
URL: http://www.hcla.org/index.html

Health Resources and Services
Administration
U.S. Department of Health and Human
Services
5600 Fishers Lane
Rockville, MD 20852-1750
(301) 443-3376
1-888-275-4772

E-mail: ask@hrsa.gov
URL: http://www.hrsa.gov/index.html/

Hospice Association of America
228 Seventh St. SE
Washington, DC 20003
(202) 546-4759
FAX: (202) 547-9559
URL: http://www.nahc.org/HAA

Joint Commission on Accreditation of
Healthcare Organizations
One Renaissance Blvd.
Oakbrook Terrace, IL 60181
(630) 792-5000
1-800-994-6610
FAX: (630) 792-5005
URL: http://www.jcaho.org/

March of Dimes Birth Defects
Foundation
1275 Mamaroneck Ave.
White Plains, NY 10605
(914) 997-4488
URL: http://www.marchofdimes.com/

Medical Group Management
Association
104 Inverness Terrace East
Englewood, CO 80112-5306
(303) 799-1111
1-877-275-6462
E-mail: service@mgma.com
URL: http://www.mgma.com/

National Association of Community
Health Centers
7200 Wisconsin Ave., Ste. 210
Bethesda, MD 20814
(301) 347-0400
URL: http://www.nachc.com/

National Association of Public Hospitals
and Health Systems
1301 Pennsylvania Ave. NW, Ste. 950
Washington, DC 20004
(202) 585-0100
FAX: (202) 585-0101
URL: http://www.naph.org/

National Association of School
Psychologists
4340 East West Hwy., Ste. 402
Bethesda, MD 20814
(301) 657-0270
1-866-331-NASP
FAX: (301) 657-0275
E-mail: center@naspweb.org
URL: http://www.nasponline.org/

National Association of Social
Workers
750 First St. NE, Ste. 700
Washington, DC 20002-4241
(202) 408-8600
URL: http://www.socialworkers.org/

National Center for Health Statistics
U.S. Department of Health and Human Services
3311 Toledo Rd.
Hyattsville, MD 20782
1-800-232-4636
URL: http://www.cdc.gov/nchs

National Committee for Quality Assurance
1100 13th St. NW, Ste. 1000
Washington, DC 20005
(202) 955-3500
1-888-275-7585
FAX: (202) 955-3599
URL: http://www.ncqa.org/

National Institute of Mental Health
Science Writing, Press, and Dissemination Branch
6001 Executive Blvd.
Rm. 8184, MSC 9663
Bethesda, MD 20892-9663
(301) 443-4513
1-866-615-6464
FAX: (301) 443-4279
E-mail: nimhinfo@nih.gov/
URL: http://www.nimh.nih.gov/

National Mental Health Association
2000 N. Beauregard St., Sixth Floor
Alexandria, VA 22311
(703) 684-7722
1-800-969-6642

FAX: (703) 684-5968
URL: http://www.nmha.org/

United Network for Organ Sharing
700 N. Fourth St.
Richmond, VA 23219
(804) 782-4800
1-888-894-6361
FAX: (804) 782-4817
URL: http://www.unos.org/

World Health Organization
Avenue Appia 20
Geneva 27, 1211Switzerland
(011-41-22) 791-2111
FAX: (011-41-22) 791-3111
URL: http://www.who.int

RESOURCES

Agencies of the U.S. Department of Health and Human Services collect, analyze, and publish a wide variety of health statistics that describe and measure the operation and effectiveness of the U.S. health care system. The Centers for Disease Control and Prevention tracks nationwide health trends and reports its findings in several periodicals, especially its *Advance Data* series, *National Ambulatory Medical Care Survey, HIV/AIDS Surveillance Reports*, and *Morbidity and Mortality Weekly Reports*. The National Center for Health Statistics provides a complete statistical overview of the nation's health in its annual *Health, United States*.

The National Institutes of Health provides definitions, epidemiological data, and research findings about a comprehensive range of medical and public health subjects. The Centers for Medicare and Medicaid Services monitors the nation's health spending. The agency's quarterly *Health Care Financing Review* and annual *Data Compendium* provide complete information on health care spending, particularly on allocations for Medicare and Medicaid. The Administration on Aging provides information about the health, welfare, and services available for older Americans.

The Agency for Healthcare Research and Quality researches and documents access to health care, quality of care, and efforts to control health care costs. It also examines the safety of health care services and ways to prevent medical errors. The Joint Commission on Accreditation of Healthcare Organizations and the National Committee for Quality Assurance are accrediting organizations that focus attention on institutional health care providers including the managed care industry.

The U.S. Census Bureau, in its *Current Population Reports* series, details the status of insurance among selected U.S. households.

Medical, public health, and nursing journals offer a wealth of health care system information and research findings. The studies cited in this edition are drawn from a range of professional publications, including *Alternative Therapies in Health and Medicine, Annals of Emergency Medicine, BMC Health Services Research, Chest, Frontiers of Health Services Management, Health Affairs, Health Care Management Review, Hospitals and Health Networks, Journal of the American Medical Association, Journal of Hospital Medicine, Modern Healthcare, New England Journal of Medicine, Pediatrics*, and *Primary Care: Clinics in Office Practice*.

Gale, Cengage Learning thanks the Gallup Organization for the use of its public opinion research about health care costs, quality, and concerns. Thanks also goes to the Organisation for Economic Cooperation and Development for permission to use information from its *Health at a Glance 2009: OECD Indicators*. Gale, Cengage Learning would also like to thank the many professional associations, voluntary medical organizations, and foundations dedicated to research, education, and advocacy about the efforts to reform and improve the health care system that were included in this edition.

INDEX

F

Families, 98

FDA (Food and Drug Administration), U.S., 65, 91, 98, 141

Financial issues. *See* Costs and expenditures

Food and Drug Administration (FDA), U.S., 65, 91, 98, 141

France, 135–136

Frappier Estate v. Wishnov, 61

G

GDP (gross domestic product), 80*t*, 119, 120*f*

Gender
access to care, 7
dentist office visits, 30*t*
emergency department visits, 46*t*–47*t*
failure to obtain care due to cost, 8*f*
hospital discharges, 48*t*–50*t*
Medicaid coverage, 113*t*–114*t*
nursing home residents, 52*t*
physicians' office visits, 23*t*–24*t*
regular sources of care, persons with, 6*f*
uninsured persons, 104, 107*t*, 108*f*

Generic drugs, 98–99

Geographic regions
children's access to care, 9*t*–10*t*, 11*t*–12*t*
health maintenance organization enrollment, 60
hospital discharges, 48*t*–50*t*
Medicare reimbursement inequalities, 108–109
uninsured persons, 103–104, 107*t*
variation in utilization and costs of health care, 101–102

Geriatricians, 18

Germany, 132, 134

Government
health care spending, 80–82, 80*t*
public opinion on role of, 149–150, 150(*f*9.2), 150(*f*9.3)

Grant programs, mental health care, 97

Gross domestic product (GDP), 80*t*, 119, 120*f*

Group HMO model, 60

Group practices, 22–23

H

H1N1 flu, 68, 70*t*

Hahnemann, Samuel, 36

Hazardous waste, 64

Health Care and Education Reconciliation Act, 2, 14, 115

Health care facilities
accreditation, 73–74
ambulatory care, 75
mental health facilities, 53–56
nursing homes, 51–53
surgical centers and urgent care centers, 48–50
See also Hospitals

Health care practitioners
access to care, 3–4
allied health care providers, 31–32, 31*t*
clinical practice guidelines, 142–143
complementary and alternative medicine, 35–38
employment trends, 38, 39*t*, 40, 40*t*
occupations, 1, 25*t*
professional societies, 75–76
See also Specific occupations

Health care reform
access to care, 8–10, 14
American Medical Association, 76
children, 112
costs and expenditures, 117
Department of Health and Human Services budget, 66
economic impact, 102
France, 136
Germany, 132, 134
health care practitioners' employment trends, 40
health insurance, 115–116
information technology, 139
managed care, 61–62
Medicaid, 93
Medicare, 92–93, 109
nurses, 29
nutrition labeling requirements, 76–77
Oregon health plan, 100
physicians' opinions, 154
prescription drugs, 88–90, 99
public opinion, 150–151, 151(*f*9.4), 151(*f*9.5), 152*f*, 152*t*, 153–154
recommendations, 1–2
spending, influence on health care, 85, 87–88

Health care settings, 1

Health care system components, 2–3

Health insurance
access to care, 5–6
American Medical Association, 76
Canada, 134
children, 8, 9*t*–10*t*, 11*t*–12*t*, 110–112, 112*f*
Children's Health Insurance Program, 64–65, 112
COBRA benefits, 66
costs, 98, 115
coverage by type, 104(*f*6.1)
coverage for core set of services, by country, 129*f*
emergency department visits, 43–44, 44*t*–45*t*, 46*t*–47*t*
factors influencing, 103
France, 135–136
Germany, 132
Health Insurance Portability and Accountability Act, 112
health maintenance organizations (HMOs), 59–61

health reform law, 115–116
health savings accounts, 112–115
international comparisons, 121, 123*f*
managed care, 58–59, 61–62
mental health care, 116–117
National Committee for Quality Assurance, 74–75
percentage of persons with public or private health insurance, 109*t*
preferred provider organizations (PPOs), 61
private health insurance, 110*t*
quality of care, 2
race/ethnicity, 9–10
senior health plans, 91–92
sources, 107, 150(*f*9.1)
U.S. health care system, 130
See also Health care reform; Uninsured persons

Health Insurance Portability and Accountability Act (HIPAA), 112

Health maintenance organizations (HMOs)
history, types, and criticism of, 59–61
Medicare, 91–92, 108
National Committee for Quality Assurance, 74–75
rationing, 100–101

Health outcomes
clinical practice guidelines, 142–143
health care report cards, 147–148
information technology, 144–145
Japan, 137
TeamSTEPPS, 141
too much care, 101–102
United Kingdom, 135
United States, 130–131

Health Plan Employer Data and Information Set (HEDIS), 74–75

Health Resources and Services Administration, 65

Health savings accounts, 112–115

Health Services Commission, Oregon, 100

Healthy People 2010 (Department of Health and Human Services), 54–56

Heart disease, 76–77, 129

Heart failure, 144

HEDIS (Health Plan Employer Data and Information Set), 74–75

HIPAA (Health Insurance Portability and Accountability Act), 112

History
Department of Health and Human Services, 63–64
health maintenance organizations, 59
March of Dimes, 77
Public Health Service, 66

HMO Act, 59

HMOs. *See* Health maintenance organizations

Holistic medicine, 17

Home health care, 56–57, 56*t*, 94

MAY - - 2011

MAY - - 2011